theclinics.com

RADIOLOGIC CLINICS OF NORTH AMERICA

Emergency Chest Imaging

Guest Editors
STUART E. MIRVIS, MD
K. SHANMUGANATHAN, MD

March 2006 • Volume 44 • Number 2

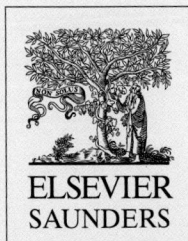

ELSEVIER
SAUNDERS

An imprint of Elsevier, Inc
PHILADELPHIA LONDON TORONTO MONTREAL SYDNEY TOKYO

W.B. SAUNDERS COMPANY
A Division of Elsevier Inc.

1600 John F. Kennedy Boulevard • Suite 1800 • Philadelphia, Pennsylvania 19103-2899

http://www.theclinics.com

RADIOLOGIC CLINICS OF NORTH AMERICA Volume 44, Number 2
March 2006 ISSN 0033-8389, ISBN 1-4160-3545-1

Editor: Barton Dudlick

Reprints: For copies of 100 or more, of articles in this publication, please contact the Commercial Reprints Department, Elsevier Inc., 360 Park Avenue South, New York, New York 10010-1710. Tel.: (+1) 212-633-3813; Fax: (+1) 212-462-1935; E-mail: reprints@elsevier.com.

The ideas and opinions expressed in *Radiologic Clinics of North America* do not necessarily reflect those of the Publisher. The Publisher does not assume any responsibility for any injury and/or damage to persons or property arising out of or related to any use of the material contained in this periodical. The reader is advised to check the appropriate medical literature and the product information currently provided by the manufacturer of each drug to be administered to verify the dosage, the method and duration of administration, or contraindications. It is the responsibility of the treating physician or other health care professional, relying on independent experience and knowledge of the patient, to determine drug dosages and the best treatment for the patient. Mention of any product in this issue should not be construed as endorsement by the contributors, editors, or the Publisher of the product or manufacturers' claims.

Radiologic Clinics of North America (ISSN 0033-8389) is published bimonthly by W.B. Saunders, 360 Park Avenue South, New York, NY 10010-1710. Business and editorial offices: 1600 John F. Kennedy Boulevard, Suite 1800, Philadelphia, Pennsylvania 19103-2899. Accounting and circulation offices: 6277 Sea Harbor Drive, Orlando, FL 32887-4800. Periodicals postage paid at New York, NY, and additional mailing offices. Subscription prices are USD 235 per year for US individuals, USD 350 per year for US institutions, USD 115 per year for US students and residents, USD 275 per year for Canadian individuals, USD 430 per year for Canadian institutions, USD 320 per year for international individuals, USD 430 per year for international institutions and USD 155 per year for Canadian and foreign students/residents. To receive student and resident rate, orders must be accompanied by name of affiliated institution, date of term, and the signature of program/residency coordinator on institution letterhead. Orders will be billed at individual rate until proof of status is received. Foreign air speed delivery is included in all Clinics subscription prices. All prices are subject to change without notice. POSTMASTER: Send address changes to *Radiologic Clinics of North America*, Elsevier Periodicals Customer Service, 6277 Sea Harbor Drive, Orlando, FL 32887-4800. **Customer Service: 1-800-654-2452 (US). From outside of the US, call (+1) 407-345-4000.**

Radiologic Clinics of North America also is published in Greek by Paschalidis Medical Publications, Athens, Greece.

Radiologic Clinics of North America is covered in *Index Medicus, EMBASE/Excerpta Medica, Current Contents/Life Sciences, Current Contents/Clinical Medicine, RSNA Index to Imaging Literature, BIOSIS, Science Citation Index,* and *ISI/BIOMED.*

Printed in the United States of America.

GOAL STATEMENT

The goal of the *Radiologic Clinics of North America* is to keep practicing radiologists and radiology residents up to date with current clinical practice in radiology by providing timely articles reviewing the state of the art in patient care.

ACCREDITATION

The *Radiologic Clinics of North America* is planned and implemented in accordance with the Essential Areas and Policies of the Accreditation Council for Continuing Medical Education (ACCME) through the joint sponsorship of the University of Virginia School of Medicine and Elsevier. The University of Virginia School of Medicine is accredited by the ACCME to provide continuing medical education for physicians.

The University of Virginia School of Medicine designates this educational activity for a maximum of 90 category 1 credits per year, 15 category 1 credits per issue, toward the AMA Physician's Recognition Award. Each physician should claim only those credits that he/she actually spent in the activity.

The American Medical Association has determined that physicians not licensed in the US who participate in this CME activity are eligible for AMA PRA category 1 credit.

AMA PRA category 1 credit can be earned by reading the text material, taking the examination online at *http://www.theclinics.com/home/cme*, and completing the evaluation. After taking the test, your will be required to review any and all incorrect answers. Following completion of the test and the evaluation, your credit will be awarded and you may print your certificate.

FACULTY DISCLOSURE/CONFLICT OF INTEREST

The University of Virginia School of Medicine, as an ACCME accredited provider, endorses and strives to comply with the Accreditation Council for Continuing Medical Education (ACCME) Standards of Commercial Support, Commonwealth of Virginia statutes, University of Virginia policies and procedures, and associated federal and private regulations and guidelines on the need for disclosure and monitoring of proprietary and financial interests that may affect the scientific integrity and balance of content delivered in continuing medical education activities under our auspices.

The University of Virginia School of Medicine requires that all CME activities accredited through this institution be developed independently and be scientifically rigorous, balanced and objective in the presentation/discussion of its content, theories and practices.

All authors/editors participating in an accredited CME activity are expected to disclose to the readers relevant financial relationships with commercial entities occurring within the past 12 months (such as grants or research support, employee, consultant, stock holder, member of speakers bureau, etc.). The University of Virginia School of Medicine will employ appropriate mechanisms to resolve potential conflicts of interest to maintain the standards of fair and balanced education to the reader. Questions about specific strategies can be directed to the Office of Continuing Medical Education, University of Virginia School of Medicine, Charlottesville, Virginia.

The authors/editors listed below have identified no financial or professional relationships for themselves or their spouse/partner:
Kenneth H. Butler, DO, FACP, FAEEM; Barton Dudlick, Acquisitions Editor; Juntima Euathrongchit, MD; Jean Jeudy, MD; Paul G. Kluetz, MD; Patrick C. Malloy, MD; Junichi Matsumoto, MD; Lisa A. Miller, MD; Stuart E. Mirvis, MD, FACR; Howard Marks Richard III, MD; Kathirkamanathan Shanmuganathan, MD; Clint W. Silker, MD; Eric J. Stern, MD; Sharon A. Swenki, MD; Nisa Thoongsuwan, MD; Stephen Waite, MD; and Charles S. White, MD.

Disclosure of Discussion of Non-FDA Approved Uses for Pharmaceutical and/or Medical Devices.
The University of Virginia School of Medicine, as an ACCME provider, requires that all authors identify and disclose any "off label" uses for pharmaceutical and medical device products. The University of Virginia School of Medicine recommends that each physician fully review all the available data on new products or procedures prior to clinical use.

TO ENROLL

To enroll in the Radiologic Clinics of North America Continuing Medical Education program, call customer service at 1-800-654-2452 or sign up online at *http://www.theclinics.com/home/cme.* The CME program is available to subscribers for an additional annual fee USD 205.

THE CLINICS ARE NOW AVAILABLE ONLINE!

Access your subscription at:
www.theclinics.com

EMERGENCY CHEST IMAGING

GUEST EDITORS

STUART E. MIRVIS, MD, FACR
Professor (Radiology), Department of Radiology, University of Maryland Medical Center; and Director, Section of Trauma and Emergency Radiology, University of Maryland Medical Center, Baltimore, Maryland

KATHIRKAMANATHAN SHANMUGANATHAN, MD
Professor, Department of Diagnostic Radiology, University of Maryland School of Medicine, Baltimore, Maryland

CONTRIBUTORS

KENNETH H. BUTLER, DO, FACEP, FAAEM
Associate Professor (Surgery), Division of Emergency Medicine, University of Maryland School of Medicine, Baltimore, Maryland

JUNTIMA EUATHRONGCHIT, MD
Research Fellow (Thoracic Imaging), Harborview Medical Center, Department of Radiology, University of Washington School of Medicine, Seattle, Washington

JEAN JEUDY, MD
Assistant Professor (Radiology), Department of Diagnostic Radiology, University of Maryland School of Medicine, Baltimore, Maryland

PAUL G. KLUETZ, MD
Resident, Department of Internal Medicine, University of Maryland, Baltimore, Maryland

PATRICK C. MALLOY, MD
Associate Professor, Department of Diagnostic Radiology; and Director, Interventional Radiology, University of Maryland Medical System, Baltimore, Maryland

JUNICHI MATSUMOTO, MD
Instructor, Department of Emergency and Critical Care Medicine, St. Marianna University School of Medicine, Kanagawa, Japan

LISA A. MILLER, MD
Assistant Professor, Department of Radiology, ShockTrauma Center, University of Maryland School of Medicine, Baltimore, Maryland

STUART E. MIRVIS, MD, FACR
Professor (Radiology), Department of Radiology, University of Maryland Medical Center; and Director, Section of Trauma and Emergency Radiology, University of Maryland Medical Center, Baltimore, Maryland

HOWARD MARKS RICHARD III, MD
Assistant Professor, Department of Diagnostic Radiology, University of Maryland Medical System, Baltimore, Maryland

KATHIRKAMANATHAN SHANMUGANATHAN, MD
Professor, Department of Diagnostic Radiology, University of Maryland School of Medicine, Baltimore, Maryland

CLINT W. SLIKER, MD
Assistant Professor, Department of Diagnostic Radiology and Nuclear Medicine, University of Maryland School of Medicine; and Diagnostic Imaging Department, University of Maryland Medical Center and R. Adams Cowley Shock Trauma Center, Baltimore, Maryland

ERIC J. STERN, MD
Professor; and Director (Thoracic Imaging), Harborview Medical Center, Department of Radiology, University of Washington School of Medicine, Seattle, Washington

SHARON A. SWENCKI, MD
Clinical Instructor (Surgery), Division of Emergency Medicine, University of Maryland School of Medicine, Baltimore, Maryland

NISA THOONGSUWAN, MD
Research Fellow (Thoracic Imaging), Harborview
Medical Center, Department of Radiology,
University of Washington School of Medicine,
Seattle, Washington

STEPHEN WAITE, MD
Assistant Professor (Radiology), Department of
Radiology, State University of New York
Downstate, Brooklyn, New York

CHARLES S. WHITE, MD
Professor (Radiology and Medicine); and Chief,
Thoracic Radiology, Department of Diagnostic
Radiology, University of Maryland School of
Medicine, Baltimore, Maryland

EMERGENCY CHEST IMAGING

Volume 44 • Number 2 • March 2006

Contents

Acute pulmonary embolism (PE) is a life-threatening condition that requires accurate diagnostic imaging. Morbidity and mortality resulting from PE can be reduced significantly if appropriate treatment is initiated early. Historically, the gold standard for the imaging of PE has been pulmonary angiography. Rapid advances in radiology and nuclear medicine have led to this modality largely being replaced by noninvasive techniques, most frequently multidetector helical CT pulmonary angiography (CTPA). For cases in which CTPA is contraindicated, other imaging modalities include nuclear ventilation-perfusion scanning, magnetic resonance pulmonary angiography, duplex Doppler ultrasonography for deep venous thrombosis, and echocardiography. This article reviews the literature on the role of these imaging modalities in the diagnosis of PE.

Acute chest pain is one of the most common complaints of patients who present to an emergency department, and accounts for up to 5% of all visits. It also is one of the most complex issues in an emergency setting because, although clinical signs and symptoms often are nonspecific, rapid diagnosis and therapy are of great importance. The chest radiograph remains an important component of the evaluation of chest pain, and usually is the first examination to be obtained. Nevertheless, cross-sectional imaging has added greatly to the ability to characterize the wide constellation of clinical findings into a distinct etiology. This article reviews how the various entities that can present as nontraumatic chest pain can manifest radiographically.

Pulmonary infections are among the most common causes of morbidity and mortality worldwide, and contribute substantially to annual medical expenditures in the United States. Despite the availability of antimicrobial agents, pneumonia constitutes the sixth most common cause of death and the number one cause of death from infection. Pneumonia can be particularly life threatening in the elderly, in individuals who have pre-existing heart and lung conditions, in patients who have suppressed or weakened immunity, and in pregnant women. This article discusses some of the important causes of acute lung infections in normal and immunocompromised hosts. Because there often is considerable overlap, infections are categorized by the host immune status that is most likely to be associated with a particular pathogen.

RADIOLOGIC
CLINICS
OF NORTH AMERICA

Radiol Clin N Am 44 (2006) xi–xii

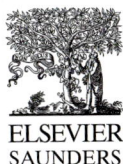

Preface
Emergency Chest Imaging

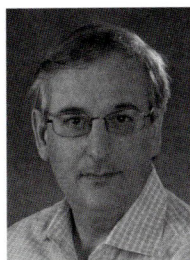

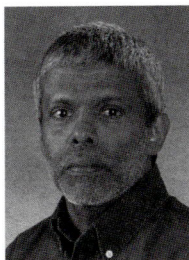

Stuart E. Mirvis, MD
Kathirkamanathan Shanmuganathan, MD

Guest Editors

Stuart E. Mirvis, MD
Professor
Department of Radiology
University of Maryland Medical Center

Director
Section of Trauma and Emergency Radiology
University of Maryland School of Medicine
Baltimore, MD, USA
E-mail address: smirvis@umm.edu

Kathirkamanathan Shanmuganathan, MD
Professor
Department of Diagnostic Radiology
University of Maryland School of Medicine
Baltimore, MD, USA
E-mail address: kshanmuganathan@umm.edu

The advent of multidetector computed tomography (MDCT) in recent years has sparked its use as a principal screening study for polytrauma patients and is increasingly commonly obtained in non-traumatic emergency department (ED) patients. The chest radiograph continues to be performed as a screening study in the polytrauma setting and for patients presenting to the ED with complaints related to the thorax. However, CT provides a significant improvement in sensitivity for detection of both traumatic and nontraumatic acute thoracic pathologies, which has fostered its common use in these settings. A thorough knowledge of the spectrum of pathology, the common and atypical CT appearances, and the influence of CT observations on management is required for contemporary imaging assessment.

In the blunt trauma patient, CT is essential to directly assess the thoracic vessels, pericardial fluid, and to potentially demonstrate airway and esophageal injuries. CT is far more sensitive than radiography for detection of pneumothorax, pleural fluid, and lung parenchymal injury. CT can document sites of active thoracic bleeding or vascular injury to direct surgical or angiographicintervention. Also, recent studies have shown that CT can play a valuable role in delineating the trajectory of penetrating thoracic injury and can help determine the need for further imaging investigation of mediastinal structures and for surgical exploration. In most poly-trauma patients multiple CT studies are usually indicated and inclusion of the chest as part of a general survey (total body CT) is being increasingly used in trauma centers. Even when the admission chest radiograph shows no definitive injury, CT can confirm the impression of normality with a higher level of accuracy or detect subtle but important pathology not revealed on the chest film. Several articles in this issue focus on traumatic chest pathology from both blunt and penetrating mechanisms.

doi:10.1016/j.rcl.2005.12.001

The use of CT for patients presenting with chest pain to the ED is increasing, because this approach can diagnose or exclude a wide variety of acute thoracic pathology. In these patients, MDCT has the potential to assess the aorta, pulmonary arteries, and coronary arteries simultaneously, the so-called "triple rule-out." It now appears that 40- or 64-slice units will be required for consistently performing high quality studies for this application. MDCT has become the definitive test to rapidly assess for pulmonary embolization being accurate, rapidly obtained, and cost-effective. Several articles in this issue discuss specific applications of MDCT in acute nontraumatic mediastinal and nonmediastinal chest pathology.

The opening article is intended to provide the radiologist with a "refresher" overview of typical clinical presentations of common nontraumatic ED emergencies to better integrate these findings with imaging observations.

RADIOLOGIC
CLINICS
OF NORTH AMERICA

Radiol Clin N Am 44 (2006) 165–179

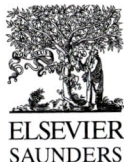

Chest Pain: A Clinical Assessment

Kenneth H. Butler, DO*, Sharon A. Swencki, MD

- Major pathologies that produce chest pain
  Pneumothorax
  Pneumonia
  Acute coronary syndrome
  Pulmonary embolism

Pericarditis
Thoracic aortic dissection
- Summary
- References

Chest pain is one of the most common chief complaints in emergency medicine. During the acute presentation of a patient who has chest pain, chest imaging is invaluable, especially in the initial stabilization of a life-threatening cardiac or pulmonary event. The initial approach to evaluating chest pain includes excluding life-threatening causes, such as aortic dissection, pulmonary embolism (PE), pneumothorax, pneumomediastinum, pericarditis, and esophageal perforation.

The evaluation of an unstable patient who has chest pain or shortness of breath begins with a primary medical survey to evaluate airway, breathing, and circulation. In tandem with this rapid assessment, the emergency physician requests radiographic images of the chest, which provide visualization of the thoracic anatomy. The first image obtained is the anteroposterior chest radiograph, using portable radiography or fixed equipment, depending on the patient's presenting clinical appearance. The initial study is invaluable in providing clinically relevant information that directs the patient's care.

Although technologic advances have improved diagnostic accuracy greatly in recent years, a thorough history and physical examination remain the most important components in the evaluation process. It is imperative to obtain as many details about the pain as possible, including its onset, location, duration, radiation, quality, and exacerbating and relieving factors. A detailed history sets in motion further diagnostic testing and management decisions.

Major pathologies that produce chest pain

Pneumothorax

Perfect coupling between the visceral and parietal pleura is required for effective ventilation. Patients who have pneumothorax have gas in the intrapleural space. This abnormality uncouples the visceral and parietal pleura and thus elevates the intrapleural pressure, which affects ventilation, gas exchange, and perfusion.

Pneumothorax commonly is divided into two types: primary spontaneous pneumothorax (PSP), which usually occurs without a precipitating event in patients who have no clinical lung disease, and secondary spontaneous pneumothorax, a complication of underlying lung disease. In actuality, most patients who have PSP have underlying lung disease, most commonly rupture of a subpleural bleb [1]. Iatrogenic pneumothorax is difficult to identify; its incidence is increasing due to the more widespread use of mechanical ventilation and interventional procedures such as central line placement and lung biopsy [2]. When pneumo-

Division of Emergency Medicine, University of Maryland School of Medicine, Baltimore, MD, USA
* Corresponding author. Division of Emergency Medicine, University of Maryland School of Medicine, 110 South Paca Street, Sixth Floor, Suite 200, Baltimore, MD 21201.
E-mail address: kbutler@smail.umaryland.edu (K.H. Butler).

doi:10.1016/j.rcl.2005.11.002

thorax is suspected, correct interpretation of chest radiographs and knowledge of the benefit of more complex imaging techniques are essential. The causes of spontaneous and iatrogenic pneumothorax and of pneumomediastinum are summarized in Box 1.

The incidence of PSP (age-adjusted) is 7.4 cases per 100,000 persons per year for men and 1.2 cases per 100,000 persons per year for women [3,4]. The incidence of secondary spontaneous pneumothorax (age-adjusted) is 6.3 cases per 100,000 persons per year for men and 2 cases per 100,000 persons per year for women [3,4]. The incidence of iatrogenic pneumothorax is not known, but it probably occurs more often than do primary and secondary spontaneous pneumothoraces combined. Pneumomediastinum occurs in approximately 1 of 10,000 hospital admissions [5].

Box 1: Causes of pneumothorax

Spontaneous pneumothorax

- Rupture of subpleural apical emphysematous blebs
- Smoking (increases the risk of a first spontaneous pneumothorax by more than 20-fold in men and by nearly 10-fold in women, compared with the risks in nonsmokers)
- Physical height (taller patients are at risk because alveoli are subjected to a greater mean distending pressure over time, which leads to subpleural bleb formation; because pleural pressure is more negative at the apex of the lung, blebs are more likely to rupture and cause pneumothorax)

Iatrogenic pneumothorax

- Transthoracic needle aspiration procedures
- Subclavian and supraclavicular needlestick
- Thoracentesis
- Mechanical ventilation (directly related to peak airway pressures)
- Pleural or transbronchial biopsy
- Cardiopulmonary resuscitation
- Tracheostomy

Pneumomediastinum

- Acute production of high intrathoracic pressures (usual cause)
- Asthma
- Smoking marijuana
- Inhalation of cocaine
- Athletic competition
- Respiratory tract infection
- Parturition
- Emesis
- Severe cough
- Mechanical ventilation

Pathogenesis

The pathogenesis of the subpleural blebs that cause PSP is related to airway inflammation that results from cigarette smoking. The risk of PSP is related directly to the level of cigarette smoking (number of pack years) [6].

Pneumothorax occurs with increasing frequency in patients who have Marfan's syndrome and homocystinuria [7]. Catamenial pneumothorax may result from thoracic endometriosis and should be considered in menstruating women who present with spontaneous pneumothorax [8].

Clinical presentation

PSP usually develops at rest. The peak age is the early 20s. The disorder is rare after age 40. Patients usually complain of the sudden onset of dyspnea and pleuritic chest pain. The severity of symptoms is related to the volume of air in the pleural space; dyspnea is more predominant if the pneumothorax is large. In patients who have a large pneumothorax, the physical findings include decreased chest excursion on the affected side, diminished breath sounds, and hyperresonant lungs. Many affected individuals do not seek medical attention for days after symptoms develop. This sequence is important, because the incidence of re-expansion pulmonary edema increases in patients whose chest tubes were placed 3 or more days after the pneumothorax occurred.

Pneumomediastinum usually occurs when intrathoracic pressures become elevated. This elevation may occur with an exacerbation of asthma, coughing, vomiting, childbirth, seizures, and a Valsalva maneuver. Patients usually complain of a sudden onset of chest pain and dyspnea.

Radiographic features

The main radiographic abnormality that is indicative of pneumothorax is a white visceral pleural line—straight or convex toward the chest wall—which is separated from the parietal pleura by an avascular collection of air. In most cases, no pulmonary vessels are visible beyond the visceral edge.

The size of a pneumothorax is difficult to estimate. The measurement of the distance between the ribs and the visceral pleura can be used to decide whether to perform a tube thoracostomy. If the distance is greater than 3 cm laterally or 4 cm at the apex, a chest tube may be needed to re-expand the lung. A pneumothorax of less than 10% will reabsorb on its own and does not require placement of a chest tube.

In upright patients who have pneumothorax, gas accumulates primarily in an apicolateral location.

As little as 50 mL of pleural gas can be seen on chest film. A lateral chest film with a 1-cm intrapleural space corresponds to a 10% pneumothorax. The size of the pneumothorax is accounted for by the collapsed lung and, to a lesser degree, the expanding chest cage.

The value of expiratory chest radiographs in detecting pneumothoraces has been overstated. In a study of 85 patients who had pneumothoraces and 93 controls, inspiratory and expiratory upright chest radiographs had equal sensitivity for pneumothorax detection [9]. Because expiratory films provide no added benefit, only inspiratory films are recommended as the initial radiograph of choice for pneumothorax.

In the supine patient, approximately 500 mL of pleural air is needed for definitive diagnosis of pneumothorax [10]. The pleural gas accumulates in the subpulmonic location and outlines the anterior pleural reflection, the costophrenic sulcus, and the anterolateral border of the mediastinum. The overall transradiancy of the entire affected hemithorax can be increased on the side of a pneumothorax in the recumbent patient.

Small pneumothoraces can be visualized more easily in the lateral decubitus view. In this position, as little as 5 mL of pleural gas is visible on the nondependent side [10].

Ultrasound detection of pneumothorax
Bedside ultrasound has become standard in most emergency departments. Focused abdominal sonography for trauma has been integrated into the assessment of the unstable patient. A key element in ultrasound assessment of the chest for pneumothorax is the presence or absence of the "sliding lung sign." On ultrasound of the normal chest, the lung surface can be seen sliding along the chest wall during inspiration and expiration. In a patient who has pneumothorax, this sign is absent, which suggests that the air adjacent to the chest wall is not contained within the lung.

Ultrasound has proven to be more sensitive than flat anteroposterior chest radiography in the diagnosis of trauma-induced pneumothorax. Ultrasound provides added benefit by allowing sonologists to differentiate between small, medium, and large pneumothoraces, with good agreement with CT results [11].

Tension pneumothorax
Tension pneumothorax shows a distinct shift of the mediastinum to the contralateral side and flattening or inversion of the ipsilateral hemidiaphragm. This is the result of accumulation of air under pressure in the pleural space. This emergent condition develops when injured tissue forms a one-way valve and allows air to enter the pleural space but prevents it from escaping naturally. Arising from numerous causes, this condition progresses rapidly to respiratory insufficiency, cardiovascular collapse, and, ultimately, death if it is unrecognized and untreated. Favorable patient outcomes require urgent clinical diagnosis and immediate management.

Conditions that mimic pneumothorax
Large subplural bullae can mimic a loculated pneumothorax. In most cases, the medial border of the bulla is concave toward the chest wall, whereas a visceral pleural contour is straight or convex laterally. Skin folds can be differentiated from a pneumothorax by density profile: they form a negative black Mach band instead of the white visceral pleural line. Skin folds increase gradually in opacity, with an abrupt drop-off at the edge, and usually extend beyond the ribcage or stop short of the ribs.

Bilateral pneumothoraces may be seen after heart/lung transplant surgery. Replacement of the heart and lungs leaves an open communication between the two sides of the thorax, which may allow air or fluid to shift from one side to the other. Extensive mediastinal dissection can disrupt the anterior junction line, allowing a unilateral pneumothorax to propagate to the contralateral hemithorax. Placement of a single thoracotomy tube decompresses and evacuates both pleural cavities.

Treatment of pneumothorax
The treatment of pneumothorax is based on its classification. A tension pneumothorax usually results in cardiopulmonary compromise (shock, bradycardia, hypoxia) and requires immediate needle decompression (thoracentesis), which can be accomplished by inserting a large-bore (16- or 18-gauge) needle (smaller needles are satisfactory for premature infants, newborns, and infants) through the second or third interspace (near the apex of the lung) in the midclavicular line. *Immediate decompression cannot wait for radiographic confirmation.* Tube thoracostomy may be required after the initial decompression if the pneumothorax reaccumulates.

Management of a simple pneumothorax depends on its size and cause. A clinically stable patient who has a small PSP (occupying <15% of the hemithorax) should be observed in the emergency department for 3 to 6 hours and discharged home if a repeat chest film demonstrates no progression of the pneumothorax. If the patient is to be admitted to the hospital, oxygen therapy may be initiated to hasten absorption of the pneumothorax. Clinically stable patients who have a large PSP should be admitted to the hospital for tube thoracostomy.

Pneumonia

Despite advances in diagnosis and treatment, pulmonary infections remain a major cause of morbidity and mortality in adult patients. An estimated 4 to 6 million cases of community-acquired pneumonia occur each year [12]. The spectrum of organisms known to cause respiratory infections is broad and constantly increasing as new pathogens are identified and the host immune response is altered by medications or other diseases or responses. In the United States, it is estimated that 1.1 million cases of community-acquired pneumonia require hospitalization each year, at an estimated cost of $8 billion [13]. Pneumonia is responsible for more than 64 million days of restricted activity from work and is the seventh leading cause of death in this country, with a mortality rate of 22.4 per 100,000 [14].

Among hospital-acquired infections, nosocomial pneumonia has the highest mortality [15]. Moreover, since the beginning of the AIDS epidemic, the lungs are identified increasingly as the source of infection.

Radiology plays a prominent role in the evaluation of pneumonia. Chest radiography is the most commonly used imaging tool in pneumonias, because of its availability and excellent cost/benefit ratio. CT should be used in unresolved cases or when complications of pneumonia are suspected [16]. The main applications of radiology in pneumonia are oriented toward detection, characterization, and follow-up, especially regarding complications.

The classic classification of pneumonias into lobar and bronchial types has been abandoned for a more clinical classification. Thus, bacterial pneumonias are divided into three main groups: community-acquired pneumonia, aspiration pneumonia, and nosocomial pneumonia. The usual pattern of community-acquired pneumonia is that of lobar pneumonia: an air-space consolidation that is limited to one lobe or segment. Nevertheless, the radiographic patterns of community-acquired pneumonia may be variable and often are related to the causative agent.

Aspiration pneumonia generally involves the lower lobes, with bilateral multicentric opacities. The most valuable information is obtained when the chest radiographs are negative and exclude pneumonia.

The criterion standard test for the diagnosis of pneumonia has been the two-view plain chest film. In a study by Courtoy and colleagues [17], however, radiologists who were blinded to culture results could not differentiate viral pneumonia from bacterial pneumonia by reviewing the chest films. Several investigative teams have concluded that no radiologic features exist that can be used to differentiate between these two major etiologic classes [17,18].

Radiographic findings that are suggestive of specific etiologic agents

Pneumococcal pneumonia Lobar consolidation, involving single or multiple lobes, is the most common radiographic pattern of community-acquired pneumococcal pneumonia in patients who require hospitalization [19]. Pleural effusions also are a common finding in pneumococcal pneumonia. The pattern of consolidation is not influenced by bacteremia or HIV status. The presence of a pneumonic process on radiography correlates with identifiable clinical signs [20,21]. Normal findings on a chest radiograph virtually exclude a diagnosis of pneumonia other than in HIV-infected patients who have *Pneumocystis carinii* or, rarely, in dehydrated, elderly, or neutropenic patients and those who were examined within 24 hours of the onset of symptoms.

Mycoplasmal pneumonia The radiographic findings in patients who are infected with *Mycoplasma pneumoniae* also are nonspecific, and in some cases, closely resemble those seen in children who have viral infections of the lower respiratory tract. Focal reticulonodular opacification confined to a single lobe is a radiographic pattern that seems to be associated more closely with *Mycoplasma* infection than with other types of pediatric respiratory illnesses. The diagnosis of *Mycoplasma* pneumonia should be considered whenever focal or bilateral reticulonodular opacification is seen. Hazy or ground-glass consolidations occur frequently; however, dense homogeneous consolidations like those seen with bacterial pneumonias are uncommon. Often, atelectasis or transient pseudo-consolidations that produce confluent interstitial shadows are seen. Radiographic findings alone are not sufficient for the definitive diagnosis of *Mycoplasma* pneumonia, but in combination with clinical findings, they can improve the accuracy of diagnosis of this disease significantly.

Guckel and colleagues [22] described three patterns of infiltration in children who have mycoplasmal pneumonia, which occur with equal frequency: peribronchial and perivascular interstitial infiltrates, patchy consolidations, and homogeneous acinar consolidations like ground glass. The infiltrates were seen primarily in the lower lungs. Enlargement of the hilar glands was a common finding among the 23 children in their series. Pleural effusion was rare. Diffuse interstitial and bilateral parahilar peribronchial patterns are common in *Mycoplasma* respiratory infections.

Viral pneumonias Viral pneumonias are located predominantly in spaces along and around the alveoli. Therefore, these pneumonias appear reticular on plain radiograph and often are bilateral and diffuse in distribution. Associated with thickening of the interlobular septa, viral pneumonias can be associated with Kerly B lines on chest radiograph. Rarely associated with complications or even pleural effusion, viral pneumonia can lead to secondary bacterial pneumonias. In viral pneumonia, four radiographic findings are common: parahilar peribronchial infiltrates, hyperexpansion, segmental or lobar atelectasis, and hilar adenopathy.

Pneumocystis carinii pneumonia Although the radiographic findings in patients who have *Pneumocystis carinii* pneumonia (PCP) vary, most chest radiographs reveal bilateral, symmetric, fine to medium reticular heterogeneous opacities [23–25]. As the disease worsens, the opacities coalesce and eventually appear as a bilateral homogeneous consolidation. Uncommonly, a more coarse reticular pattern or a miliary pattern may be noted [25,26].

Unilateral or unilobar involvement may occur, but the radiographic pattern remains fine reticular opacities. Predominant upper lobe involvement occurs with increased frequency in patients who have used aerosolized pentamidine for prophylaxis [21,27,28]; however, because the use of this form of prophylaxis has waned, the incidence of this appearance has decreased. The presence of hilar or mediastinal adenopathy as well as pleural fluid is rare and suggests another disease process. Usually, these findings are seen in patients who have been taking aerosolized pentamidine and have developed disseminated pneumocystosis [29,30]. Cases of pneumocystosis following the use of dapsone prophylaxis have been reported [31]. Calcified hilar and mediastinal lymph nodes have been reported but are rare [32]. Approximately 10% of patients who have HIV disease and subsequently proven PCP have had normal chest radiographs. In some circumstances, gallium scanning or high-resolution CT may demonstrate lung abnormalities, particularly ground-glass opacities [33]. In many institutions, however, treatment is recommended empirically, without a request for further imaging [34,35].

Legionella Virtually all patients who have Legionnaire's disease have abnormal chest radiography that shows pulmonary infiltrates at the time of clinical presentation. In a few cases of nosocomial disease, fever and respiratory tract symptoms have preceded the appearance of the infiltrate on chest radiography. Findings on chest films are nonspecific and do not distinguish *Legionella* from causes of pneumonia. Pleural effusion is evident in one third of cases.

In immunosuppressed patients, distinctive, rounded, nodular opacities may be seen; these lesions may expand or cavitate. Pulmonary abscesses may occur in the immunosuppressed host. Infiltration that progresses on chest radiography, despite appropriate antibiotic therapy, is common, and radiographic improvement lags behind clinical improvement by several days. Complete clearing of infiltrates requires 1 to 4 months.

Acute coronary syndrome

Acute coronary syndrome (ACS) is a spectrum of acute myocardial ischemia that spans acute myocardial infarction (AMI) and unstable angina [36]. Less than 25% of patients who are admitted with suspicion of ACS still have this diagnosis at discharge [37].

History and physical examination
Chest pain or discomfort is the most common presenting complaint in patients who have ACS [37]. The character and radiation of the pain are important for the diagnosis [38]. The pain usually is described as a deep visceral discomfort and may be difficult to localize to one region of the chest [38]. The character of the pain often is described as pressure, a weight on the chest, tightness, constriction about the throat, or an aching feeling. The pain is not affected by respiration or movement. Beginning gradually and reaching maximum severity after 2 or 3 minutes, the pain lasts for minutes or longer [38]. Physical exertion or emotional stress may be associated with the onset of pain, and the pain may subside with rest [36]. Radiation of the pain to the arm or neck increases the likelihood of AMI [38]. The patient may have associated symptoms of shortness of breath, nausea, vomiting, profound weakness, dizziness, palpitations, and diaphoresis [36].

Chest pain is absent in up to 6.2% of patients who have ACS and 9.8% of patients who have AMI [39]. Atypical presentations are more likely in elderly patients and diabetics, who have an altered ability to localize symptoms [38], and in women and younger people [36]. Atypical symptoms include epigastric pain, indigestion, stabbing chest pain, pleuritic chest pain, chest pain that is reproducible on palpation, and isolated dyspnea [36].

Risk factors for cardiac disease are elicited during the history. Traditional risk factors for coronary artery disease (CAD) include hypertension, hypercholesterolemia, cigarette smoking, diabetes, peripheral vascular disease, family history of CAD, personal history of CAD, male gender, and increasing age [36–38]. These are long-term risk factors for

CAD; the absence of risk factors for CAD should not be used to exclude the diagnosis of ACS [37,38].

The physical examination of a patient in whom ACS is suspected generally is not helpful unless it reveals an alternate diagnosis [37]. Thus, the physical examination should focus on excluding other diagnoses; identifying causes of myocardial ischemia, such as uncontrolled hypertension or thyroid disease; and searching for signs of hemodynamic instability [36]. Caution should be taken in automatically attributing chest pain that is reproducible on examination to musculoskeletal causes, because 11% of cases of partially or fully reproducible chest pain may be attributable to ACS [37]. Any degree of pulmonary rales on examination is associated with ACS; however, an S3 gallop on cardiac auscultation is nonspecific [37].

Pope and colleagues [37] found that patients who had a final diagnosis of ACS were more likely to have a lower pulse rate and higher blood pressure than patients who had other diagnoses; this probably is associated with adrenergic excess or lower compliance of an ischemic left ventricle. The clinician would need to know the patient's baseline vital signs; usually, that information is not available in the emergency department setting, which limits the usefulness of this observation [38]. The probability of AMI is increased if the patient is diaphoretic and is decreased if the respiratory rate is normal [37].

Laboratory studies

Because myocytes lose their membrane integrity in response to ischemia, they release molecules into the peripheral circulation [36]. These molecules, known as cardiac biomarkers, are useful in the diagnosis of AMI. The biomarkers that can be detected do not aid in the diagnosis of unstable angina, which accounts for roughly half of all cases of ACS [38,40,41]. The cardiac biomarkers that are in widespread use are creatinine kinase (CK), creatinine kinase MB fraction (CK-MB), myoglobin, cardiac troponin I (cTnI), and cardiac troponin T (cTnT).

Creatinine kinase and creatinine kinase MB fraction   CK and CK-MB are nonspecific biomarkers that can be found in any case of muscle damage [36]. Until recently, CK-MB had been the principal serum marker of cardiac myocyte damage [36]. The sensitivity of serum CK and CK-MB concentrations for detection of ischemia increases with the duration of the patient's symptoms [38]. Serial measurements of both biomarkers increase sensitivity and specificity when performed over 4 to 9 hours [38]. Serial CK-MB has a sensitivity of 87% and a specificity of 96% for AMI [38]. These serial tests should be performed over 4 to 9 hours.

Myoglobin   Serum myoglobin is another nonspecific biomarker that appears in the peripheral circulation as early as 1 to 2 hours after muscle damage [36]. Again, the sensitivity of myoglobin measurements in the diagnosis of AMI increases with serial measurements [38,41]. Serum myoglobin levels should not be used in isolation for the diagnosis of ACS [36]; however, there is some evidence that a normal myoglobin concentration 2 hours after presentation can exclude AMI [38,42].

Troponin   cTnI and cTnT are specific for myocardial damage and have supplanted CK-MB as the preferred biomarker for myocardial ischemia [36]. These biomarkers are not found in the blood of healthy individuals [36]. As with the other cardiac biomarkers, the sensitivity of cTnI and cTnT increases with serial measurements and with duration of symptoms [38]. Elevated levels of cTnI and cTnT are associated with increased mortality, even when the ECG is inconclusive for ACS and CK-MB concentrations are normal [36,42].

Electrocardiography

Electrocardiography is a safe, inexpensive, and readily available bedside test that represents the standard of care for patients who have expected ACS. When possible, the ECG should be obtained while the patient is symptomatic [36]. Although the ECG is highly sensitive for AMI, it is neither highly sensitive nor specific for ACS in general [38]. Pope and colleagues [37] found that up to 20% of patients who had AMI and 37% of patients who had the diagnosis of unstable angina had a normal ECG at presentation. The ECG should be interpreted with consideration of the patient's presentation. Thus, in a patient with a clinical picture that is consistent with ACS and a normal ECG, the probability of ischemia is not reduced substantially [38].

ST-segment and T-wave abnormalities are the quintessential electrocardiographic abnormalities in the diagnosis of ACS [37,38]. ST-segment elevation indicates transmural ischemia [36], whereas ST-segment depression indicates subendocardial ischemia [38]. Inverted T waves indicate acute ischemia [38]. Q waves are diagnostic of infarction but could represent previous infarction [38]. Obtaining an old ECG can aid in determining if any abnormalities have developed acutely.

Radiology

Chest radiography   A chest film usually is obtained during the initial assessment of the patient who has ACS. This imaging study is used to search for other causes of the patient's symptoms and to assess for contraindications to heparin therapy (eg, aortic dissection). The presence of pulmonary edema, which could indicate acute heart failure, also is evaluated using plain chest radiography.

Echocardiography For the patient who has a low risk for ACS, resting echocardiography has a high sensitivity (93%), although only a moderate specificity (66%), for diagnosing AMI [43]. Echocardiography does not distinguish between acute and chronic abnormalities and requires skilled technicians and interpreters, which often limits its use in the acute setting [40]. Echocardiography is useful in providing information about the patient's hemodynamic status and may help to identify other causes of disease, such as PE and pericarditis [40].

Nuclear imaging Thallium-201 (^{201}Tl) and technetium-99m sestamibi (^{99m}Tc-sestamibi) are radionucleotides used commonly in nuclear cardiac imaging. Noninvasive tests based on those isotopes detect ischemic or infarcted myocardium. Both imaging modalities can detect perfusion abnormalities for several hours after the last symptomatic episode of chest pain [36]. Abnormal results of myocardial perfusion imaging studies done with the patient at rest indicate risk for AMI and death and the need for revascularization, whereas normal images at rest indicate the patient has a low risk for cardiac complications [36]. ^{201}Tl images must be taken within 15 to 20 minutes of injection, which limits the usefulness of this modality in the acute setting [40]. Imaging with ^{99m}Tc sestamibi is advantageous because serial imaging can be done, and left ventricular wall motion abnormalities can be evaluated using gated single photon emission CT (SPECT) imaging [36]. Nuclear cardiac imaging is most useful in patients who have low to moderate risk for ACS and no acute ECG changes [43].

Pulmonary embolism

PE must be considered in every patient who has chest pain and dyspnea. PE is the third most common cause of cardiovascular death among Americans, accounting for 50,000 to 100,000 deaths per year [44,45]. Only 30% of PE are diagnosed before death [46]. Alternatively, less than 35% of patients who are suspected of having a PE actually have one [45,47–49]. PE is a challenging diagnosis to reach, it often is missed, and it often is sought but not found.

History and physical examination

The history and physical examination are notoriously insensitive for PE. The classic presentation of PE is chest pain, dyspnea, and hemoptysis; however, this triad is present in less than 20% of patients [48]. Patients who have significant PE may remain asymptomatic if the obstruction of pulmonary circulation is less than 50% [50].

The Prospective Investigation of Pulmonary Embolism Diagnosis (PIOPED) study found that in patients who were diagnosed with PE, one or more risk factors for PE were likely to be present [47]. Risk factors for venous thromboembolism are listed in Box 2.

The most common symptom of acute PE is unexplained dyspnea of acute onset [48,51]. Dyspnea is present in more than 70% of patients who are diagnosed with PE [44]. Palpitations, cough, anxiety, lightheadedness, abdominal pain, back pain, atrial fibrillation, and hiccoughs are nonspecific symptoms [48,51]. Syncope occurs in 8% to 13% of patients who have PE [52].

The presentation of the patient who has PE depends on the degree of obstruction of the pulmonary circulation, the speed of accumulation of the clot burden, and the patient's underlying health [50]. Three clinical syndromes have been described in the patient who has PE: pulmonary infarction, isolated dyspnea, and circulatory collapse [48,53]. Signs and symptoms of PE vary according to the clinical syndrome that is present. For patients who have pulmonary infarction, pleuritic chest pain and hemoptysis may predominate [53]. Patients who have underlying cardiovascular disease, such as elderly patients, are more likely to have pulmonary infarction [48].

Box 2: Risk factors for pulmonary embolism

Inherited hematologic risk factors

- Antithrombin III deficiency
- Factor V Leiden mutation
- Proteins C and S deficiency
- Lupus anticoagulant
- Abnormalities in fibrinolysis

Acquired risk factors

- Advanced age
- Smoking
- Immobilization
- Surgery
- Malignancy
- Trauma
- Oral contraceptives/hormone replacement
- Pregnancy
- Central venous catheters
- Obesity
- Myocardial infarction
- Congestive heart failure

Data from Refs. [44,48,53].

For patients who have isolated dyspnea, the degree of dyspnea varies with the degree of pulmonary vascular infarction [48]. For patients who have no underlying cardiovascular disease, the extent of embolism correlates with the degree of arterial hypoxemia [50]. Patients who have circulatory collapse may present following syncope, be hemodynamically unstable, or present in cardiac arrest [53].

No specific or sensitive physical examination finding is indicative of PE [53]. The most common signs of PE on examination are tachypnea and tachycardia [51]; however, normal vital signs should not discourage the physician from searching for a PE [53]. Fever, wheezing, rales, pleural rub, a loud pulmonic component of the second heart sound, right ventricular lift, right-sided fourth heart sound, cyanosis, and evidence of phlebitis may be present [45,51,53].

Clinical scoring systems

Clinical scoring systems attempt to help the clinician estimate the probability of PE. The best known of the clinical scoring systems is Well's criteria for prediction of PE [Table 1]. This scoring system combines the assessment of risk factors, presenting signs and symptoms, as well as the clinician's suspicion of an alternate diagnosis [54]. This scoring system is vulnerable because it relies heavily on the subjective judgment of the clinician as to the presence of alternate diagnoses [53].

Laboratory studies

Although arterial blood gas analysis (ABG) is a widely available and rapid laboratory study, it lacks the sensitivity to diagnose or exclude PE [53,55]. Patients who do not have underlying cardiopulmonary disease may have normal PaO_2, nor-

mal $PaCO_2$, and normal $P(Aa)O_2$ gradients in the face of angiographically proven PE [55].

D-dimer, a breakdown product of fibrin, is found in the blood when plasmin acts on a fibrin clot. As a marker of clot lysis, D-dimer is found in any condition in which there is formation or dissolution of clot. Thus, D-dimer can be found in elevated levels in association with PE, trauma, cancer, disseminated intravascular coagulation, myocardial infarction, sepsis, and preeclampsia and following surgery. Therefore, D-dimer is more useful in excluding PE than in diagnosing it [53,55,56,58]. Wells and colleagues [56] concluded that in a patient with a low clinical probability of PE using the Well's clinical scoring system and a negative D-dimer assay, PE can be ruled out safely without any imaging study [55].

ECG

Most patients who have PE have some abnormality on ECG, but ECG abnormalities in patients who have PE are nonspecific [51]. The ECG is most helpful to exclude other causes of the patient's symptoms, such as myocardial ischemia or pericarditis. The characteristic ECG abnormality of PE is the S1Q3T3 pattern; however, this is found in less than 20% of ECGs from patients who have proven PE [53]. T-wave inversion in the precordial leads is the most common electrocardiographic finding and is present in 68% of patients who have PE [48]. Tachycardia and incomplete right bundle branch block also have been found more often in patients who have PE than in patients who have other diagnoses [45].

Imaging

Chest radiography   Like electrocardiography, chest radiography often is abnormal, but nonspecific, and may elucidate other diagnoses. The PIOPED study found that the most sensitive radiographic finding for PE is atelectasis or parenchymal abnormality, with a sensitivity of 68% [47]. Other common abnormalities that are found on chest radiography include pleural effusion, pulmonary infiltrates, mild elevation of the hemidiaphragm, enlargement of the pulmonary artery, and cardiomegaly [51,53]. It is important not to exclude the diagnosis of PE based on radiographic evidence of pneumonia or congestive heart failure, because these entities may coexist with PE [48]. The classic signs of relative oligemia (Westermark's sign) and wedge-shaped pulmonary opacity (Hampton's hump) are rare [53].

Ventilation–perfusion scintigraphy   Historically, ventilation-perfusion (V/Q) lung scanning has been the initial imaging modality of choice in

Table 1: Wells' criteria for assigning pretest probability for pulmonary embolism

Criteria	Points
Clinical symptoms or signs of DVT	3
PE more likely than other diagnosis	3
Heart rate >100 bpm	1.5
Immobilization or surgery within last 4 wk	1.5
History of DVT or PE	1.5
Hemoptysis	1
Malignancy	1

Clinical probability of PE	Points
Low	<2
Moderate	2–5
High	>6

Data from Refs. [56–58].

patients suspected of having PE. The results of the V/Q scan are interpreted in association with the patient's assigned pretest probability [48,53]. A high-probability V/Q scan in a patient who has a high pretest probability has an 85% to 90% positive predictive value of PE; a normal V/Q scan in a patient who has a low pretest probability essentially excludes the diagnosis of PE [47,59]. Most V/Q scans fall into the category of nondiagnostic, however, which severely limits the usefulness of this imaging modality [45]. Patients who have underlying lung disease also have abnormal baseline studies [48].

Multidetector CT angiography Multidetector CT angiography (MDCT-A) is becoming the initial study of choice in the acute setting for the diagnosis of PE, primarily because of its widespread availability, speed, and noninvasive nature. In comparison with V/Q scanning, CT is more accurate [45] and is more likely to show another cause of the patient's symptoms if PE is not present. There has been some question as to the sensitivity of CT for PE. Pooled data show a wide range of sensitivities (53–100%) and specificities (81–100%) [60]; however, for central PE, the sensitivity of CT increases to 94% [45]. Subsegmental emboli and horizontal vessels are not well visualized on CT [48]. Other drawbacks of CT imaging include the use of nephrotoxic contrast and radiation exposure; in addition, the study requires a cooperative patient, because motion artifact limits the quality of the images [45].

Magnetic resonance angiography Magnetic resonance angiography (MRA) may be used to visualize PE and lower extremity deep vein thrombosis (DVT) and offers the advantages of safer contrast material, noninvasive nature, and no ionizing radiation [48,53]. MRA is limited in its use by expense and availability. In addition, MR imaging is time consuming and allows only limited access to patients who become unstable [48].

Pulmonary angiography Pulmonary angiography is considered the gold standard for the diagnosis of PE [47]. Often, this procedure is not readily available; requires nephrotoxic contrast; and is invasive, time-consuming, and expensive. In addition, the patient must be transported away from the emergency department, and the images rarely elucidate an alternate diagnosis [53].

Echocardiography Transthoracic echocardiography (TTE) is noninvasive and can be performed at the bedside. Findings on echocardiography that suggest PE include right-sided thrombus; dilation of the right ventricle, pulmonary artery, or inferior vena cava; decreased right ventricular function; loss of right ventricular contractility; tricuspid regurgitation;

and abnormal septal wall motion [53]. Transesophageal echocardiography (TEE) is more invasive—usually requiring sedation—but is more sensitive than TTE for detection of these hemodynamic abnormalities [51,53].

Ultrasound Lower extremity ultrasound imaging for the detection of DVT has the greatest usefulness in the patient who has signs and symptoms of DVT and PE [45]. This test should not be used as an initial imaging modality for the patient who has suspected acute PE [45], but it may be useful as an adjunct test to detect the source of PE.

Pericarditis

Pericarditis is inflammation of the pericardium, the fibrous sac surrounding the heart and great vessels [61,62]. The many causes of pericarditis include collagen vascular disease, renal insufficiency, neoplasm, viral infections, tuberculosis, and bacterial infections [63]. In many cases, the exact etiology remains unknown [63,64]. The diagnosis of pericarditis is suspected in the patient who has chest pain, pericardial rub on physical examination, and characteristic ECG changes [65].

History and physical examination

By history alone, pericarditis may be difficult to differentiate from myocardial ischemia, because the patient may complain of retrosternal chest pain with a radiation pattern similar to that of myocardial ischemia [65,66]. Classically, pericarditis presents with a retrosternal location of pain, but the patient may complain of pain anywhere in the chest [66]. The pain often is described as sharp or stabbing [61]. A pleuritic component of the pain, including increasing pain with inspiration, an increase in pain with supine position, and some relief with upright posture or sitting forward, is described often [61,65]. The pain may radiate to the neck, arms, or left shoulder [61]. Pain that radiates to either trapezius muscle ridge is likely to be pericarditis secondary to phrenic nerve innervation of the anterior pericardium and both trapezius ridges [61,65,66]. Onset of pain is sudden and progressive over hours to days [61,65].

Fever or other features of a nonspecific prodrome may precede pericarditis of infectious etiology [65,67]. A medical history of renal failure, known neoplasm, collagen vascular disease, or thyroid disorder may aid in the diagnosis, because these are common causes of pericarditis [68]. Temperature higher than 38°C is rare, but when present, may indicate purulent pericarditis [61].

A pericardial friction rub is pathognomic for pericarditis and is 100% specific for the disease [65,66]. The pericardial friction rub may come and go with time; thus, the patient should be examined repeatedly [61,66]. The rub is best heard at the left lower sternal border with the patient leaning forward at the end of expiration [5,6,61]. Generally, the rub is described as rasping, creaking, harsh, or high pitched. Classically, it is triphasic, but it may be biphasic or monophasic [62,65]. The stereotypic triphasic rub that corresponds to the motion of the heart during ventricular systole, diastolic ventricular filling, and atrial contraction is present in only half of patients [69].

The presence of muffled heart sounds, tachycardia, distended neck veins, hypotension, and pulsus paradoxus suggests cardiac tamponade. The patient may be in acute respiratory distress, but the lungs generally will be clear [67].

Laboratory studies

Laboratory studies are obtained to exclude other causes of chest pain and to elucidate the possible cause of the pericarditis. Markers of inflammation, such as leukocytosis, elevated C-reactive protein, and elevated erythrocyte sedimentation rate, usually are found in patients who have acute pericarditis [61]. Plasma electrolytes should be measured, and renal function should be evaluated [65].

The patient's clinical picture should guide additional testing, which might include blood cultures, tuberculin skin test, antinuclear antibodies, rheumatoid factor, thyroid function tests, viral throat swabs, and specific viral and bacterial serologies [63–65,68].

Pericardiocentesis should be considered in patients who have tamponade or suspected neoplastic or purulent pericarditis [61,65]. Routine pericardiocentesis for purely diagnostic purposes is not recommended [70].

Cardiac biomarker levels may be abnormal in patients who have pericarditis. Specifically, cTnI is elevated in more than 30% of patients who have acute pericarditis [71–73]. Men and younger patients are more likely to have elevated cTnI levels [71]. Elevation of cTnI is seen only in patients who have elevated ST segment on ECG and indicates myocardial cell damage [72]; however, cTnI levels do not indicate poor prognosis [71,72]. Serum CK and CK-MB levels also may be elevated [61].

Electrocardiography

Diffuse elevation of the ST segments in the precordial and limb leads that is associated with PR segment depression is a classic electrocardiographic indication of acute pericarditis [74]. Historically, electrocardiographic abnormalities of acute pericarditis have been said to evolve over time, with four distinct stages described [75–78]. In stage I, ST elevation is diffuse, with PR segment depression.

Stage II is normalization of the ST and PR segments, whereas stage III is characterized by widespread T-wave inversions. The ECG normalizes again in stage IV. With the exception of purulent pericarditis, if the patient is treated promptly, stage I may be the only electrocardiographic abnormality seen [66]. The diffuse ST segment elevation of pericarditis can be differentiated from myocardial ischemia by the absence of reciprocal ST depression [7] and by the concave shape of the ST-segment elevations [61]. The presence of cardiac tamponade is characterized by low-voltage ECG with electrical alternans [77].

Radiography

Radiologic studies may exclude other causes of chest pain. Chest radiography for pericarditis is aimed primarily at evaluation of the mediastinum and lungs for possible causes of the inflammation [61]. Cardiomegaly may be seen when an effusion of more than 250 mL has accumulated [61,65, 67,69].

CT and MR imaging

CT and MR imaging may be used to image the pericardium and pericardial space but are obtained most commonly to exclude other causes of chest pain or shortness of breath. CT and MR imaging evidence of thickened pericardium, enhancement of the pericardium that indicates inflammation, and visualization of pericardial effusion support the diagnosis of pericarditis [79,80].

Echocardiography

Often, TTE is performed in patients who have suspected pericarditis. The presence of an effusion will help to confirm the diagnosis [61]. Evidence of tamponade on echocardiogram indicates the need for pericardiocentesis.

Thoracic aortic dissection

Thoracic aortic dissection (TAD) is the most common aortic emergency that requires immediate surgery [81]. A dissection occurs when there is a tear in the intimal layer of the vessel wall. Blood passes through the tear, separates the intima from the vessel media or adventitia, and results in a false channel. Shear forces lead to dissection propagation as blood continues to flow through this false channel [82].

TAD can be difficult to diagnose. In the patient who presents to the emergency department and has acute chest or back pain, ACSs are 80 times more common than are aortic dissections [83]. Given that TADs occur most commonly in men who are aged 50 to 70 years and have a history of hypertension, it is not surprising that myocardial ischemia is the most common misdiagnosis [84].

History and physical examination

The acute onset of severe pain, which is maximal at symptom onset, is the most common initial symptom [85]. Usually, the pain is in the midline, may be present in the back, and rarely radiates [85]. A tearing or ripping quality of pain is classic and highly specific for TAD [86]; however, the International Registry of Acute Aortic Dissection (IRAD) found that most often, the pain was described as "sharp" [81]. Migratory pain has been considered classic for TAD, with pain corresponding to the propagation of the dissection, but was found in only 14% of patients in the IRAD [81]. Hypertension is the most common predisposing risk factor for TAD [81]. Inherited disorders, such as Marfan's syndrome and Ehler-Danlos' syndrome, associated with abnormal connective tissue structure have high rates of TAD [87,88]. Among women who are younger than 40 years who experience TAD, half are pregnant [85,87]. Cocaine use has been associated with TAD [89]. A history of syncope, with or without chest pain, was documented in 12% of patients who had TAD [81].

Pulse deficits or blood pressure differentials are independent predictive variables for TAD [83]; however, pulse deficits were documented in only 20% of patients in the IRAD [81]. Shear injury of the left carotid artery or compression of the aortic branches that supply the spinal cord may produce focal neurologic deficits [87,88]. When these deficits are present on examination, there is an increased likelihood of TAD [86]. A pulsatile sternoclavicular joint is rare but may indicate dissection [87].

When the dissection is proximal, an aortic regurgitation murmur may be heard. The IRAD study found this murmur in 44% of patients who had proximal TAD [81]. Cardiac tamponade with resultant physical examination findings of muffled heart sounds, elevated jugular venous distention, and narrow pulse pressure may be found when blood fills the pericardium [82].

Laboratory studies

Generally, routine laboratory studies are not helpful in the diagnosis of TAD [87]. Often, laboratory studies are obtained to assess other causes of chest pain. Recent studies suggest that D-dimer concentration may be useful as a diagnostic tool for the diagnosis of TAD [90]. Serum biomarkers of smooth muscle myosin heavy chain and soluble elastin fragments have been found in higher concentrations in patients who had aortic dissection,

but the means of assessing these markers is not widely available in most clinical settings [91,92].

Electrocardiography

In the patient who has TAD, the ECG may be normal or show left ventricular hypertrophy from long-standing hypertension [87]. Changes suggestive of myocardial ischemia related to coronary artery involvement in the dissection or occlusion of the artery may be present in up to one third of patients [87,93]. Two thirds of patients who have TAD have nonspecific ECG abnormalities of nonspecific ST-segment or T-wave changes [85].

Imaging

Chest radiography Chest radiography is not specific for aortic dissection but is useful in combination with the history and physical examination. In approximately 50% of cases of dissection, the classic radiographic sign of widened mediastinal shadow is seen [85]. Some type of chest film abnormality [Box 3] is present in 90% of patients [86].

CT In the IRAD study, CT often was the initial imaging test for patients who have suspected aortic dissection, likely secondary to its widespread availability and noninvasive nature [81]. CT has a sensitivity of 93.8% and a specificity of 87% for TAD [96]. A positive contrast CT for TAD shows the raised intimal flap of the dissection between the true and false lumens of the aorta [96]. Thrombus also may be visualized within the false lumen [96]. If a dissection is not present, CT images may identify another cause of the patient's symptoms. Drawbacks of CT imaging include relative difficulty in identifying the origin of the intimal tear, inability to assess involvement of the aortic branch ves-

---

Box 3: Common abnormalities found on chest radiography for aortic dissection

- Widened mediastinal shadow
- Altered configuration of the aorta
- Localized hump on the aortic arch
- Widening of the distal aortic knob past the origin of the left subclavian artery
- Aortic wall thickness indicated by the width of the aortic shadow beyond intimal calcification
- Displacement of the calcification in the aortic knob
- Double aortic shadow
- Disparity in the sizes of the ascending and descending aorta
- Presence of a pleural effusion, most commonly on the left

Data from Refs. [85,94,95].

sels, and lack of information about aortic valve regurgitation [85,96].

MR imaging   MR imaging has a reported sensitivity and specificity of 98% for TAD [96]. This imaging modality provides quality images of the entire aorta, showing extent of the dissection, site of the tear, involvement of branch vessels, and involvement of the aortic valve [85,97]. However, MR imaging is expensive, time consuming, and not widely available and limits access to the potentially unstable patient [87]. Because of this, MR imaging rarely is obtained in the emergent setting.

Echocardiography   The sensitivity and specificity of TTE for the detection of TAD vary widely, depending on the location of the dissection [85]. TTE does not visualize the aortic arch well and is virtually useless for the descending aorta [97]; however, TTE is useful for detection of tamponade or aortic insufficiency, which are complications of proximal dissections [87].

TEE is much better than TTE in the detection of TAD. TEE has a reported sensitivity of up to 98%, with a specificity of 77% [96]. A positive TEE may show a double-lumen aorta separated by the dissection membrane, which moves with the differential flow through the lumens [87]. TEE also can identify the site of dissection, sense abnormal flow, visualize a thrombus, assess for involvement of aortic valve and aortic branch vessels, and detect pericardial effusion [85]. The advantages of TEE are that it can be performed at the patient's bedside in a swift manner [85]. In many centers, TEE represents the noninvasive study of choice for the patient suspected of having TAD [85]. TEE requires esophageal intubation, which often necessitates sedation, and may not be available in some centers, especially in the evening and on weekends.

Aortography   Traditionally, aortography has been considered the gold standard for the diagnosis of TAD, but it has been replaced by less invasive and more readily available radiologic studies. Findings on aortography that are indicative of TAD include distortion of contrast flow, flow reversal, flow stasis, failure of major vessels to fill with contrast, and aortic valve insufficiency [85]. Aortography may underestimate the size of the dissection if a thrombus is present [97]. The procedure is invasive and requires mobilization of an angiographic team. Aortography rarely is obtained for the acute diagnosis of TAD [81].

Summary

The use of radiographic imaging remains vital in the assessment of patients who present with chest pain.

Despite advances in medical care, cardiopulmonary emergencies remain a major cause of morbidity and mortality in the United States. Rapid bedside radiographic detection of intrathoracic disorders is critical in clinical decision making related to these potentially life-threatening emergencies.

References

[1] Tamura M, Ohta Y, Sato H. Thoracoscopic appearance of bilateral spontaneous pneumothorax. Chest 2003;124(6):2368–71.

[2] Steele R, Irvin CB. Central line mechanical complication rate in emergency medicine patients. Acad Emerg Med 2001;8(2):204–7.

[3] National Healthcare Quality Report. Agency for Healthcare Research and Quality, Department of Health and Human Services, 2003.

[4] Chang AK, Barton ED. Pneumothorax, iatrogenic, spontaneous and pneumomediastinum. Available at http://www.emedicine.com/EMERG/topic469.htm. Accessed November 4, 2005.

[5] Ferraro P, Beauchamp G, Lord F, et al. Spontaneous primary and secondary pneumothorax: a 10-year study of management alternatives. Can J Surg 1994;37(3):197–202.

[6] Cottin V, Streichenberger N, Gamondes JP, et al. Respiratory bronchiolitis in smokers with spontaneous pneumothorax. Eur Respir J 1998;12(3):702–4.

[7] Yellin A, Shiner RJ, Lieberman Y. Familial multiple bilateral pneumothorax associated with Marfan syndrome. Chest 1991;100(2):577–8.

[8] Alifano M, Roth T, Broet SC, et al. Catamenial pneumothorax: a prospective study. Chest 2003;124(3):781–2.

[9] Seow A, Kazerooni EA, Pernicano PG, et al. Comparison of upright inspiratory and expiratory chest radiographs for detecting pneumothoraces. AJR Am J Roentgenol 1996;166(2):313–6.

[10] Carr JJ, Reed JC, Choplin RH, et al. Plain and computed radiography for detecting experimentally induced pneumothorax in cadavers: implications for detection in patients. Radiology 1992;183(1):193–9.

[11] Blaivas M, Lyon M, Duggal S. A prospective comparison of supine chest radiography and bedside ultrasound for the diagnosis of traumatic pneumothorax. Acad Emerg Med 2005;12(9):844–9.

[12] Mandell LA. Epidemiology and etiology of community-acquired pneumonia. Infect Dis Clin North Am 2004;18:761–76.

[13] Niederman MS, McCombs JS, Unger AN, et al. The cost of treating community-acquired pneumonia. Clin Ther 1998;20(4):820–37.

[14] Hoyert DL, Heron M, Murphy SL, et al. Deaths: final data for 2003. Hyattsville (MD): US Department of Health and Human Services, Centers for Disease Control and Prevention, National Center for Health Statistics; January

19, 2006. Available at: http://www.cdc.gov/nchs. Accessed on January 24, 2006.

[15] Vincent JL, Bihari DJ, Suter PM, et al. The prevalence of nosocomial infection in intensive care units in Europe. Results of the European Prevalence of Infection in Intensive Care (EPIC) Study. EPIC International Advisory Committee. JAMA 1995;274(8):639–44.

[16] Franquet T. Imaging of pneumonia: trends and algorithms. Eur Resp J 2001;18:196–208.

[17] Courtoy I, Lande AE, Turner RB. Accuracy of radiographic differentiation of bacterial from nonbacterial pneumonia. Clin Pediatr (Phila) 1989;28(6):261–4.

[18] Ponka A, Sarna S. Differential diagnosis of viral, mycoplasmal and bacteraemic pneumococcal pneumonias on admission to hospital. Eur J Respir Dis 1983;64(5):360–8.

[19] Van Mieghem IM, De Wever WF, Verschakelen JA. Lung infection in radiology: a summary of frequently depicted signs. JBR-BTR 2005;88(2): 66–71.

[20] Murray JF, Mills J. Pulmonary infectious complications of human immunodeficiency virus infection. Am Rev Respir Dis 1990;141:1356–72.

[21] Lyon R, Haque AK, Asmuth DM, et al. Changing patterns of infections in patients with AIDS: a study of 279 autopsies of prison inmates and nonincarcerated patients at a university hospital in eastern Texas, 1984–1993. Clin Infect Dis 1996; 23:241–7.

[22] Guckel C, Benz-Bohm G, Widemann B. Mycoplasmal pneumonias in childhood. Roentgen features, differential diagnosis and review of literature. Pediatr Radiol 1989;19(8):499–503.

[23] Goodman PC. Pneumocystis carinii pneumonia. J Thorac Imaging 1991;6(4):16–21.

[24] Goodman PC. The chest film in AIDS. In: Sande MA, Volberding P, editors. The medical management of AIDS. 4th edition. Philadelphia: Saunders; 1995. p. 592–613.

[25] Moe AA, Hardy WD. Pneumocystis carinii infection in the HIV-seropositive patient. Infect Dis Clin North Am 1994;8:331–64.

[26] Wasser LS, Brown E, Talavera W. Miliary PCP in AIDS. Chest 1989;96(3):693–5.

[27] Chaffey MH, Klein JS, Gamsu G, et al. Radiographic distribution of Pneumocystis carinii pneumonia in patients with AIDS treated with prophylactic inhaled pentamidine. Radiology 1990;175(3):715–9.

[28] Baughman RP, Dohn MN, Shipley R, et al. Increased Pneumocystis carinii recovery from the upper lobes in Pneumocystis pneumonia: the effect of aerosol pentamidine prophylaxis. Chest 1993;103(2):426–32.

[29] Hanson DL, Chu SY, Farizo KM, et al. Distribution of CD4 lymphocytes at diagnosis of acquired immunodeficiency syndrome-defining and other human immunodeficiency virus-related illnesses. Arch Intern Med 1995;155:1537–42.

[30] Primack SL, Müller NL. HRCT in acute diffuse lung disease in the immunocompromised patient. Radiol Clin North Am 1994;32:731–44.

[31] Boiselle PM, Tocino I, Hooley RJ, et al. Chest radiograph interpretation pf Pneumocystis carinii pneumonia, bacterial pneumonia, and pulmonary tuberculosis in HIV-positive patients: accuracy, distinguishing features, and mimics. J Thorac Imaging 1997;12:47–53.

[32] Janzen DL, Padley SPG, Adler BD, et al. Acute pulmonary complications in immunocompromised non-AIDS patients: comparison of diagnostic accuracy of CT and chest radiography. Clin Radiol 1993;47:159–65.

[33] Chastre J, Trouillet JL, Vuagnat A, et al. Nosocomial pneumonia in patients with acute respiratory distress syndrome. Am J Respir Crit Care Med 1998;157:1165–72.

[34] Seidenfeld JJ, Pohl DF, Bell RD, et al. Incidence, site and outcome of infections in patients with adult respiratory distress syndrome. Am Rev Respir Dis 1986;134:12–6.

[35] Niederman MS, Fein AM. Sepsis syndrome, the adult respiratory distress syndrome and nosocomial pneumonia: a common clinical sequence. Clin Chest Med 1990;11:633–56.

[36] Kamineni R, Alpert JS. Acute coronary syndromes: initial evaluation and risk stratification. Prog Cardiovasc Dis 2004;46:379–92.

[37] Pope JH, Ruthazer R, Beshansky JR, et al. Clinical features of emergency department patients presenting with symptoms suggestive of acute cardiac ischemia; a multicenter study. J Thromb Thrombolysis 1998;6:63–74.

[38] Pope JH, Selker HP. Diagnosis of acute cardiac ischemia. Emerg Med Clin North Am 2003;21: 27–59.

[39] Coronado BE, Pope JH, Griffith JL, et al. Clinical features, triage, and outcome of patients presenting to the ED with suspected acute coronary syndromes but without pain: a multicenter study. Am J Emerg Med 2004;22:568–74.

[40] Selker HP, Zalenski RJ, Antman EM, et al. An evaluation of technologies for identifying acute cardiac ischemia in the emergency department: executive summary of a national heart attack alert program working group report. Ann Emerg Med 1997;29:1–12.

[41] Balk EM, Ioannidis JPA, Salem D, et al. Accuracy of biomarkers to diagnose acute cardiac ischemia in the emergency department: a meta-analysis. Ann Emerg Med 2001;37:478–94.

[42] Newby LK. Markers of cardiac ischemia, injury, and inflammation. Prog Cardiovasc Dis 2004; 46:404–16.

[43] Ioannidis JPA, Salem D, Chew PW, et al. Accuracy of imaging technologies in the diagnosis of acute cardiac ischemia in the emergency department: a meta-analysis. Ann Emerg Med 2001;37: 471–7.

[44] Lee LC, Shah K. Clinical manifestation of pulmonary embolism. Emerg Med Clin North Am 2001;19:925–42.

[45] Rodger M, Wells PS. Diagnosis of pulmonary embolism. Thromb Res 2001;103:V225–38.

[46] Morgenthaler TI, Ryu JH. Clinical characteristics of fatal pulmonary embolism in a referral hospital. Mayo Clin Proc 1995;70:417–24.

[47] Investigators PIOPED. Value of the ventilation/perfusion scan in acute pulmonary embolism. Results of the Prospective Investigation of Pulmonary Embolism Diagnosis study (PIOPED). JAMA 1990;263:2753–9.

[48] Laack TA, Goyal DG. Pulmonary embolism: an unsuspected killer. Emerg Med Clin North Am 2004;22:961–83.

[49] Perrier A, Howarth N, Didier D, et al. Performance of helical computed tomography in unselected outpatients with suspected pulmonary embolism. Ann Intern Med 2001;135:88–97.

[50] Riedel M. Acute pulmonary embolism: pathophysiology, clinical presentation, and diagnosis. Heart 2001;85:229–40.

[51] Tapson VF. Acute pulmonary embolism. Cardiol Clin 2004;22:353–65.

[52] Brilakis ES, Tajik AJ. 82-year-old man with recurrent syncope. Mayo Clin Proc 1999;74:609–12.

[53] Sadosty AT, Boie ET, Stead LG. Pulmonary embolism. Emerg Med Clin North Am 2003;21:363–84.

[54] Wells PS, Ginsberg JS, Anderson DR, et al. Use of a clinical model for safe management of patients with suspected pulmonary embolism. Ann Intern Med 1998;129:997–1005.

[55] Weiner SG, Burstein JL. Nonspecific tests for pulmonary embolism. Emerg Med Clin North Am 2001;19:943–55.

[56] Wells PS, Anderson DR, Rodger M, et al. Excluding pulmonary embolism at the bedside without diagnostic imaging: management of patients with suspected pulmonary embolism presenting to the emergency department by using a simple clinical model and D-dimer. Ann Intern Med 2001;135:98–107.

[57] Wicki J, Perneger TW, Junod AF, et al. Assessing clinical probability of pulmonary embolism in the emergency ward: a simple score. Arch Intern Med 2001;161:92–7.

[58] Carrier M, Wells PS, Rodger MA. Excluding pulmonary embolism at the bedside with low pretest probability and D-dimer: safety and clinical utility of 4 methods to assign pre-test probability. Thromb Res 2005, in press.

[59] Hull RD, Hirsh J, Carter CJ, et al. Pulmonary angiography, ventilation lung scanning, and venography for clinically suspected pulmonary embolism with abnormal perfusion lung scan. Ann Intern Med 1983;98:891–9.

[60] Rathbun SW, Rashkob GE, Whitsett TL. Sensitivity and specificity of helical computed tomography in the diagnosis of pulmonary embolism: a systematic review. Ann Intern Med 2000; 132(3):227–32.

[61] Lange RA, Hillis LD. Acute pericarditis. N Engl J Med 2004;351:2195–202.

[62] Ross AM, Grauer SE, Acute pericarditis: evaluation and treatment of infectious and other causes. Postgrad Med 2004;115(3):67–70, 73–5.

[63] Levy PY, Corey R, Berger P, et al. Etiologic diagnosis of 204 pericardial effusions. Medicine 2003;82:385–91.

[64] Zayas R, Anguita M, Torres F, et al. Incidence of specific etiology and role of methods for specific etiologic diagnosis of primary acute pericarditis. Am J Cardiol 1995;75:378–82.

[65] Troughton RW, Asher CR, Klein AL. Pericarditis. Lancet 2004;363:717–27.

[66] Spodick DH. Acute pericarditis: current concepts and practice. JAMA 2003;289:1150–3.

[67] Goyle KK, Walling AD. Diagnosing pericarditis. Am Fam Phys 2002;66:1695–702.

[68] Levy PY, Maotti JP, Gauduchon V, et al. Comparison of intuitive versus systematic strategies for aetiological diagnosis of pericardial effusion. Scand J Infect Dis 2005;37:216–20.

[69] Spodick DH. Pericardial rub: prospective, multiple observer investigation of pericardial friction in 100 patients. Am J Cardiol 1975;35:357–62.

[70] Permanyer-Miralda G. Acute pericardial disease: approach to the aetiologic diagnosis. Heart 2004; 90(3):252–4.

[71] Imazio M, Brunella D, Cacchi E, et al. Cardiac troponin I in acute pericarditis. J Am Coll Cardiol 2003;42:2144–8.

[72] Bonnefoy E, Godon G, Kirkorian M, et al. Serum cardiac troponin I and ST-segment elevation in patients with acute pericarditis. Eur Heart J 2000; 21:832–6.

[73] Brandt RR, Filzmaier K, Hanrath P. Circulating cardiac troponin I in acute pericarditis. Am J Cardiol 2001;87:1326–8.

[74] Wang K, Asinger RW, Marriott HJL. ST-Segment elevation in conditions other than acute myocardial infarction. N Engl J Med 2003;349: 2128–35.

[75] Ginzton LE, Laks MM. The differential diagnosis or acute pericarditis from the normal variant: new electrocardiographic criteria. Circulation 1982;65:1004–9.

[76] Spodick DH. Diagnostic electrocardiographic sequences in acute pericarditis: significance of PR segment and PR vector changes. Circulation 1973; 48:575–80.

[77] Surawicz B, Lasseter KC. Electrocardiogram in pericarditis. Am J Cardiol 1970;26:471–4.

[78] Bruce MA, Spodick DH. Atypical electrocardiogram in acute pericarditis: characteristics and prevalence. J Electrocardiol 1980;13:61–6.

[79] Rienmüller R, Gröll R, Lipton MJ. CT and MR imaging of pericardial disease. Radiol Clin North Am 2004;42:587–601.

[80] Wang ZJ, Reddy GP, Gotway MB, et al. CT and MR imaging of pericardial disease. Radiographics 2003;23:S167–80.

[81] Hagan PG, Nienaber CA, Isselbacher EM, et al. The international registry of acute ortic dissection (IRAD): new insights into an old disease. JAMA 2000;283:897–903.

[82] Klein DG. Thoracic aortic aneurysms. J Cardiovasc Nurs 2005;20:245–50.

[83] von Kodolitsch Y, Schwartz AG, Nienaber CA. Clinical prediction of acute aortic dissection. Arch Intern Med 2000;160:2977–82.

[84] Rogers RL, McCormack R. Aortic disasters. Emerg Med Clin North Am 2004;22:887–908.

[85] Khan IA, Nair CK. Clinical, diagnostic, and management perspectives of aortic dissection. Chest 2002;122:311–28.

[86] Bushnell J, Brown J. Clinical assessment for acute thoracic aortic dissection. Ann Emerg Med 2005;46:90–2.

[87] Chan K, Varon J, Wenker OC, et al. Acute thoracic aortic dissection: the basics. J Emerg Med 1997;15:859–67.

[88] Prêtre R, von Segesser LK. Aortic dissection. Lancet 1997;349:1461–4.

[89] Perron AD, Gibbs M. Thoracic aortic dissection secondary to crack cocaine ingestion. Am J Emerg Med 1997;15:507–9.

[90] Hazui H, Fukumoto H, Negoro N, et al. Simple and useful tests for discriminating between acute aortic dissection of the ascending aorta and acute myocardial infarction in the emergency setting. Circ J 2005;69:677–82.

[91] Suzuki T, Katoh H, Watanabe M, et al. Novel biochemical diagnostic method for acute aortic dissection: results of a prospective study using an immunoassay of smooth muscle myosin heavy chain. Circulation 1996;93:1244–9.

[92] Shinohara T, Suzuki K, Okada M, et al. Soluble elastin fragments in serum are elevated in acute aortic dissection. Arterioscler Thromb Vasc Biol 2003;23:1839–44.

[93] Armstrong WF, Bach DS, Carey LM, et al. Clinical and echocardiographic findings in patients with suspected acute aortic dissection. Am Heart J 1998;136:1051–60.

[94] Earnest F, Muhm JR, Sheedy PF. Roentgenographic findings in thoracic aortic dissection. Mayo Clin Proc 1979;54:43–50.

[95] Jagannath AS, Sos TA, Lockhart SH, et al. Aortic dissection: a statistical analysis of the usefulness of plain chest radiographic findings. AJR Am J Roentgenol 1986;147:1123–6.

[96] Nienaber CA, von Kodolitsch Y, Nicholas V, et al. The diagnosis of thoracic aortic dissection by noninvasive imaging procedures. N Engl J Med 1993;328:1–9.

[97] Nienaber CA, von Kodolitsch Y. Diseases of the aorta. Cardiol Clin 1998;16:295–314.

RADIOLOGIC
CLINICS
OF NORTH AMERICA

Radiol Clin N Am 44 (2006) 181–197

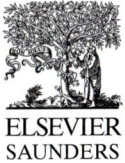

Thoracic Vascular Injury

Stuart E. Mirvis, MD[a,b,*]

- Mediastinal hemorrhage and thoracic vascular injury
- Traumatic aortic injury in blunt trauma
  Multirow detector CT technique
  CT findings of traumatic aortic injury
  Pitfalls in diagnosis
- Penetrating aortic injury
- Nonaortic major thoracic arterial injuries
  Thoracic aortic branches
- Major venous thoracic injuries
- Summary
- References

The role of CT in the diagnosis of traumatic injury of the thoracic aorta has been debated for at least 2 decades [1–5]. Thoracic CT has been applied to diagnose or exclude traumatic aortic injury from blunt trauma since the middle to late 1980s, and continually has challenged the more well established use of thoracic angiography as the "reference standard" for diagnosis [6–9].

Several trends have increased the preference for CT over angiography: (1) the overall greater reliance on CT in the assessment of the patient who has sustained polytrauma; (2) the steady improvement in the technologic sophistication of CT, first with the introduction of helical scanning, and later, multirow detector CT (MDCT); and (3) the development of advanced CT workstations that allow rapid generation of tailored multiplanar, three-dimensional (3-D) volume, and endovascular presentations of aortic anatomy to improve diagnostic accuracy. Over the same period, it has been recognized increasingly that angiography is more time consuming to perform, less available than CT on an acute basis, and significantly more expensive than CT as a screening study. Today, most institutions that admit numerous patients who have experienced blunt chest trauma use MDCT with CT-angiography as the screening study of choice for aortic injury; it has replaced thoracic angiography almost completely for screening patients who have sustained chest trauma. Angiography remains a potential problem solver for uncertain CT results, and for planning and guiding endovascular aortic stent-graft placement.

MDCT is the diagnostic study of choice for blunt chest trauma in general. It has far greater accuracy than does radiography for detecting many thoracic traumatic injuries, some of which are life threatening or have a high potential for morbidity if not diagnosed and treated acutely. Thin-slice MDCT with rapid scanning and contrast-bolus timing also has shown great promise in detecting and localizing a variety of nonaortic vascular thoracic injuries, including active bleeding, which can lead to early surgical or angiographic intervention to control blood loss.

Mediastinal hemorrhage and thoracic vascular injury

The presence of mediastinal hemorrhage is an important clue to potential major thoracic vascular

[a] Department of Radiology, University of Maryland Medical Center, Baltimore, MD, USA
[b] Section of Trauma and Emergency Radiology, University of Maryland School of Medicine, Baltimore, MD, USA
* Department of Radiology, University of Maryland Medical Center, 22 South Greene Street, Baltimore, MD 21201.
E-mail address: smirvis@umm.edu

doi:10.1016/j.rcl.2005.10.007

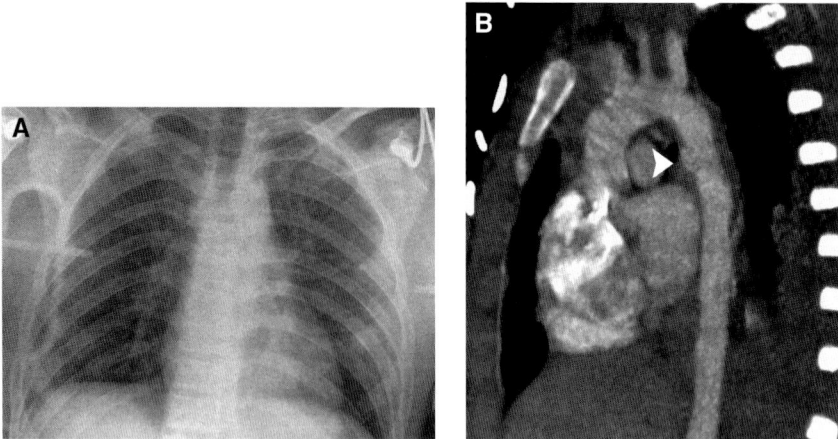

Fig. 1. Near normal chest radiograph in a patient who has aortic injury. (A) Anteroposterior supine admission study shows an essentially normal mediastinal contour. There is slight enlargement of the proximal descending aortic shadow. (B) MPR through the long axis of the aorta shows pseudoaneurysm (*arrowhead*) at typical site. Mediastinal blood tracks along aorta and around the arch branches.

injury, which most commonly involves the proximal descending thoracic aorta at the level of the left mainstem bronchus and left pulmonary artery. Chest radiography provides the initial assessment of mediastinal contour. Although several articles have described apparently reliable radiographic signs of hemomediastinum [10–13] and potential aortic injury, subsequent larger series reported that many of these signs are less accurate than was suggested originally [14–16]. Although it is true that most patients who have hemomediastinum display a "widened mediastinum" on chest radiography, this finding does not indicate the presence or absence of vascular injury. Patients who have narrow mediastinal widths or mediastinal/cardiac width ratios can have traumatic aortic injury [TAI; Figs. 1 and 2]. Patients who have mediastinal hemorrhage have less than a 20% probability of having major thoracic vascular injury [8]. The precise analysis of the mediastinal contour offers the best chance of diagnosing or excluding mediastinal hemorrhage, based upon radiologic screening. Radio-

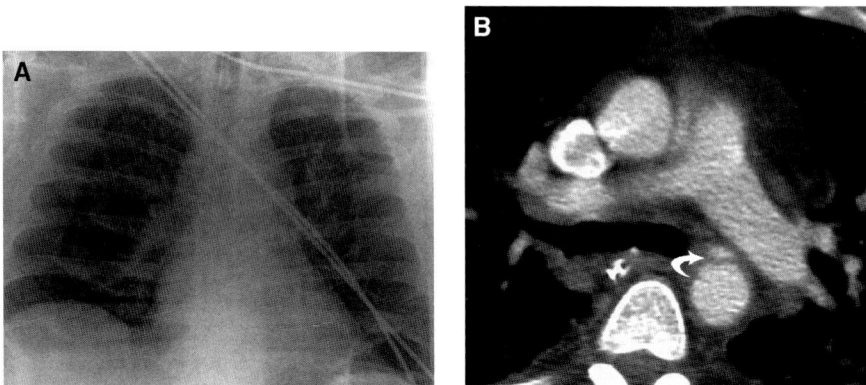

Fig. 2. Near normal chest radiograph in a patient who has aortic injury. (A) Anteroposterior supine admission radiograph in has abnormal mediastinal contours. The descending aortic arch is ill-defined, slight nasogastric tube bowing to the right is observed, and there is too much soft tissue density in the right paratracheal region. (B) CT image shows typical pseudoaneurysm (*curved arrow*) in proximal descending aorta with slight nasogastric tube displacement to the right.

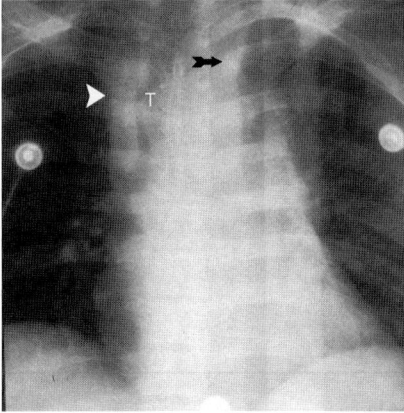

Fig. 3. Markedly abnormal mediastinal contour in a patient who has aortic injury. Supine chest radiography shows right paratracheal soft tissue density (*arrowhead*), a widened left paraspinal stripe that extends to the apex of the hemithorax (*arrow*), tracheal deviation to the right (T) and enlarged, poorly defined aortic contour.

logic signs that serve as markers for mediastinal hemorrhage that is associated with TAI include:

An obscured, abnormal, or absent aortic arch and descending aorta shadow [Fig. 3]

Right paratracheal soft tissue density [Fig. 3]

Rightward displacement of the esophagus and trachea in a patient who is nonrotated [see Fig. 3]

A widened left paraspinal stripe (greater than half the diameter of the adjacent aorta) or extension of the stripe above the aortic arch [see Fig. 3]

Radiographic evaluation often is falsely positive for evidence of mediastinal blood, and therefore, for potential great vessel injury. Some causes of falsely positive diagnoses include:

Supine positioning that often widens and distorts the mediastinal contour

Atelectasis, pleural effusions, lung contusions, lung hematoma, and other traumatic or nontraumatic lung pathology that obscures the mediastinal margins

Limited technical quality of studies, motion artifacts, overlying support tubes and lines, and so forth

Mediastinal lipomatosis or pre-existing mediastinal masses

Acquired and congenital vascular anomalies, marked thoracic scoliosis

Mediastinal hemorrhage without vascular injury

Unless the mediastinal contours can be defined clearly and unequivocally, mediastinal hemorrhage cannot be excluded. Given that aortic and other major thoracic arterial injuries have a high incidence of rupture and mortality within hours to days of admission, the injury must be excluded quickly and definitively [17]. Generally, arteriography has provided the diagnostic standard for this purpose, but this study is costly, invasive, and time consuming, and may delay other diagnostic or therapeutic procedures. In rare cases of equivocal MDCT results for aortic injury, arteriography or transesophageal echo may be required. Therefore, emergency centers must provide immediate diagnostic arteriography on a 24-hour basis; however, in some cases, the results of arteriography are atypical or nondiagnostic [18].

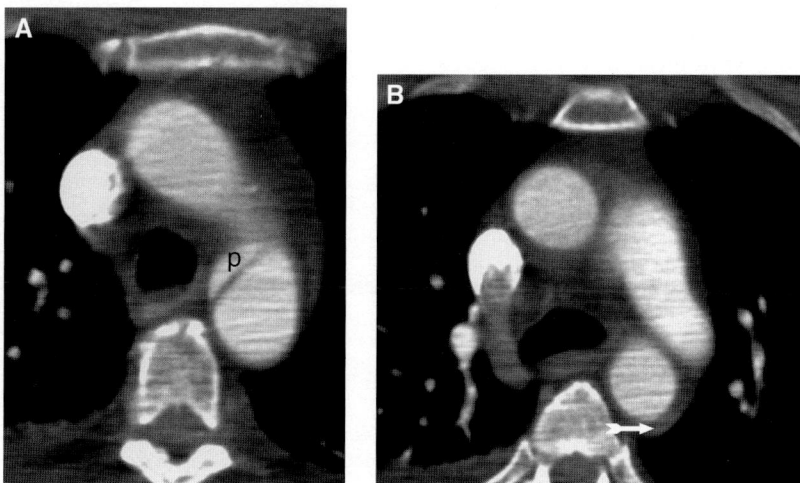

Fig. 4. Aortic injury with minimal hemomediastinum. (*A*) CT images shows a pseudoaneurysm (p) arising from anterior proximal descending aorta just beyond arch. (*B*) There is only a small amount of periaortic mediastinal hemorrhage (*arrow*).

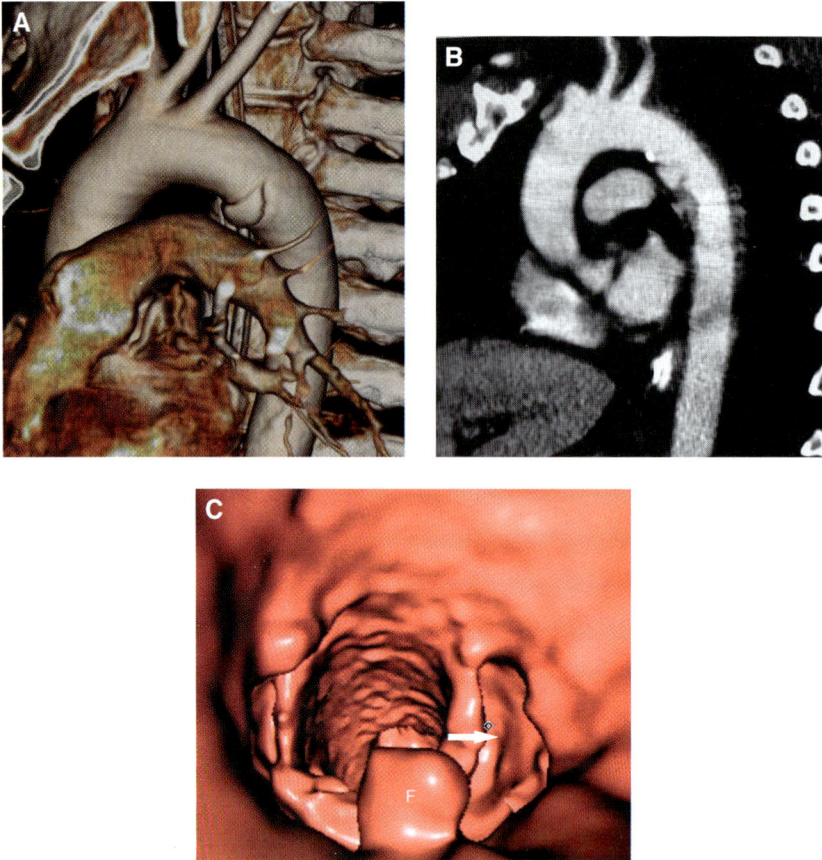

Fig. 5. Postprocessing of aortic injuries. (*A*) Volume rendered image of aortic pseudoaneurysm shows relationship to branch vessels. (*B*) MPR view along long axis of aorta shows pseudoaneurysm and adjacent intimal flaps in a different patient. (*C*) Endovascular view of same patient as B showing pseudoaneurysm (*arrow*) and intimal flap (F).

In recent years, the Maryland Shock-Trauma center mostly has abandoned thoracic angiography in favor of MDCT when there is possible mediastinal hematoma radiographically. Because aortic injuries may occur with minimal surrounding mediastinal hematoma [Fig. 4], and therefore, with minimal distortion of the mediastinal contour, the center is relying increasingly on MDCT as the major "screening" study for this injury. Although the author still "clears" many adequate chest radiographs on the supine or erect view, the threshold has been lowered to proceed to MDCT in any questionable case.

Traumatic aortic injury in blunt trauma

Multirow detector CT technique

In general, MDCT is more sensitive than is chest radiograph for the diagnosis of most traumatic tho-

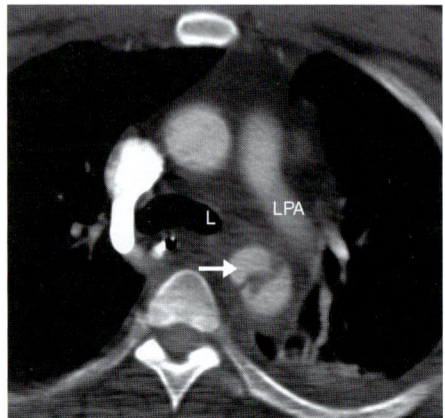

Fig. 6. Typical aortic pseudoaneurysm. CT shows a pseudoaneurysm (*arrow*) arising from the antero-medial aspect of proximal descending aorta at level of left mainstem bronchus (L) and left pulmonary artery (LPA). Mediastinal blood surrounds aorta. An intimal flap and adherent thrombus are noted.

maximum intenstity projection (MIP), volumetric, and endovascular reformations [Fig. 5].

CT findings of traumatic aortic injury

Most patients who have TAI have clear and diagnostic findings, such as a pseudoaneurysm, typically in the anterior aspect of the proximal descending aorta at the level of the left main pulmonary artery and left mainstem bronchus [Fig. 6] [20]. The pseudoaneurysm is an incomplete tear in the wall in which arterial blood is contained by the adventia of the artery alone, and therefore, is unstable. Other findings on CT that typically are seen in TAI include one or more of the features that are listed in Box 1.

Intraluminal thrombus can develop on intimal tears and provides a source for distal arterial embolization [Figs. 6 and 7]. Traumatic coarctation of the aorta, with a resulting decrease in downstream blood flow and blood pressure, can be caused by large pseudoaneurysms that compress the aortic lumen or intimal flaps that project into the lumen and impede flow [Fig. 8] [21]. Rarely, the aortic wall can dissect as a result of blunt force injury; this begins at the typical injury site in the proximal descending aorta with potential propagation of the tear into the abdominal aorta, as seen with typical atherosclerotic dissection [Fig. 9] [22]. On rare occasions, the aorta is bleeding actively at the time of the CT; this is an unstable circumstance that seldom permits an opportunity for salvage [23]. In some cases, the injury to the aorta is manifest on CT in more subtle ways, such as an abnormal contour to the aortic lumen, sudden change in lumen shape, or diameter variation over a short distance [Fig. 10] [24,25].

racic pathology [19], and typically it is indicated for patients who have experienced blunt polytrauma. Using bolus tracking with a threshold of 90 Hounsfield units (HU) set in the proximal ascending aorta, the author performs a 16 × 0.75–mm or 16 × 1.5–mm scan (in large patients) of the entire chest, and reconstructs data at 3- or 5-mm intervals. If needed in questionable cases, the raw data are reconstructed at 1- to 2-mm intervals with 50% overlap. This thin-section reconstructed data set is used for all multiplanar reformation (MPR),

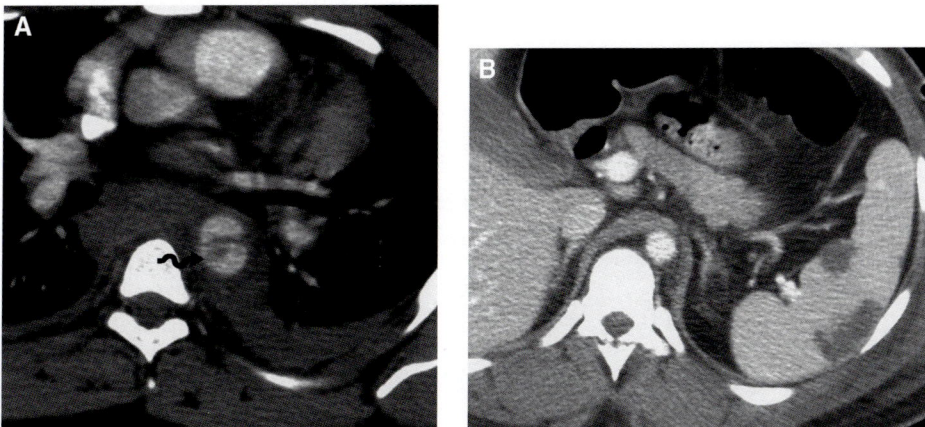

Fig. 7. Aortic injury with luminal thrombus and embolization. (*A*) CT reveals intimal flap between aortic lumen and pseudoaneurysm with adherent thrombus (*arrow*). (*B*) Two well-defined peripheral infarcts are observed in the spleen, most likely from embolized clot.

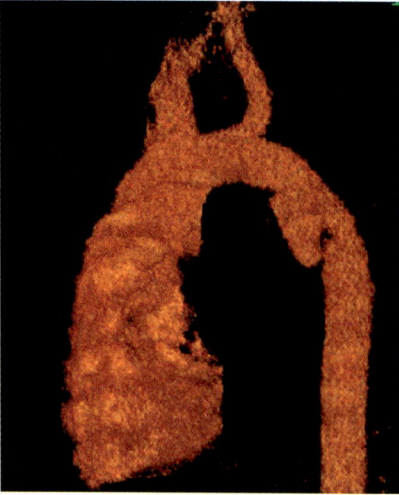

Fig. 8. Pseudoaneurysm compressing aortic lumen. MDCT shows a large pseudoaneurysm narrowing lumen of aorta and decreasing flow distal to narrowed segment.

In all cases, one must search for other sites of aortic injury that may be isolated or concurrent with injury at the proximal descending aorta such as the ascending aorta [26], the aortic arch, the peridiaphragmatic aorta, and the great vessel origins [Figs. 11–13]. In some cases, the aortic injury may be subtle [Fig. 14], and consist of a small intimal tear and possible attached thrombus. Use of MPR, MIP, volumetric, and virtual angioscopic 3-D views can help to convey the precise anatomy of the aortic injury to the vascular or chest surgeon

and interventional radiologist [Figs. 5, 15 and 16]. Once an aortic injury is diagnosed on CT, it rarely is necessary to perform angiography; this procedure introduces an unnecessary delay in treatment when time is of the essence [27]. Only if the CT study is equivocal, despite use of thin-slice collimation, a well-opacified lumen, and use of image reformations, should thoracic angiography or transesophageal sonography be performed [27]. Information in positive cases of TAI should include location and length of the injury; proximity to the nearest major branch vessel; any anomalies of thoracic anatomy, particularly vessel branching patterns; size and orientation of the pseudoaneurysm; presence of adherent thrombus; and the diameter of intact aorta above and below the area of injury. Evidence of active bleeding from the aorta constitutes a "hyperemergent" finding that requires immediate notification of the responsible clinical service [Fig. 17].

Given the emergence of potential stent-graft placement for aortic injury, characterization of aortic injury is more crucial than ever to permit the planning of appropriate therapy [28,29]. In cases of minor intimal injury, blood pressure regulation may be most appropriate with regular follow-up imaging. In other cases, the particular anatomy of the injury may lend itself to stent-graft management [Fig. 18] to temporize and treat other injuries before surgery or as definitive care. In other cases, traditional thoracotomy may be necessitated by the particular anatomy or evidence of ongoing hemorrhage. Further research is needed to correlate the anatomy of particular aortic injuries with optimal treatment.

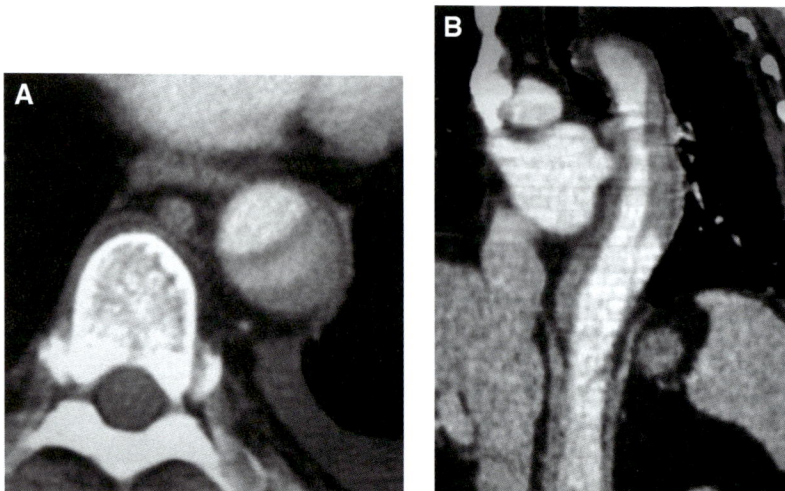

Fig. 9. Traumatic aortic dissection. Axial (*A*) and coronal (*B*) chest CT images show true and false lumens of traumatic dissection. Tear started in the proximal descending aorta and continued into distal abdominal aorta.

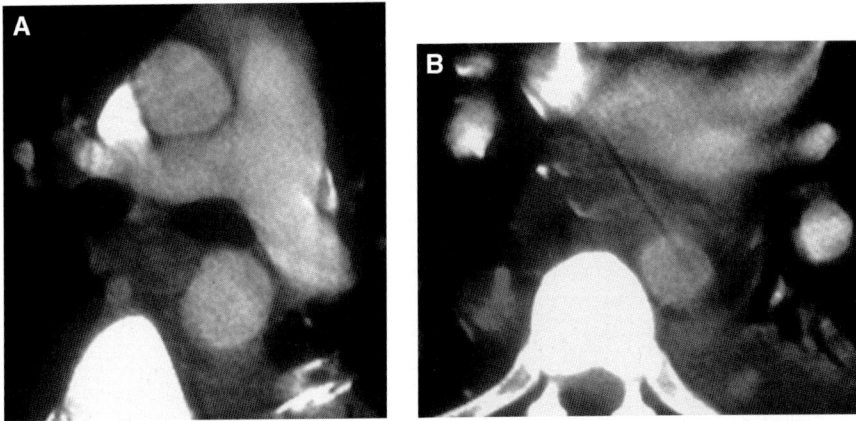

Fig. 10. Sudden variation in aortic diameter—aortic injury. (*A* and *B*) Two images of descending aorta show rapid change in aortic diameter over short distance without intervening vascular branches. This finding suggests a subtle pseudoaneurysm or flow volume decrease. Mediastinal blood surrounds aorta.

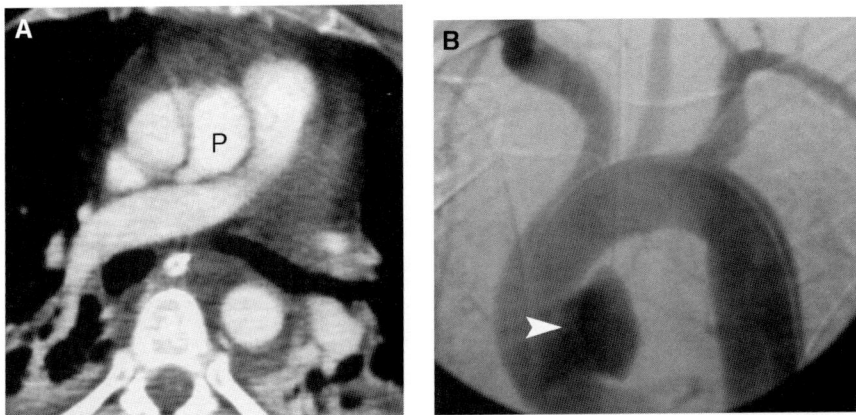

Fig. 11. Ascending aortic pseudoaneurysm. (*A*) CT shows appearance of three vessels arising from base of the heart. The middle "vessel" is a pseudoaneurysm (P) of the proximal aorta in this patient who sustained blunt trauma. (*B*) Angiogram verifies the diagnosis (*arrowhead*).

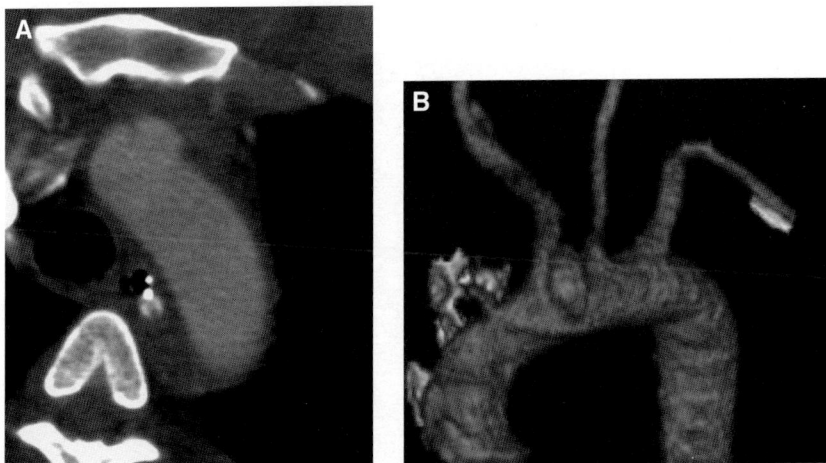

Fig. 12. Aortic arch pseudoaneurysm. (*A*) CT in a patient who sustained blunt trauma shows defect in aorta arch adjacent to innominate artery origin with surrounding mediastinal hemorrhage. (*B*) Volume rendering shows size of pseudoaneurysm and its relation to branch vessel to better advantage.

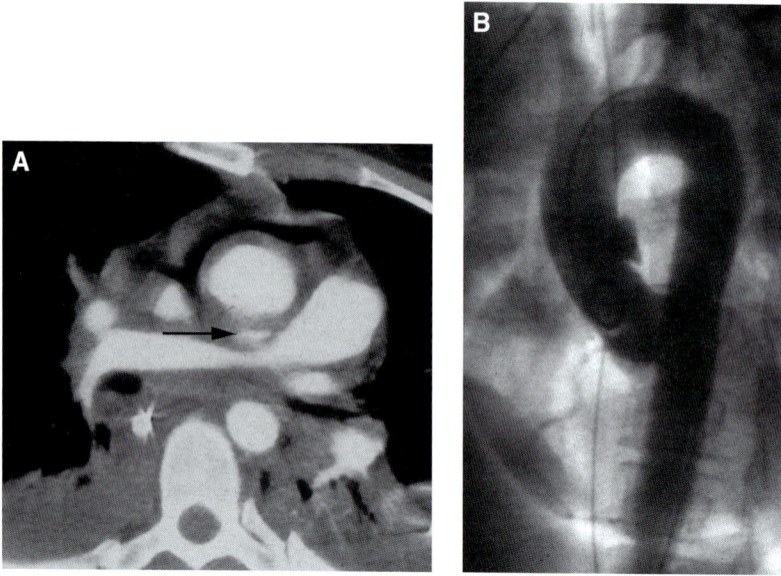

Fig. 13. Ascending aortic pseudoaneurysm. (*A*) CT shows small pseudoaneurysm arises from proximal ascending aorta in a patient who fell 75 feet (*arrow*). (*B*) Angiogram verifies the diagnosis.

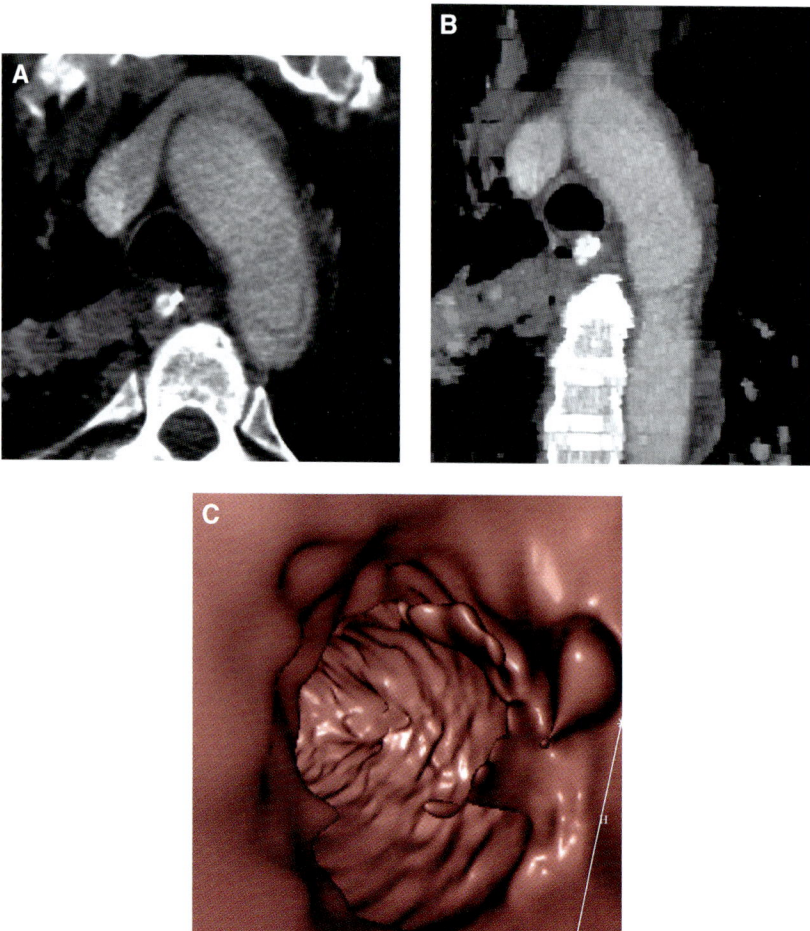

Fig. 14. Intimal defects in aortic injury. Axial (*A*) and coronal (*B*) CT views reveal thin lucent intimal flaps indicating aortic injury. (*C*) Endoluminal view shows flaps projecting into lumen of aorta.

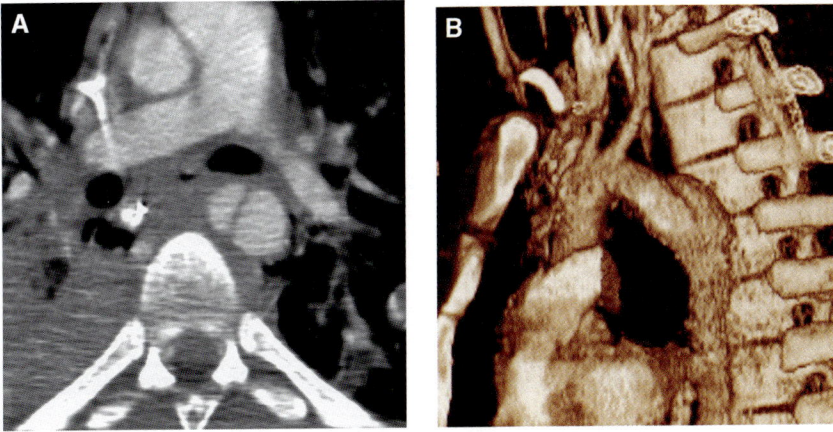

Fig. 15. Typical aortic pseudoaneurysm. (*A*) Axial CT shows pseudoaneurysm projecting anteromedially from lumen at level of left mainstem bronchus and left pulmonary artery. Mediastinal blood pushes esophagus and carina to the right. (*B*) 3-D volume-rendered injury.

Pitfalls in diagnosis

The variation of normal aortic anatomy must be well understood when assessing the aorta for potential injuries. As thin-section MDCT has become performed more routinely on greater numbers of patients, these normal variants are recognized increasingly, and therefore, become sources of diagnostic confusion [30]. This is particularly true when mediastinal hemorrhage also is present. The aortic isthmus in adults has a variable appearance on thoracic aortogram and CT. Its configuration may show a concavity, a straightening or slight convexity, or a discrete focal bulge. The last finding represents a ductus diverticulum, and was present in 9% of patients in a review of 103 aortograms [31].

The ductus diverticulum and ductus arteriosus remnant can cause confusion with aortic injury [Figs. 19 and 20]. Classically, the ductus diverticulum is a smooth, broad-based anteromedial outpouching of the aortic isthmus that points toward the left pulmonary artery–main pulmonary artery junction. The ductus remnant is a fibrotic cordlike, possibly calcified, linear structure that may be seen in the aortico-pulmonary window; it represents a part of the atrophic ductus arteriosus [Fig. 21]. In the author's experience, the remnant usually con-

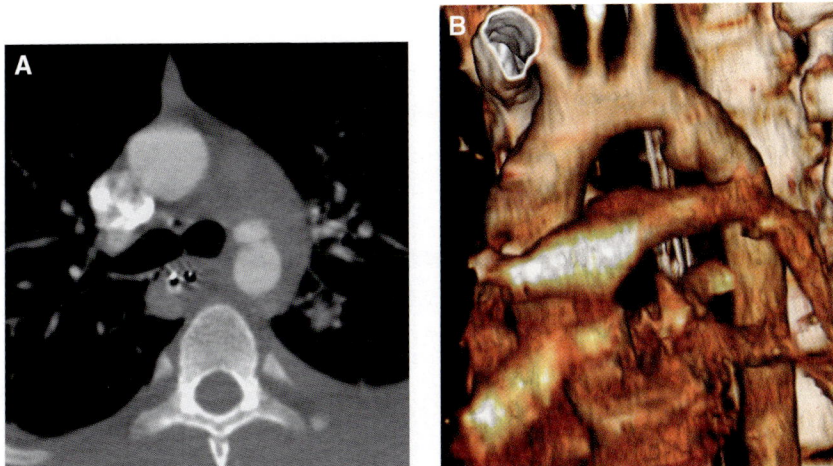

Fig. 16. Typical aortic pseudoaneurysm. (*A*) Axial CT shows pseudoaneurysm projecting anteriorly from aorta with surrounding mediastinal hemorrhage. Carina and nasogastric tube are displaced to the right. (*B*) 3-D volume rendering of injury shows relationship to major arch branches.

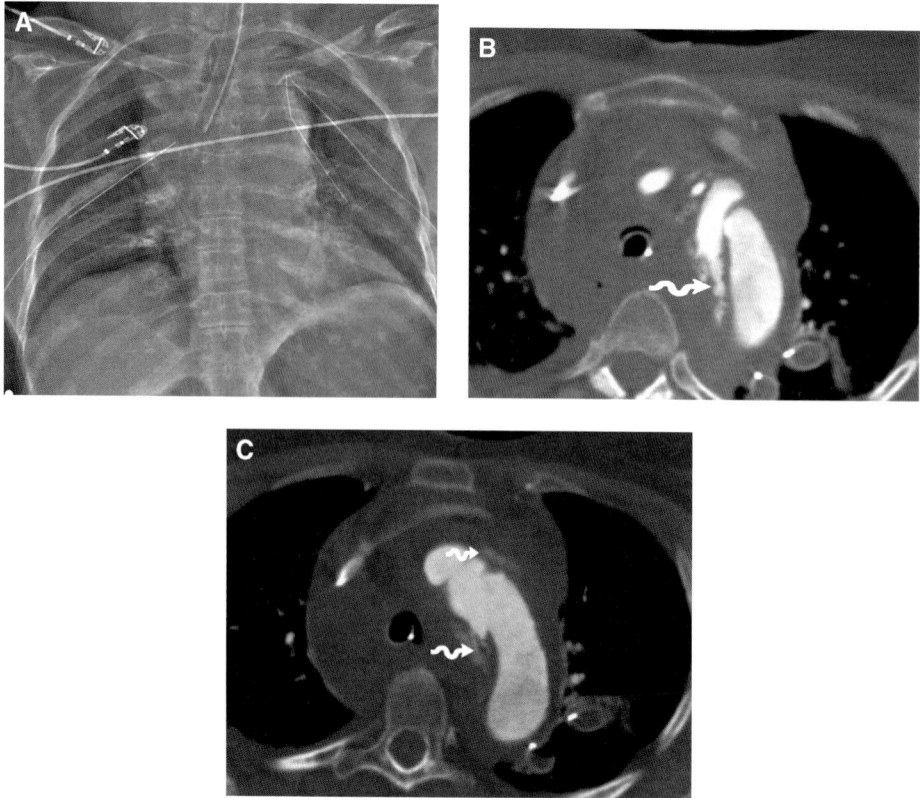

Fig. 17. Actively bleeding aortic injury. (*A*) Admission supine chest radiography of a patient who sustained blunt trauma shows markedly abnormal mediastinal contour. (*B, C*) CT images show contrast leaking from pseudoaneurysm (*arrows*) and extensive mediastinal hematoma.

nects to the thoracic aorta, rather than the left pulmonary artery, although it extends in that direction. On occasion, ductus variants may have irregular contours with a sharp edge or even an acute margin with the aortic lumen, which makes distinction from an injury difficult [32,33].

In addition, in some patients the contour of the proximal descending aorta is atypical [Fig. 22]. Some of these cases may represent slight congenital variations in the formation of the proximal descending aorta, such as a mild pseudocoarctation. Another normal aortic contour variant in the aorta

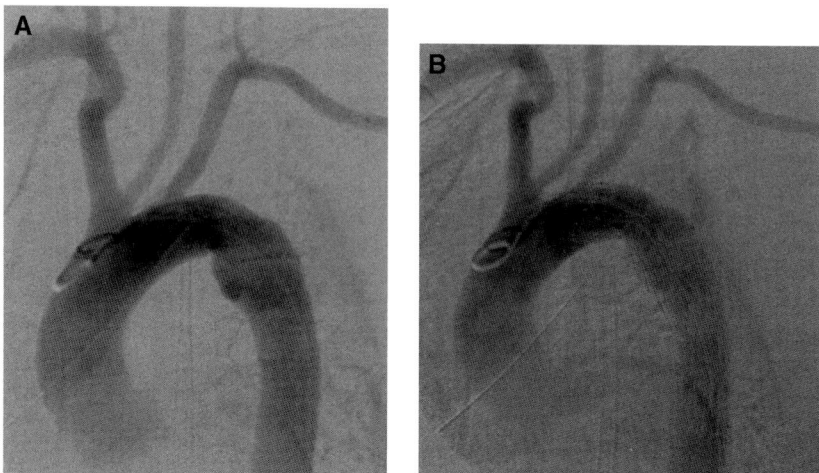

Fig. 18. Stenting aortic injury. (*A*) Angiogram of typical aortic injury. (*B*) Overlapping stent grafts cover injured area, and permit contrast to flow into left subclavian artery.

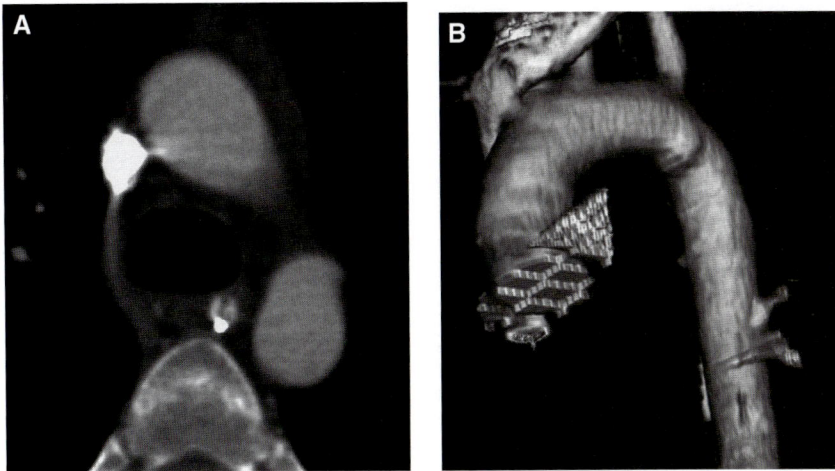

Fig. 19. CT angiography of ductus diverticulum. (*A*) A smooth outpouching arises from anterior aorta above the level of the left pulmonary artery and left mainstem bronchus. No mediastinal blood is present. (*B*) 3-D volume image shows the smooth outpouching with obtuse margins with aortic lumen is directly opposite the left subclavian origin, an atypical location for a traumatic pseudoaneurysm.

is a fusiform enlargement or prominence immediately beyond the ductus arteriosus. His (Wilhelm His, Swiss anatomist and embryologist 1831–1904) named this the *aortic spindle*: the point of junction of the two parts is marked in the concavity of the arch by an indentation or angle. This condition persists, to some extent, in the adult, where the average diameter of the spindle exceeds that of the isthmus by 3 mm. Again, the aortic walls should have smooth surfaces in these circumstances.

In approaching these difficult cases, the use of MPR, 3-D volume, and endovascular views is paramount. The MPR and 3-D images help to establish the exact location and contour of the anatomy that can assist in the distinction between a ductus variant and an injury [see Fig. 22]. Also, endoluminal views can help in showing the presence or absence of an intimal flap or tear, a component that is nearly always present in blunt aortic injuries. In all cases of congenital variants of aortic anatomy,

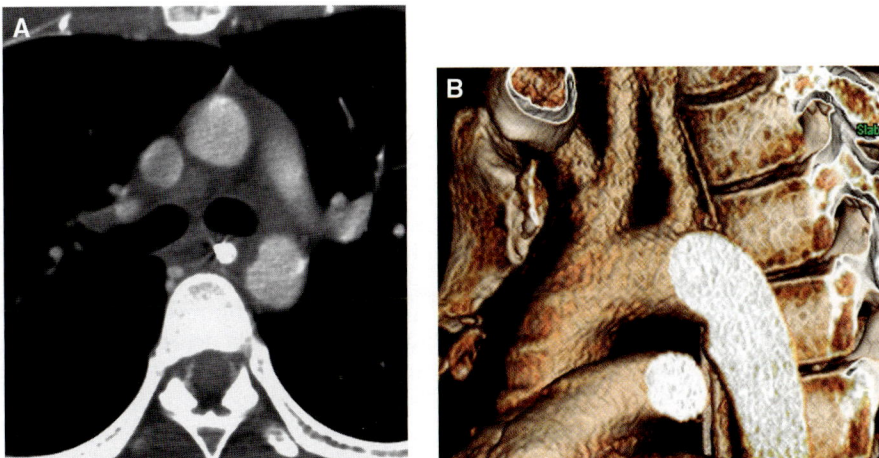

Fig. 20. Atypical aortic contour. (*A*) A smooth outpouching arises from the anterior aorta at the level of the left mainstem bronchus without adjacent mediastinal blood. (*B*) Volume-rendered image through outpouching shows smooth internal contours and obtuse margins with aorta. No further procedures were performed.

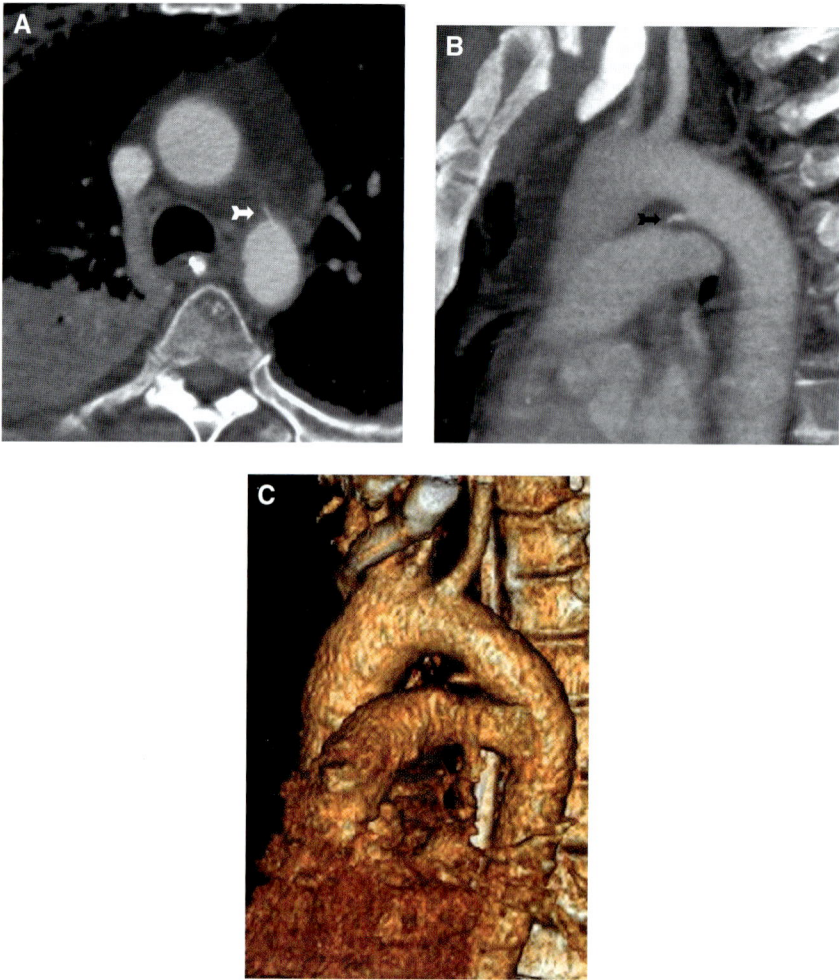

Fig. 21. Ductus remnant. (*A*) CT shows atypical contour to aortic lumen at level just above carina with linear density (*arrow*) arising from focal bulge in aorta. No mediastinal blood is observed. (*B*) MPR along the long axis of the aorta shows the calcified ductus remnant (*arrow*) pointing to the pulmonary artery. (*C*) Volume CT view shows slight focal bulge in aorta and linear structure directed toward pulmonary artery bifurcation. No further procedure concerning the aorta was performed.

mediastinal hemorrhage will be absent, which supports a benign characterization of the anomaly. Rarely, there is little to no perivascular mediastinal blood in patients who have acute aortic injury.

In other cases, the CT findings of TAI are subtle. This has a much greater potential to occur when using conventional or single-detector helical CT, or with suboptimal contrast boluses or patient motion. In general, confusion is likely to be greatest when relying solely on axial place CT images. Small pseudoaneurysms are often better observed using a sagittal or coronal MPR or a plane along the major axis of the thoracic aorta. Again, the author has found that in selected cases, the 3-D volume rendered projection, maximum intensity projection, and endoluminal views can enhance analysis of the aorta and lead to a more confident diagnosis.

In cases that remain equivocal despite a complete CT analysis, or in patients in whom a technically high-quality study cannot be obtained, other modalities, such as thoracic angiography or sonography, should be performed expeditiously. The choice of modality should depend on the availability and expertise of the performing physicians and the overall clinical setting.

In some patients who sustain blunt trauma, the abdominal CT may be obtained and the chest CT may be delayed or not be performed. It is important to appreciate potential signs of thoracic aortic injury that may be seen on the abdominal study,

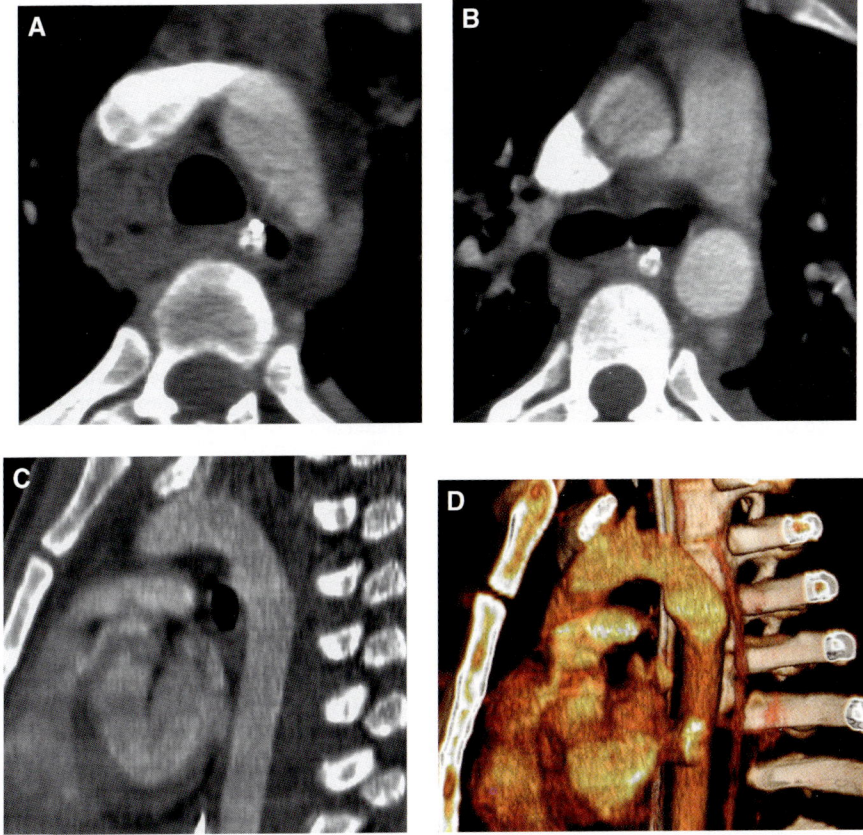

Fig. 22. Atypical aortic contour. (*A*) Axial CT in a patient who sustained blunt trauma shows hemorrhage in the right paratracheal region. Axial (*B*), sagittal (*C*), and 3-D (*D*) sagittal images show atypical configuration of aorta, but no irregularities to lumen. Endovascular view (not shown) revealed no intimal defects. Because of the mediastinal blood, the clinical team obtained angiography of aorta with equivocal result. Transesophageal sonogram was interpreted as aortic injury. At surgery, the aorta had no injury.

including a small caliber aorta that results from coarctation of the lumen by clot, intimal flaps, or a compressing pseudoaneurysm [see Figs. 8 and 23]. It is the author's impression that this phenomenon occurs, to some degree, in up to 25% of all traumatic aortic injuries. Also, it is common for mediastinal blood to dissect down along the aorta and accumulate in the retrocrural space at the aortic hiatus [Fig. 24] [34].

Penetrating aortic injury

In general, the concepts that apply to CT imaging in blunt aortic trauma are not valid regarding penetrating injury. The major role of CT (as described elsewhere in this issue) is determination of the presence or absence of mediastinal involvement along or near the course of the penetrating object. In some cases, however, in the pursuit of this goal, direct findings of injury to major mediastinal structures can be diagnosed. Aortic or major arterial injuries can be detected, and appear as irregular vascular contours, luminal narrowing or irregularity, pseudoaneurysms, dissections, and acute bleeding. In some cases, because of the external nature of the injury, the luminal side of the vessel may appear completely normal by CT or

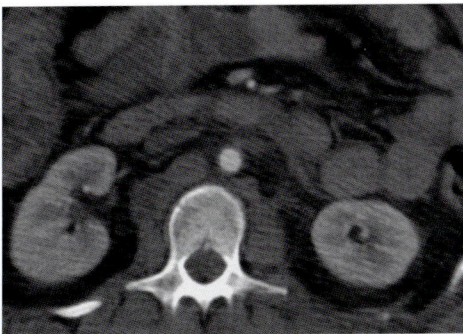

Fig. 23. Small aorta sign. Abdominal image in a patient who sustained blunt trauma shows subjectively small caliber of aorta that is due to coarctation of thoracic lumen from injury.

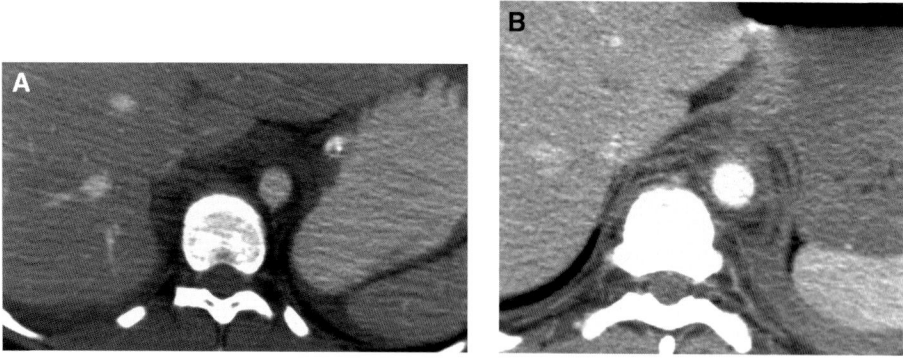

Fig. 24. Peridiaphragmatic hemorrhage in aortic injury. (*A* and *B*) Two different patients who sustained trauma show retrocrural hemorrhage at the level of the aortic hiatus—an indirect, but important, sign of potential aortic injury. Also observed in *A* and *B* is a smaller than normal caliber of the aorta at level of aortic diaphragmatic hiatus.

arteriography. Perivascular hemorrhage should be present in most cases. Following the course of the missile or knife track also should help to determine the likelihood of direct vascular involvement [Fig. 25].

Nonaortic major thoracic arterial injuries

Thoracic aortic branches

Injuries of the primary branches of the aorta are uncommon relative to the proximal descending aorta, but represent a significant potential isolated injury or one that is concurrent with aortic injury [Figs. 11 and 26] [35]. Chen and colleagues [36] studied 85 patients who had either aortic, isolated branch vessel, or both concurrently in 71 (83.5%), 11 (13%), and 3 (3.5%) patients, respectively.

Ahrar and colleagues [37] identified 81 patients who had angiographic evidence of traumatic injury to the thoracic aorta or its branches; 66 (81.5%) had only aortic rupture. Fifteen patients (18.5%) had injuries of the aortic branch vessels.

These branch injuries are potentially fatal of their own accord, but their identification also is key in determining an appropriate approach for surgical repair. Whereas the more common isolated proximal descending aortic injury usually is approached by way of a posterolateral thoracotomy, a proximal innominate artery injury requires a median sternotomy. The latter could be used to access both injuries if concurrent, but adequate exposure to the innominate injury is not be possible from the left thoracotomy. Thus, all injuries to the aorta and its proximal branches must be identified before any surgery is undertaken.

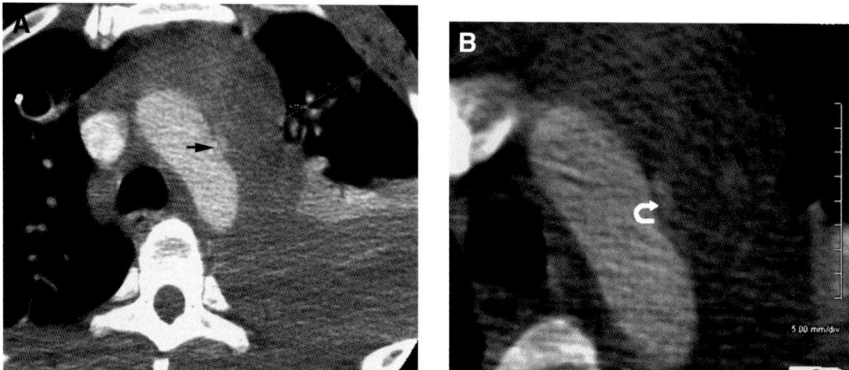

Fig. 25. Penetrating aortic injury. Axial CT (*A*) and magnified axial view (*B*) show knife track extending to aortic arch with small amount of blood extravasating from lumen (*arrows*) and surrounding hematoma.

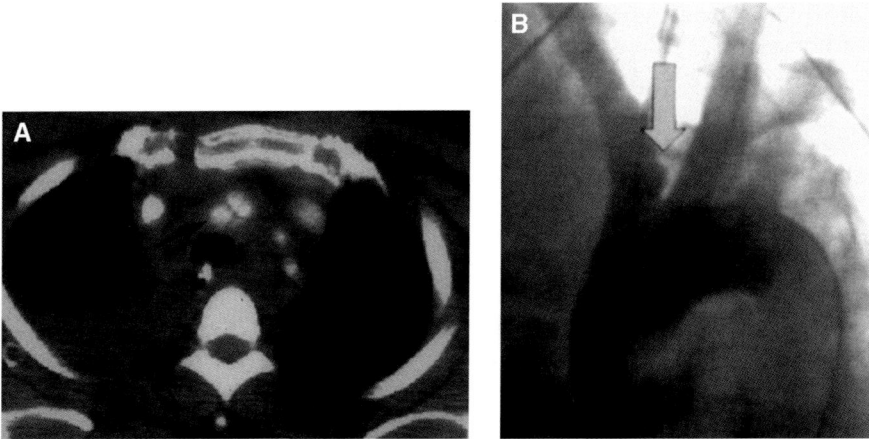

Fig. 26. Aortic branch vessel injury. (*A*) CT shows pseudoaneurysm arising from proximal innominate artery (*arrow*) with surrounding hemorrhage. (*B*) Angiogram verifies injury (*arrow*).

There is little published information on the use or accuracy of CT for diagnosis of proximal (intrathoracic) branch vessel injuries. A careful search for these injuries must be made. If an injury clearly involves the major branch vessels this should not require confirmation. Conversely, if there is blood around the great vessel origins and superior mediastinum without CT evidence of a major branch artery injury, confirmation by angiogram should be considered. It is hoped that in the near future, the published experience with MDCT for primary aortic branches is adequate to verify its accuracy. The CT identification of lung and chest wall vascular injures is discussed elsewhere in this issue.

Major venous thoracic injuries

Based on a literature review, injuries to the major thoracic veins from blunt trauma seem to be extremely rare. Most likely, these injuries often are fatal, and therefore, rarely are imaged.

Intrapericardial inferior vena cava injury should be considered in cases of major hepatic injury, particularly if there is blood around the intrahepatic inferior vena cava or extravasation of contrast material. Superior and inferior vena cava injury also should be considered in cases of pericardial tamponade when an arterial bleeding site is not identified. Potential signs of injury include intravenous

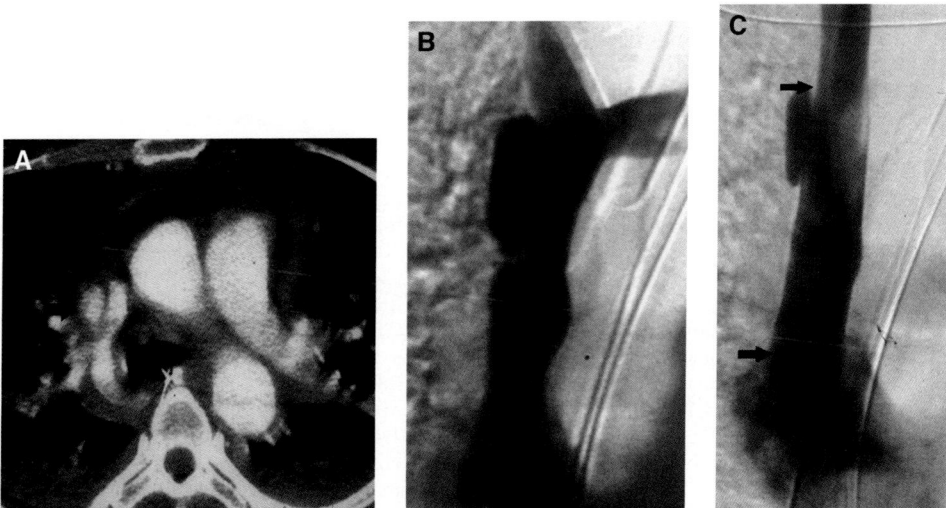

Fig. 27. Superior vena cava injury in blunt trauma. (*A*) Axial CT image in a patient who sustained blunt trauma shows a linear tear in the superior vena cava at level of azygous vein entry. (*B*) Vena cavagram verifies pseudoaneurysm. (*C*) Appearance of injury after stent placement (*arrows*).

thrombus, dissection, contrast extravasation, and pericaval hematoma [Fig. 27] [38–40].

Summary

The availability of MDCT has increased the use of CT and its accuracy as a screening study for traumatic aortic injuries. In general, CT has become much more commonly used in screening for major injuries in patients who have experienced blunt polytrauma. Therefore, an understanding of the CT signs of TAI and pitfalls in the diagnosis need to be well recognized by all radiologists and other physicians who view this study. Angiography (see elsewhere in this issue) and transesophageal sonography provide valuable adjunct studies to solve problems when the CT study is technically limited or, in rare cases, equivocal. One or both of these alternative modalities need to be available quickly in institutions that receive patients who have sustained major trauma.

Treatment of TAI by medical management (blood pressure regulation) or endovascular stenting as a temporizing or definitive therapy requires excellent image quality, preferably with display of multiplanar and volumetric views. To assist in treatment planning, details of aortic anatomy (ie, size, exact location and type [characteristics] of injury; proximity of branch vessels; proximal and distal aortic diameter; atypical vascular or thoracic anatomy) need to be described routinely as part of the imaging report.

References

[1] Patel NH, Stephens Jr KE, Mirvis SE, et al. Imaging of acute thoracic aortic injury due to blunt trauma: a review. Radiology 1998;209(2):335–48.

[2] Nagy K, Fabian T, Rodman G, et al. Guidelines for the diagnosis and management of blunt aortic injury: an EAST Practice Management Guidelines Work Group. J Trauma 2000;48(6):1128–43.

[3] Graham AN, McManus KG, McGuigan JA, et al. Traumatic rupture of the thoracic aorta: computed tomography may be a dangerous waste of time. Ann R Coll Surg Engl 1995;77(2):154–5.

[4] Fisher RG, Chasen MH, Lamki N. Diagnosis of injuries of the aorta and brachiocephalic arteries caused by blunt chest trauma: CT vs aortography. AJR Am J Roentgenol 1994;162(5):1047–52.

[5] Merine D, Brody WR. Role of CT in excluding major arterial injury after blunt thoracic trauma. Invest Radiol 1989;24(9):733–4.

[6] Sinclair DS. Traumatic aortic injury: an imaging review. Emerg Radiol 2002;9(1):13–20.

[7] Melton SM, Kerby JD, McGiffin D, et al. The evolution of chest computed tomography for the definitive diagnosis of blunt aortic injury: a single-center experience. J Trauma 2004;56(2):243–50.

[8] Mirvis SE, Shanmuganathan K, Buell J, et al. Use of spiral computed tomography for the assessment of blunt trauma patients with potential aortic injury. J Trauma 1998;45(5):922–30.

[9] Demetriades D, Gomez H, Velmahos GC, et al. Routine helical computed tomographic evaluation of the mediastinum in high-risk blunt trauma patients. Arch Surg 1998;133(10):1084–9.

[10] Wales LR, Morishima MS, Reay D, et al. Nasogastric tube displacement in acute traumatic rupture of the thoracic aorta: a postmortem study. AJR Am J Roentgenol 1982;138:821–3.

[11] Peters DR, Gamsu G. Displacement of the right paraspinous interface. A radiologic sign of acute traumatic rupture of the thoracic aorta. Radiology 1980;134:599–603.

[12] Seltzer SE, D'Orsi C, Kirshner R, et al. Traumatic aortic rupture: plain radiographic findings. AJR Am J Roentgenol 1981;137:1011–4.

[13] Marnocha KE, Maglinte DD, Woods J, et al. Blunt chest trauma and suspected aortic rupture: reliability of chest radiograph findings. Ann Emerg Med 1985;14(7):644–9.

[14] Mirvis SE, Bidwell JK, Buddemeyer EU, et al. Value of chest radiography in excluding traumatic aortic rupture. Radiology 1987;163:487–93.

[15] Marnocha KE, Maglinte DD, Woods J, et al. Mediastinal-width/chest-width ratio in blunt chest trauma: a reappraisal. AJR Am J Roentgenol 1984;142:275–7.

[16] Woodring JH, King JG. The potential effects of radiographic criteria to exclude aortography in patients with blunt chest trauma. Results of a study of 32 patients with proved aortic or brachiocephalic arterial injury. J Thorac Cardiovasc Surg 1989;97:456–60.

[17] Parmley LF, Marion WC, Jahnke EJ. Nonpenetrating traumatic injury of the aorta. Circulation 1958;17:1086–91.

[18] Mirvis SE, Pais SO, Shanmuganathan K. Atypical results of thoracic aortography to exclude aortic rupture. Emerg Radiol 1988;1:42–8.

[19] Lomoschitz FM, Eisenhuber E, Linnau KF, et al. Imaging of chest trauma: radiological patterns of injury and diagnostic algorithms. Eur J Radiol 2003;48:61–70.

[20] Cleverley JR, Barrie JR, Raymond GS, et al. Direct findings of aortic injury on contrast-enhanced CT in surgically proven traumatic aortic injury: a multi-centre review. Clin Radiol 2002;57(4):281–6.

[21] Mirvis SE, Shanmuganathan K, Miller BH, et al. Traumatic aortic injury: diagnosis with contrast-enhanced thoracic CT–five-year experience at a major trauma center. Radiology 1996;200(2):413–22.

[22] Berthet JP, Marty-Ane CH, Veerapen R, et al. Dissection of the abdominal aorta in blunt

trauma: endovascular or conventional surgical management? J Vasc Surg 2003;38(5):997–1003 [discussion 1004].

[23] Scaglione M, Pinto A, Pinto F, et al. Role of contrast-enhanced helical CT in the evaluation of acute thoracic aortic injuries after blunt chest trauma. Eur Radiol 2001;11(12):2444–8.

[24] Mirvis SE. Diagnostic imaging of acute thoracic injury. Semin Ultrasound CT MR 2004;25(2): 156–79.

[25] Losanoff JE, Richman BW, Amiridze N, et al. Floating thrombus of the thoracic aorta: a rare consequence of blunt trauma. J Trauma 2004; 57(4):892–4.

[26] Cressman EN, Winer-Muram HT, Farber J. Traumatic intrapericardial ascending aortic rupture: CT appearance. J Thorac Imaging 2004;19(1): 45–7.

[27] Downing SW, Sperling JS, Mirvis SE, et al. Experience with spiral computed tomography as the sole diagnostic method for traumatic aortic rupture. Ann Thorac Surg 2001;72:495–501.

[28] Wellons ED, Milner R, Solis M, et al. Stent-graft repair of traumatic thoracic aortic disruptions. J Vasc Surg 2004;40:1095–100.

[29] Amabile P, Collart F, Gariboldi V, et al. Surgical versus endovascular treatment of traumatic thoracic aortic rupture. J Vasc Surg 2004;40:873–9.

[30] Fisher RG, Sanchez-Torres M, Whigham CJ, et al. "Lumps" and "bumps" that mimic acute aortic and brachiocephalic vessel injury. Radiographics 1997;17(4):825–34.

[31] Jeffrey RB, Minagi H, Federle MP, et al. Angiographic evaluation of the ductus diverticulum. Cardiovasc Intervent Radiol 1982;5(1):1–4.

[32] Morse SS, Glickman MG, Greenwood LH, et al. Traumatic aortic rupture: false-positive aorto-graphic diagnosis due to atypical ductus diverticulum. AJR Am J Roentgenol 1988;150(4): 793–6.

[33] Patel NH, Hahn D, Comess KA. Blunt chest trauma victims: role of intravascular ultrasound and transesophageal echocardiography in cases of abnormal thoracic aortogram. J Trauma 2003; 55(2):330–7.

[34] Wong H, Gotway MB, Sasson AD, et al. Periaortic hematoma at diaphragmatic crura at helical CT: sign of blunt aortic injury in patients with mediastinal hematoma. Radiology 2004;231(1): 185–9.

[35] Holdgate A, Dunlop S. Review of branch aortic injuries in blunt chest trauma. Emerg Med Australas 2005;17(1):49–56.

[36] Chen MYM, Miller PR, McLaughlin CA, et al. The trend of using computed tomography in the detection of acute thoracic aortic and branch vessel injury after blunt thoracic trauma: single-center experience over 13 years. J Trauma 2004; 56(4):783–5.

[37] Ahrar K, Smith DC, Bansal RC, et al. Angiography in blunt thoracic aortic injury. J Trauma 1997;42(4):665–9.

[38] Graham CA, McLeod LS, Mitchell RG, et al. Survival after laceration of the superior vena cava from blunt chest trauma. Eur J Emerg Med 1996; 3(3):191–3.

[39] Fey GL, Deren MM, Wesolek JH. Intrapericardial caval injury due to blunt trauma. Conn Med 1999;63(5):259–60.

[40] Chaumoitre K, Zappa M, Portier F, et al. Rupture of the right atrium-superior vena cava junction from blunt thoracic trauma: helical CT diagnosis. AJR Am J Roentgenol 1997;169(6):1753.

RADIOLOGIC
CLINICS
OF NORTH AMERICA

Radiol Clin N Am 44 (2006) 199–211

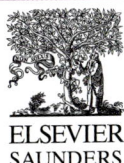

Imaging of Diaphragm Injuries

Clint W. Sliker, MD[a,b,*]

- Anatomy
- Location and mechanism of diaphragm injury
- Clinical diagnosis
- Imaging diagnosis
  Chest radiography
  CT

- Blunt diaphragm rupture
  Penetrating diaphragm injury
  Diagnostic pitfalls of CT
  MR imaging
  Other imaging modalities
- Summary
- References

Diaphragm injury may result from blunt and penetrating trauma. Blunt diaphragm rupture (BDR) is an uncommon injury with an overall reported incidence of 0.16% to 5% [1–4] in patients who experience blunt trauma, although it may occur in up to 8% of patients who have experienced blunt trauma who undergo emergent celiotomy [5]. BDR is even less common in the pediatric population; in one series, it occurred in only 0.07% of patients who were admitted over a 21-year period [6]. Most blunt injuries, 77% to 95% [1,3,7,8], result from road traffic accidents. Penetrating trauma has been reported to cause 12.3% to 20% [1,9] of diaphragm injuries, although it has been suggested that penetrating trauma causes diaphragm injury more commonly than does blunt trauma [5]. Differences in the reported frequencies of different mechanisms of injury may reflect varying geographic regions and socioeconomic strata that are served by the hospital where the studies were based [10].

Acute diaphragm injury is associated with widely ranging mortality of 5.5% to 51% [1,3,9,11], with death typically resulting from associated injuries [1,3,11] or in-hospital complications, such as adult respiratory distress syndrome [1]. With BDR,

there is a high rate of associated severe injuries, most commonly splenic and hepatic injuries, as well as pelvic fractures [1,3,8,11]. Liver and pulmonary injuries frequently occur in conjunction with penetrating diaphragmatic injuries (PDIs) [9]. An animal study that was conducted by Shatney and colleagues [12] suggested that some small traumatic defects may spontaneously heal without surgery; however, it is generally believed that over time, persistent negative intrathoracic pressure pulls abdominal contents into the thoracic cavity, and thereby, prevents healing [4,10]. At times, the delayed diagnosis of diaphragm injury may result from incidental findings on studies that were performed to evaluate unrelated conditions (eg, malignancy) [13]. Nevertheless, up to 7.2% [14] of injuries that are missed acutely may manifest delayed complications in a period that ranges from days [7] to 50 years [15]. Complications usually relate to visceral herniation through the diaphragmatic defect, and include respiratory compromise that is due to impaired pulmonary inflation [7,10,15–18] and visceral incarceration with or without strangulation or perforation [7,14,16–19]. Late presentation of diaphragm injury carries a

a Department of Diagnostic Radiology and Nuclear Medicine, University of Maryland School of Medicine, Baltimore, MD, USA
b Diagnostic Imaging Department, University of Maryland Medical Center and R. Adams Cowley Shock Trauma Center, Baltimore, MD, USA
* Diagnostic Imaging Department, University of Maryland Medical Center and R. Adams Cowley Shock Trauma Center, 22 South Greene Street, Baltimore, MD 21201.
E-mail address: csliker@umm.edu

doi:10.1016/j.rcl.2005.10.003
radiologic.theclinics.com

mortality that approaches 30% to 80% in the presence of visceral strangulation [4,10]. Given the risks of visceral herniation and strangulation, surgical repair of most diaphragm injuries is standard, although many cases of penetrating right hemidiaphragm injury can be treated nonoperatively, because of the small defect size, with a low risk of hepatic herniation and consequent complications [10].

Anatomy

The diaphragm is a dome-shaped musculoskeletal structure that partitions the thoracic and abdominal cavities, and serves as the primary muscle of respiration [4]. It can be divided into several fibromuscular components that converge onto a central tendon. The anterior part attaches to the posterior margins of the lower sternum and xiphoid process. The lateral, or costal, parts attach to the inner margins of the sixth through twelfth ribs. Finally, the posterior lumbar part attaches to the medial and lateral arcuate ligaments. In addition, the regions of more prominent posterior diaphragm thickening, the crura, attach to the first through third lumbar vertebrae on the right and second lumbar vertebra on the left. The thoracic surface of the diaphragm is covered by parietal pleura, whereas the abdominal surface is covered by the peritoneum, with the exception of the portion that is in contact with the bare area of the liver. Three normal openings interrupt diaphragmatic continuity: the aortic hiatus at the thoracoabdominal junction, the esophageal hiatus at the tenth thoracic vertebral level, and the inferior vena caval hiatus at the eighth thoracic vertebral level [4,5,20].

Several normal characteristics may contribute to difficulties with assessing the diaphragm. Portions of the diaphragm may abut structures of similar attenuation (eg, liver, spleen) normally, and thereby, render direct visualization of diaphragm abnormalities difficult [20]. Segments of the diaphragm dome are parallel to the normal axial planes that are used in CT [20], the current standard in diagnostic imaging of patients who have experienced blunt trauma. In addition, several normal variants may lead to diagnostic confusion. Among them are incidental posterolateral diaphragmatic defects that are associated with herniation of abdominal contents (Bochdalek hernias) [Fig. 1] that occur in 0.17% to 6% of otherwise normal patients [4,21]. Next, areas of apparent discontinuity can be seen where the diaphragm inserts on the costal margins [Fig. 2] [20]. There may be areas of marked localized thinning (ie, eventration) with maintenance of diaphragmatic continuity, or areas of diaphragmatic discontinuity [Fig. 3] that can range in size from 5 mm to nearly the entire hemidiaphragm [4,22]. These defects are uncommon in younger age groups, but are progressively more common after the third decade [22]. In addition to areas of diaphragm deficiency, advancing age also predisposes to increasing areas of nodularity and contour irregularity [4,22].

Location and mechanism of diaphragm injury

The left hemidiaphragm is injured in 50% to 88% of patients who have BDR, whereas right-sided injuries are less frequent and occur in 12% to 40% of cases [1,3,8,11,23–27]. In adults, bilateral and central tendon injuries are uncommon and are observed in only 2% to 6% of patients who present with BDR [3,5,8,11,27]. Children manifest an approximately even rate of right- and left-sided injuries that may be due to the increased mobility

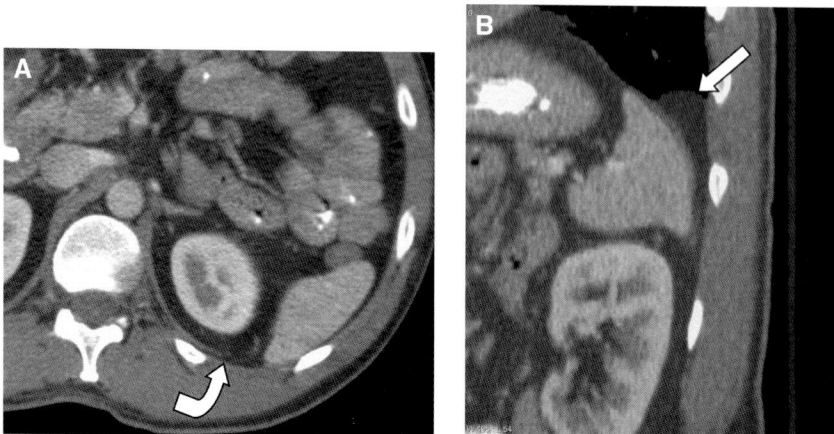

Fig. 1. Incidental Bochdalek hernia. (*A*) Axial abdominal CT demonstrates a posterior left diaphragm defect (*curved arrow*). (*B*) Sagittal reconstructed image shows small retroperitoneal fat herniation (*arrow*) through defect.

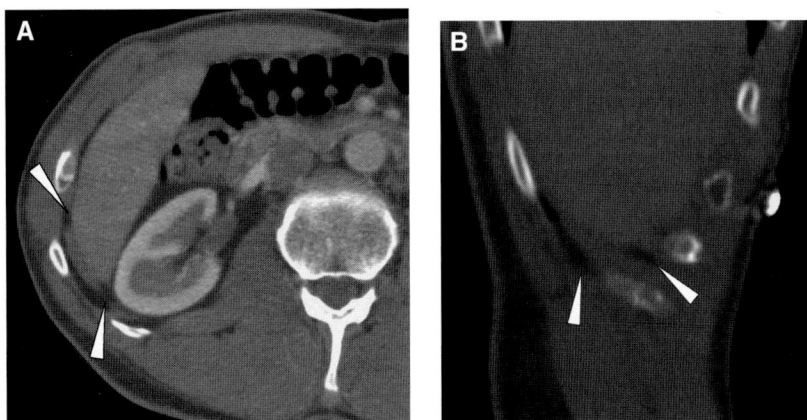

Fig. 2. Normal variant diaphragm insertions. Axial (*A*) and sagittal (*B*) reconstructed CT images demonstrate thinned diaphragm muscle and fat (*arrowheads*) between costal insertions.

of the liver that affords less protection to the right hemidiaphragm than in the adult [6]. In the setting of penetrating trauma, there is an overall equal prevalence of injury on each side [1,5], although it has been suggested that stab wounds are more common on the left side because of the predominance of right-handed attackers [4].

The higher frequency of left-sided BDR has been attributed to an area of congenital posterolateral weakness [20]. Most injuries occur in this location and spread centrally in a radial fashion, although injuries also may occur primarily more centrally or at the sites of diaphragmatic attachment. The relative infrequency of right-sided BDR also may be due to the inherently stronger right hemidiaphragm [11]. In addition, the mass of the liver may afford protective effects [11,20] by sealing the diaphragm defect [24], and thereby, preventing herniation of viscera into the chest and limiting specific features of injury that are seen with diag-

nostic imaging. Moreover, the lower frequency of right-sided injury may be due to underdiagnosis [11,28], and therefore, may not reflect the true incidence of injury. Whereas PDI tends to be small (length ≤1–2 cm) [20,25], BDR tends to be large (length frequently ≥10 cm) [1,3,8,11,24,29].

Proposed mechanisms for blunt injury include lateral impact, with the resulting distortion of the thoracoabdominal wall causing shearing of the diaphragm or disruption of its attachments, and sudden increased intra-abdominal pressure that results from frontal impact [11,20]. The threefold greater frequency of diaphragm injuries in lateral impact motor vehicle collisions relative to frontal impact collisions [11] should increase the radiologist's suspicion for BDR in cases of severe side-impact injury.

Clinical diagnosis

Clinical diagnosis of acute diaphragm injury can be challenging. Symptoms may be nonspecific and include dyspnea, chest pain, shoulder pain, and cyanosis [4,5]. Typically, symptoms are secondary to visceral herniation through the diaphragm defect [5]. Bowel sounds over the hemithorax are suggestive, although other physical findings, such as decreased or absent breath sounds, contralateral mediastinal shift, abdominal tenderness, and guarding, are nonspecific and are obscured easily by signs of other more obvious life-threatening injuries [5]. Consequently, a high index of suspicion is required.

Although diaphragmatic injuries are diagnosed readily by celiotomy or thoracotomy, unless needed for other therapeutic or diagnostic purposes, less invasive means of diagnosis are more desirable. Historically, diagnostic peritoneal lavage (DPL)

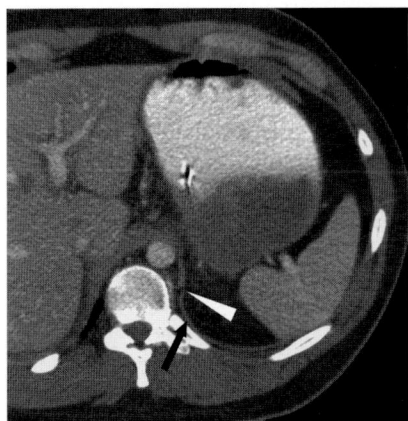

Fig. 3. Normal variant focal discontinuity (*arrowhead*) interrupts typical normal diaphragm (*arrow*).

has served as a minimally invasive means of diagnosing intra-abdominal injury. Whereas DPL results may be diagnostic for diaphragm injury when lavage fluid drains from a chest tube [1,11], it is only 64% to 87% sensitive [1,3,25]. Laparoscopy and thoracoscopy have been proposed as minimally invasive means to diagnose and treat diaphragm injuries, particular in the setting of penetrating trauma [19,30–32], although their role as first-line diagnostic tools remains incompletely explored in the medical literature.

Imaging diagnosis

Historically, the imaging diagnosis of diaphragm injury has proven difficult. Similar to the clinical setting, imaging signs may be subtle and easily overlooked in the face of other more obvious injuries.

Chest radiography

Frequently, chest radiographs are the initial diagnostic imaging examination that is performed in patients who have suspected injuries to the thoracoabdominal region. Although they are useful initial tools in the evaluation for diaphragm injury, supine positioning, portable technique, and reduced patient cooperation can limit diagnostic quality [20], and they may prove unreliable when evaluating the integrity of the diaphragms. The sensitivity of chest radiography for diagnosing diaphragm injury in the setting of blunt trauma has been investigated more thoroughly than in the setting of penetrating trauma. When limited to BDR, initial radiographs are diagnostic or highly suggestive in 27% to 73% of patients [3,25–27,33]. With the addition of serial chest radiographs, an addi-

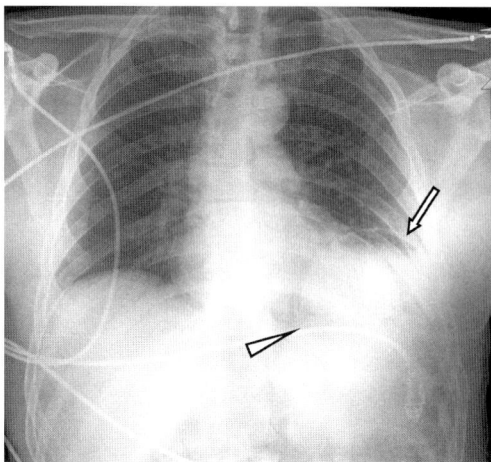

Fig. 5. Left-sided diaphragm rupture. Admission chest radiograph shows nasogastric tube (*arrow*) in intrathoracic stomach (*arrowheads*).

tional 8.3% to 25% [3,25] of BDRs may be identified within the first 24 hours. Serial radiographs may be particularly useful in ventilated patients in whom positive-pressure support overcomes the natural negative pressure gradient that normally would facilitate herniation of abdominal contents into the chest by way of the diaphragm defect [3,5]. When limited to diagnosis of left-sided BDR, admission chest radiographs identify or strongly suggest 52% to 79% of injuries [25–27]. Generally, radiographic diagnosis of right-sided BDR is more difficult, with radiographs demonstrating 0% to 17% of injuries [25,26], although in one study of 16 patients, BDR was radiographically apparent in 63% [27].

Specific radiographic signs of diaphragm injury include: intrathoracic location of abdominal viscera, with or without a site of focal constriction (ie, "collar sign") [Fig. 4], and clear demonstration of a nasogastric tube tip above the left hemidiaphragm [Fig. 5] [20,25]. Although the left hemidiaphragm may be higher than usual in supine patients, in 90% of normal patients, the left diaphragm dome is 1 to 3 cm lower than the right [4]; marked elevation of the hemidiaphragm (>4 cm than the right) without associated atelectasis is another highly suggestive sign [25]. Other sensitive, but nonspecific, findings include obscuration or distortion of the diaphragm margin and diaphragm elevation with contralateral mediastinal shift [20,25]. Elevation of the right diaphragm apex with shift of the apex to a point midway between the mediastinal margin and the lateral chest wall secondary to hepatic herniation is suggestive of right-sided BDR [Fig. 6] [27]. This is in contrast to a superolateral shift, which typically indicates a subpulmonic pleural effusion. In addition to positive ventilatory support, concurrent abnormalities, such as pulmonary contusion, atelectasis, and pleural effusion, may mask diaphragm injury [20,27].

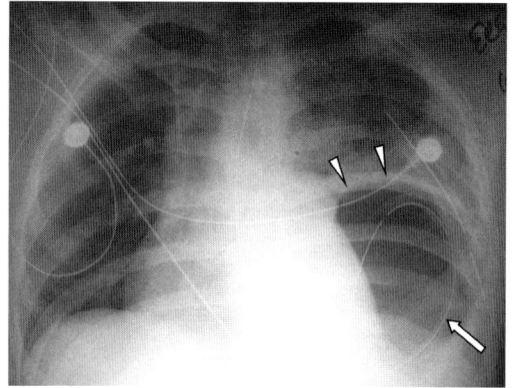

Fig. 4. Left-sided diaphragm rupture with collar sign. Admission chest radiograph demonstrates intrathoracic stomach (*arrow*) with subtle medial constriction or "collar" (*arrowhead*).

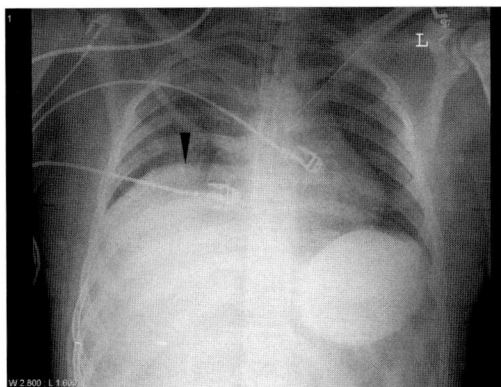

Fig. 6. Right-sided diaphragm rupture. Admission chest radiograph shows elevated right hemidia-phragm apex (*arrowhead*) to left of point midway between lateral chest wall and right mediastinal margin.

CT

Helical CT and the newer, increasingly prevalent multidetector CT (MDCT) techniques are main-stays in the assessment of the patient who has polytrauma patient. Mainly because of the high likelihood of concomitant injuries, at most trauma centers, CT is used to assess hemodynamically stable patients who have experienced blunt trauma with potential diaphragm injury. With the trend toward nonoperative management of solid organ injuries, the recognition of other injuries that pre-viously would have been diagnosed at laparotomy, including diaphragm injuries, has taken on increas-ing importance [10,28]. Moreover, nonoperative management has expanded into the arena of pene-trating trauma with the advent of CT assessment for nonflank torso injuries [34] that previously would have been addressed with exploratory laparotomy or serial clinical and radiographic examinations.

Helical CT protocols that are described in the literature routinely incorporated intravenous con-trast and yielded 5- to 10-mm thick contiguous images. MDCT allows for greater flexibility in regards to the choice of optimum image reconstruc-tion. At the University of Maryland Shock Trauma Center (STC), routine admission chest–abdomen–pelvis scans are obtained on a 16-channel MD-CT (MX8000 IDT, Philips; Best, the Netherlands) with the following scanning parameters (16 × 0.75 mm detector configuration, rotation time 0.75 sec, and pitch 1.2). Typically, 5-mm thick axial images are reconstructed at 5-mm intervals, although the recent trend has been to reconstruct 3-mm thick images at 3-mm intervals. Because associated vis-ceral injuries are the immediate concern, intrave-nous contrast is administered routinely (150 mL of iohexol [300 mgI/mL] at 3 mL/sec with a 45-sec scan delay). Typically, oral contrast is administered,

although it is not mandatory. When necessary, the raw data is reconstructed into thin section axial and multiplanar reconstructed images. Although the use of multiplanar reconstructions (MPRs) is not standard at the STC in all patients who have experi-enced blunt trauma, they are used routinely when diaphragm injury is a concern. Although the useful-ness of MPRs in this setting has been questioned [35], case reports and small series advocate the use of MPRs to solidify the diagnosis [28,36–38], with particular value demonstrated when assessing right-sided injury [28]. To the author's knowledge, no large published series supports the routine use of MPRs to assess for BDR; however, recent work with 40-channel MDCT demonstrates significantly better visualization of the diaphragm with high-quality MPRs, relative to axial images [39,40]. The clinical experience with 16-channel MDCT at the STC sup-ports the use of MPRs to improve the accuracy of CT for diagnosing diaphragm injury and the delineation of injuries that are demonstrated by axial images.

Blunt diaphragm rupture

Reports of conventional CT diagnosis of BDR yield sensitivity of 14% to 82% [8,25,26,33,41] and specificity of 87% [33]. Subsequent studies of heli-cal CT detection of BDR reveal improved sensitivity of 71% to 100% [28,35,42] and specificity of 75% to 100% [28,35]. Sensitivity for left-sided injuries is greater (78–100%) than for right-sided inju-ries (50–79%) [28,35]. The diagnostic accuracy of MDCT, when used to detect diaphragm injury, remains unexplored; however, MDCT's advan-tages over helical CT, including the ability to obtain thinner images with improved z-axis resolution and less respiratory motion, suggest that detection of injury will continue to improve.

Reported CT signs of diaphragm injury include direct visualization of injury, segmental diaphragm nonvisualization, intrathoracic herniation of vis-cera, the collar sign, the dependent viscera sign, diaphragm thickening, and peridiaphragmatic ac-tive contrast extravasation. Commonly, hemo-thorax, hemoperitoneum, atelectasis, and adjacent visceral injury accompany the CT signs of dia-phragm injury.

Directly visualization of injury

The sensitivity and specificity of a directly visu-alized diaphragm tear are 36% to 82.7% and 88.1% to 95%, respectively [33,35,41,42]. Typically, images demonstrate the free edge of the disrupted dia-phragm demarcating the defect [Fig. 7]. This is in contrast with nonvisualization of the diaphragm without demonstration of the torn diaphragm mar-gin. The free margin may be central or peripheral at

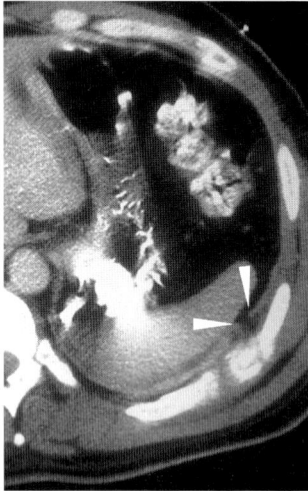

Fig. 7. Posttraumatic defect. Margins of diaphragm tear (*arrowheads*) demarcate fat-containing defect.

the site of diaphragm insertion. At times, the muscle edge doubles back upon itself or is thickened by muscle retraction or hemorrhage [Fig. 8].

Segmental diaphragm nonvisualization
Isolated segmental nonvisualization of the diaphragm is up to 85.9% sensitive and 67.7% specific for BDR [42]; however, this sign must be used with caution when seen in isolation, especially in the elderly, in whom it can be a normal variant [20,28]. In the absence of visceral herniation, hemothorax and atelectasis may blur the diaphragm margins, and thereby, yield a false positive examination [28]. The usefulness of this sign increases when other signs of injury are present,

or when there are other local intra-abdominal abnormalities, such as hemoperitoneum or retroperitoneal hematoma [42].

Intrathoracic herniation of viscera
Although the specificity of clearly demonstrated intrathoracic herniation of abdominal viscera into the chest is high at 94.1% to 100% [33,35,42], its sensitivity varies widely from 8% to 81% [6,23,33,35,41,42]. When limited to left-sided injury, sensitivity is high at 90.9% [42]. On the left, the stomach and colon frequently herniate. Although its size and contour limit the value of the sign, the liver typically herniates with right-sided lesions [see Fig. 8]. Other intra-abdominal contents, including small bowel, omentum [Fig. 9], and spleen, also may herniate. Factors that may hinder intrathoracic herniation include the presence of intrathoracic space-occupying abnormalities, such as a large hemothorax, or increased intrathoracic pressure secondary to positive pressure ventilation. Consequently, this abnormality can be recognized on follow-up examinations after drainage of pleural fluid or discontinuance of positive pressure ventilatory support.

Collar sign
If an abdominal structure herniates through a diaphragm rent, the free edges of the diaphragm can constrict the herniated organ, and thereby, result in a "collar." Even when its relative level does not clearly suggest so, the collar sign is an indication of intrathoracic herniation of abdominal contents [Figs. 10 and 11]. Several organs may combine to manifest the collar-like constriction [Fig. 12]. This sign also demonstrates a widely ranging sensitiv-

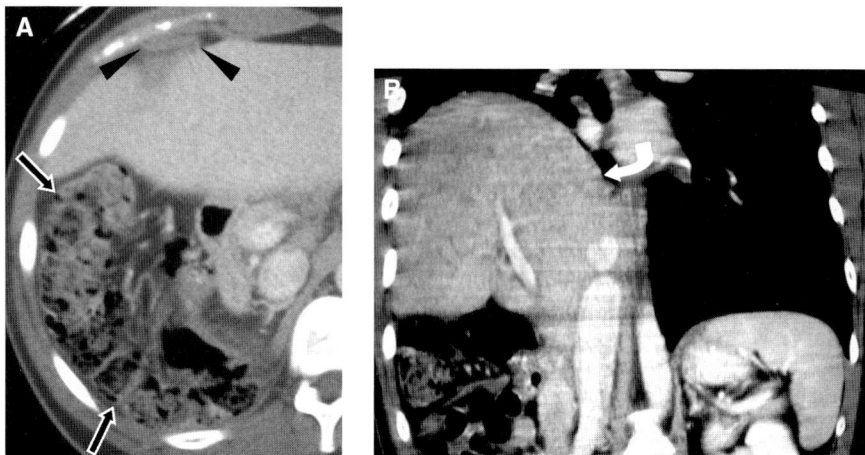

Fig. 8. Right-sided diaphragm rupture. Axial (*A*) and coronal (*B*) MPR CT. Anterior free diaphragm edge curls onto itself (*arrowheads*). Segment of colon (*arrows*) is posteroinferior to the liver, which is herniated into the chest (*curved arrow*).

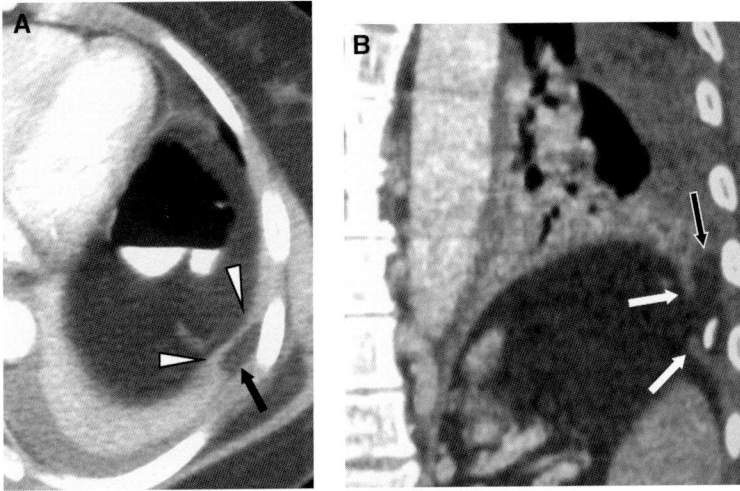

Fig. 9. Peritoneal fat herniation. Axial (*A*) and coronal (*B*) MPR CT images. Atelectatic lung (*arrowheads*) partially surrounds peritoneal fat (*black arrow*) that herniated through a blunt diaphragm tear (*white arrows*).

ity, 24% to 85% [28,33,35,41,42], although there is a consistently high specificity, 80.7% to 100% [28,33,35,42]. The size and consistency of the liver make this a less valuable sign for right-sided injuries, with sensitivities of 16.7% to 40% [28,42], although the addition of MPRs can increase sensitivity to 50% [Fig. 13] [28].

Dependent viscera sign

Normally, the intact diaphragm prevents the upper abdominal viscera from contacting the posterior chest wall in the supine patient. When the diaphragm is torn, its constraints are released, and the viscera may lie "dependent" against the posterior chest wall. On the left, this sign is present when the stomach [Fig. 14] or bowel abuts the posterior ribs or is situated posterior to the spleen; on the right, it is present when the upper third of the liver contacts the posterior chest wall [43]. In the initial

reporting of this sign by Bergin and colleagues [43], an overall sensitivity of 90% was reported; however, subsequent studies [35,42] yielded lower sensitivity (46.6%–52%), with high specificity (71%–96.5%) [35,42]. At times, a large pleural effusion or hemothorax may hinder the dependent migration of viscera in the presence of BDR, and the dependent viscera sign should be sought on follow-up examinations after fluid drainage [35].

Abnormally thick diaphragm and active diaphragmatic hemorrhage

The diaphragm is considered abnormally thickened by subjective comparison with the contralateral side [44]. To limit the influence of normal variability in diaphragmatic crus thickness, the point of reference should be 10 mm from the midline [42]. In the presence of injury, intramuscular hematoma

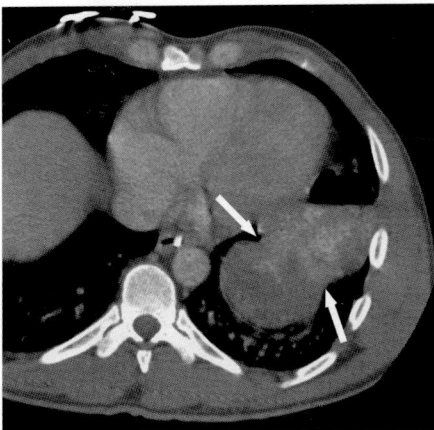

Fig. 10. Axial CT shows gastric collar sign (*arrows*).

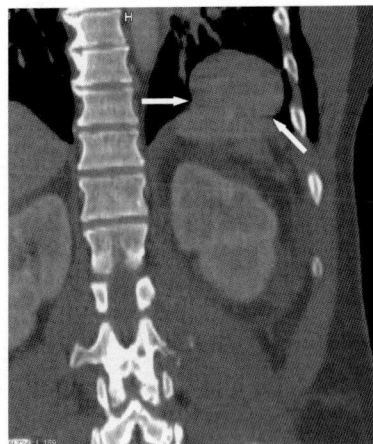

Fig. 11. Coronal CT MPR shows splenic collar sign (*arrows*).

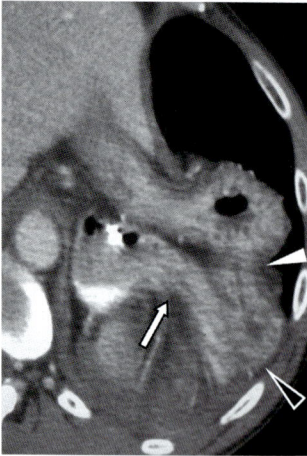

Fig. 12. Axial CT shows collar sign involving small bowel (*white arrowhead*) and stomach (*white arrow*). Note contiguous small bowel (*black arrowhead*).

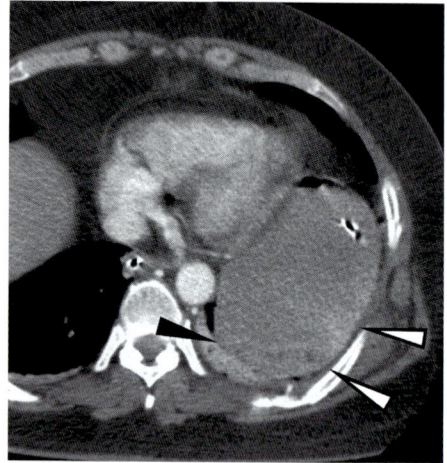

Fig. 14. Dependent viscera sign. The stomach (*arrowheads*) abuts the posterior chest wall on axial CT.

or edema or muscle retraction accounts for the abnormally thick diaphragm [42,44]. An abnormally thickened diaphragm was reported to be 100% [42] sensitive for right-sided diaphragm injuries, although overall sensitivity is only 36% to 60% [35,42]. Specificity also is low, 58.4% to 77% [35,42]. One of the sign's limitations is that it does not allow the radiologist to distinguish a full-thickness diaphragmatic rupture that warrants repair from a partial-thickness tear [Fig. 15] that does not merit surgery [42,44]. Moreover, hemorrhage secondary to injuries to adjacent structures can track to the diaphragm and mimic intrasubstance diaphragmatic hemorrhage [42,44]. Therefore, although it may prompt rigorous investigation for BDR, an abnormally thick diaphragm should

not be used as the sole criterion to diagnose diaphragm rupture.

Active contrast extravasation (hemorrhage) at the diaphragm is another nonspecific sign that can be the only indication of injury [35]. Like diaphragm thickening, the use of this sign as the sole indicator of injury should be made with great caution. The site of hemorrhage may not be the diaphragm, and, in fact, it may be related to injury to adjacent organs, such the liver, spleen [42], or intercostal arteries.

Multiple signs of injury
Frequently, multiple signs of injury are present in the same patient [Fig. 16], and, when used together, can elevate the sensitivity of CT to 100% [42]. Nevertheless, the luxury of multiple signs of

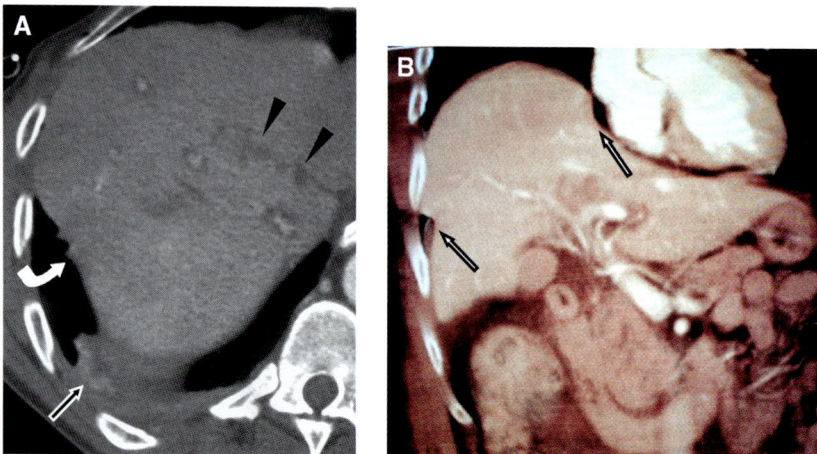

Fig. 13. Right-sided collar sign. (*A*) Axial CT demonstrates liver laceration (*black arrowheads*), atelectasis (*black arrow*), and subtle abnormal liver contour (*curved arrow*). (*B*) Coronal volume rendered MPR reveals obvious hepatic collar sign (*white arrows*) due to blunt diaphragm rupture.

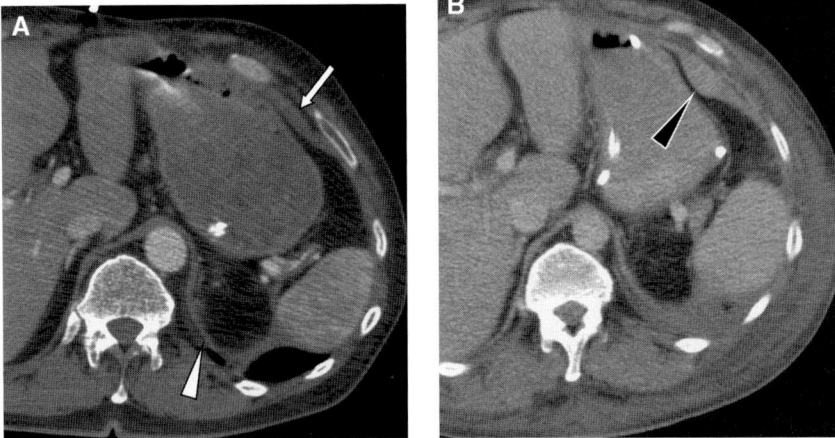

Fig. 15. Thickened diaphragm. (*A*) Admission CT demonstrates anterior diaphragm thickening (*arrow*) compared with normal posterior diaphragm (*white arrowhead*) thickness. (*B*) CT obtained 3 days later shows prominent focal thickening (*black arrowhead*) that is due to organized hematoma in intact diaphragm.

injury is not universal. In their review of the accuracy of helical CT for the detection of diaphragm injury (blunt and penetrating), Larici and colleagues [35] found that CT was 84% sensitive, although no individual sign of injury exhibited a sensitivity that was greater than 52%; this clearly demonstrates the importance of each manifestation of injury.

Penetrating diaphragm injury

Little has been reported about the accuracy of CT in diagnosing penetrating diaphragmatic injury. In their series of 14 patients who had PDIs, Larici and colleagues [35] reported that helical CT's sensitivity

and specificity were 86% and 79%, respectively. In their series of patients who had suffered penetrating trauma to the torso, Shanmuganathan and colleagues [34] suggested that helical CT may be an accurate means of diagnosing PDI, although only 34% of subjects had surgically documented injuries.

Because the signs of BDR generally result from the large defect size, they are less helpful when assessing potential PDI. Nevertheless, the signs of BDR remain valuable in the setting of PDI. For example, despite the small size of injuries, herniation of abdominal contents, especially fat [Fig. 17]

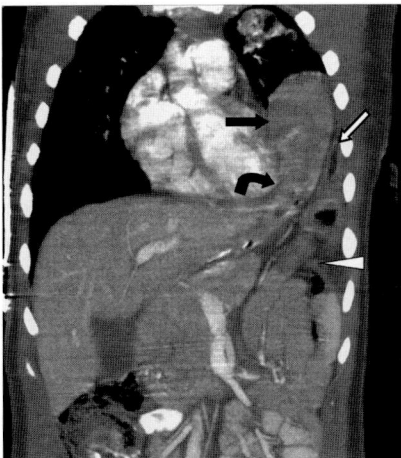

Fig. 16. Multiple signs of blunt diaphragm rupture. Coronal MPR CT demonstrates intrathoracic herniation of stomach (*black arrow*) and colon (*white arrow*), gastric collar sign (*curved arrow*), and free edge of ruptured left hemidiaphragm (*arrowhead*).

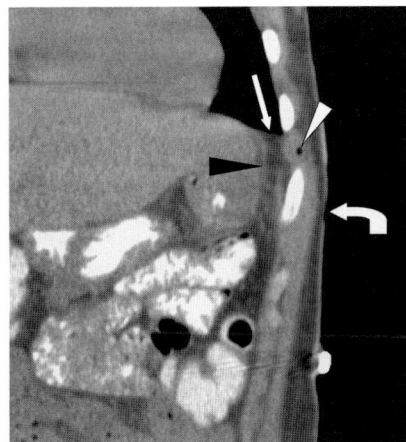

Fig. 17. Penetrating diaphragm injury from stab to lateral left thoracoabdominal region. Coronal MPR CT image reveals omental fat (*arrow*) herniating through a small diaphragmatic hole. Note the free diaphragm edge (*black arrowhead*), air in knife tract (*white arrowhead*), and cutaneous defect (*curved arrow*) that delineate the tract.

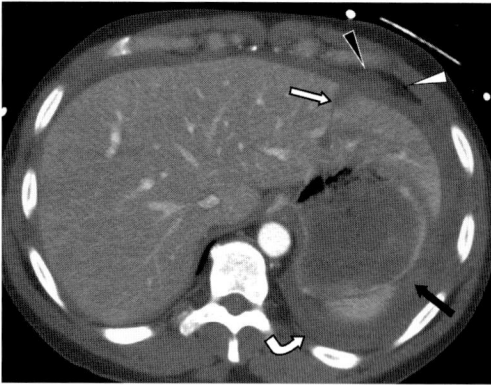

Fig. 18. CT of inferred penetrating diaphragm injury in victim of single left subcostal stab wound. Hematoma (*black arrowhead*) and gas (*white arrowhead*) anterior to the diaphragm and a contiguous liver laceration (*white arrow*) indicate that the knife penetrated the diaphragm. Hemoperitoneum (*black arrow*) and hemothorax (*curved arrow*) result from violation of the peritoneal and pleural diaphragmatic surfaces.

[34], can occur early, and is a specific sign of PDI. Clearly, familiarity with subtle signs of diaphragm injury is particularly important in this challenging clinical setting.

A wound tract (from knife, bullet, and so forth) that extends along both sides of the diaphragm is a sign of diaphragm injury that is specific to penetrating trauma [Fig. 18] [34,35]. This sign has a sensitivity of only 36% but a specificity of 100% [35], even without demonstration of the actual defect. In such cases in which PDI is inferred, its characteristically small size hinders visualization of the defect. When combined with diaphragmatic motility, it is unlikely that the hole will align with the trajectory during CT scanning, unless herniation already has occurred. Given the reliability of a wound tract as an indicator of injury and the propensity for delayed complications in untreated PDI, Shackleton and colleagues [23] recommend follow-up imaging of patients who do not undergo open or videoscopic exploration, and who have previous CT scans that show a wound trajectory that involves the diaphragm.

Diagnostic pitfalls of CT

Causes of confusion and misdiagnosis include failure to recognize normal variations, overemphasis of nonspecific signs of injury, failure to recognize subtle signs of injury, and scanning artifacts. When nonspecific signs of injury or suspected normal variants are present, the liberal use of multiplanar reconstructions can be helpful. At times, repeat scanning with oral contrast and thinner image reconstruction, or follow-up scanning after several days, may improve diagnostic confidence. Occasionally, motion artifacts can degrade study quality. If there are no signs of thoracoabdominal injury, the likelihood of a diaphragm injury is miniscule and the injury can be excluded confidently; however, when signs of injury are evident, repeat scanning with a greater pitch may be required.

MR imaging

Through its ability to provide direct sagittal and coronal images, MR imaging is well suited to imaging the entire diaphragm. Moreover, its excellent contrast resolution typically allows clear discrimination between the diaphragm and adjacent structures, such as the liver and atelectatic lung [20]. Despite its benefits, the MR environment introduces difficulties into the management of patients who have polytrauma who may harbor diaphragm injury; among them, the strong magnetic field is incompatible with some monitoring devices, and poor access to the patient may hinder treatment of hemodynamic instability. At some institutions, staffing issues may limit scanner availability.

Nevertheless, in hemodynamically stable patients, rapid and focused scanning protocols can facilitate fast scanning. Shanmuganathan and colleagues [45] use a simple protocol that consists of sagittal and coronal spin-echo T1-weighted images; they no longer include gradient echo sequences in their protocol because of potential chemical shift artifact that may mimic an intact diaphragm. Iochum and colleagues [20] advocate a protocol that includes a single-shot fast spin-echo sequence that uses a short echo time and half-Fourier acquisition, as well as a fat-suppressed gadolinium-enhanced fast spoiled gradient-echo sequence. Regardless of the sequences, cardiac gating and respiratory gating are mandatory to limit motion artifacts [46].

Because of its fibromuscular composition, the normal diaphragm is demonstrated as a continuous hypointense band on T1 and spoiled gradient-echo images [20,45]. Signs of injury are comparable to those on CT [13,45,46]. Specifically, there typically is demonstration of abrupt discontinuity of the normal low-signal diaphragm that can be associated with herniation of abdominal fat or viscera into the chest [Fig. 19].

Its advantages not withstanding, the limitations of MR imaging in the setting of acute trauma, in addition to currently available MDCT technology and videoscopic techniques, have relegated it to ancillary status at the STC. In cases of suspected delayed presentation or equivocal diagnosis by CT, MR imaging can play a valuable role as a noninvasive means to assess diaphragm integrity.

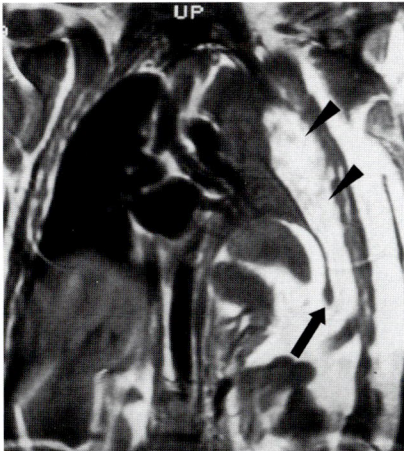

Fig. 19. MR imaging of blunt diaphragm rupture. Coronal T1-weighted spin echo image demonstrates omental herniation (*arrowheads*) through a large peripheral tear (*arrow*) at the lateral diaphragm insertion (Courtesy of Charles White, MD, Baltimore, MD.)

Other imaging modalities

Hepatobiliary scanning, barium studies, and fluoroscopy have been described as means to diagnose diaphragm injury [7,11,14,24]. Given current CT and MR imaging technology, none plays an active role in the acute management of the patient who has experienced blunt trauma or the diagnosis of diaphragm injuries.

Sonographic diagnosis of diaphragm injury has been described [47–49]. Sonographic signs of injury include herniation of viscera through the diaphragm [47,48], diaphragm disruption, diaphragm nonvisualization [48], and absent diaphragm excursion during the respiratory cycle [49]. Ultrasound had a positive predictive value of 88% among the eight patients who were described by Kim and colleagues [48]. Nevertheless, in addition to the congenital and developmental diaphragm variations that may limit other imaging examinations, ultrasound assessment of the diaphragm can be compromised by pulmonary aeration, gastric and colonic gas, subcutaneous emphysema, bandages and support appliances, abdominal pain, and obesity [48,50].

Given its limitations, ultrasound is not recommended as a primary tool for diagnosing diaphragm injuries. Yet, at many institutions, focused abdominal sonography for trauma (FAST) is an integral part of the initial diagnostic evaluation of patients who have experienced trauma. The FAST technique involves scanning the dependent peritoneal reflections for fluid (ie, hemoperitoneum) [50]. Several of these areas, including the right and left subphrenic spaces, are bounded by the diaphragm. At some institutions, other areas that are bordered by the diaphragm, including the pericardial sac [50] and the pleural spaces [49], are scanned. Recognition of sonographic signs of diaphragm injury while surveying these regions during the initial FAST examination may facilitate more rapid diagnosis of injury, although a normal appearance should not eliminate diaphragm injury as a potential diagnostic consideration.

Summary

Because of potentially devastating delayed complications, early diagnosis of diaphragm injuries should be an important goal for radiologists who are involved in the care of patients who have experienced trauma. Despite the increasing availability of MR imaging and advancing videoscopic techniques, routine chest radiography and helical thoracoabdominal CT usually lead to the correct diagnosis, as long as the radiologist maintains a high index of suspicion and recognizes the subtle signs of diaphragm injury.

References

[1] Mihos P, Potaris K, Gakidis J, et al. Traumatic rupture of the diaphragm: experience with 65 patients. Injury 2003;34:169–72.

[2] Barsness KA, Bensard DD, Ciesla D, et al. Blunt diaphragmatic rupture in children. J Trauma 2004;56(1):80–2.

[3] Rodriguez-Morales G, Rodriguez A, Shatney CH. Acute rupture of the diaphragm in blunt trauma: analysis of 60 patients. J Trauma 1986;26(5): 438–44.

[4] Tarver RD, Conces DJ, Cory DA, et al. Imaging the diaphragm and its disorders. J Thorac Imaging 1989;4(1):1–18.

[5] Shanmuganathan K, Killeen K, Mirvis SE, et al. Imaging of diaphragmatic injuries. J Thorac Imaging 2000;15(2):104–11.

[6] Koplewitz BZ, Ramos C, Manson DE, et al. Traumatic diaphragmatic injuries in infants and children: imaging findings. Pediatr Radiol 2000; 30:471–9.

[7] Patselas TN, Gallagher EG. The diagnostic dilemma of diaphragm injury. Am Surg 2002; 68(7):633–9.

[8] Athanassiadi K, Kalavrouziotis G, Athanassiou M, et al. Blunt diaphragmatic rupture. Eur J Cardiothorac Surg 1999;5:469–74.

[9] Haciibrahimoglu G, Solak O, Olcmen A, et al. Management of traumatic diaphragmatic rupture. Surg Today 2004;34:111–4.

[10] Reber PU, Schmied B, Seiler CA, et al. Missed diaphragmatic injuries and their long-term sequelae. J Trauma 1998;44(1):183–8.

[11] Kearney PA, Rouhana SW, Burney RE. Blunt rupture of the diaphragm: mechanism, diagno-

sis, and treatment. Ann Emerg Med 1989;18: 1326–30.

[12] Shatney CH, Sensaki K, Morgan L. The natural history of stab wounds of the diaphragm: implications for a new management scheme for patients with penetrating thoracoabdominal trauma. Am Surg 2003;69(6):508–13.

[13] Barbiera F, Nicastro N, Finazzo M, et al. The role of MRI in traumatic rupture of the diaphragm. Our experience in three cases and review of the literature. Radiol Med (Torino) 2003;105: 188–94.

[14] Saber WL, Moore EE, Hopeman AR, et al. Delayed presentation of traumatic diaphragmatic hernia. J Emerg Med 1986;4:1–7.

[15] Singh S, Kalan MMH, Moreyra CE, et al. Diaphragmatic rupture presenting 50 years after the traumatic event. J Trauma 2000;49(1):156–9.

[16] Kanowitz A, Marx JA. Delayed traumatic diaphragmatic hernia simulating acute tension pneumothorax. J Emerg Med 1989;7:619–22.

[17] Faul JL. Diaphragmatic rupture presenting forty years after injury. Injury 1998;29(6):479–80.

[18] Vermillion JM, Wilson EB, Smith RW. Traumatic diaphragmatic hernia presenting as a tension fecopneumothorax. Hernia 2001;5:158–60.

[19] Leppaniemi A, Haapiainen R. Occult diaphragmatic injuries caused by stab wounds. J Trauma 2003;55(4):646–50.

[20] Iochum S, Ludig T, Walter F, et al. Imaging of diaphragmatic injury: a diagnostic challenge? Radiographics 2002;22:S103–18.

[21] Mullins ME, Stein J, Saini SS, et al. Prevalence of incidental Bochdalek's hernia in a large adult population. AJR Am J Roentgenol 2001;177: 63–6.

[22] Caskey CI, Zerhouni EA, Fishman EK, et al. Aging of the diaphragm: a CT study. Radiology 1989; 171:385–9.

[23] Shackleton KL, Stewart ET, Taylor AJ. Traumatic diaphragmatic injuries: spectrum of radiographic findings. Radiographics 1998;18:49–59.

[24] Estrera AS, Landay MJ, McClelland RN. Blunt traumatic rupture of the right hemidiaphragm: experience in 12 patients. Ann Thorac Surg 1985; 39(6):525–30.

[25] Gelman R, Mirvis SE, Gens D. Diaphragmatic rupture due to blunt trauma: sensitivity of plain chest radiographs. AJR Am J Roentgenol 1991; 156:51–7.

[26] Shapiro MJ, Heiberg E, Durham RM, et al. The unreliability of CT scans and initial chest radiographs in evaluating blunt trauma induced diaphragmatic rupture. Clin Radiol 1996;51:27–30.

[27] Baron B, Daffner RH. Traumatic rupture of the right hemidiaphragm: diagnosis by chest radiography. Emerg Radiol 1994;1(5):231–5.

[28] Killeen KL, Mirvis SE, Shanmuganathan K. Helical CT of diaphragmatic rupture caused by blunt trauma. AJR Am J Roentgenol 1999;173: 1611–6.

[29] Leaman PL. Rupture of the right hemidiaphragm

[30] Matz A, Alis M, Charuzi I, et al. The role of laparoscopy in the diagnosis and treatment of missed diaphragmatic rupture. Surg Endosc 2000;14:537–9.

[31] McQuay Jr N, Britt LD. Laparoscopy in the evaluation of penetrating thoracoabdominal trauma. Am Surg 2003;69(9):788–91.

[32] Martinez M, Briz JE, Carillo EH. Video thoracoscopy expedites the diagnosis and treatment of penetrating diaphragmatic injuries. Surg Endosc 2001;15:28–32.

[33] Murray JG, Caoili E, Gruden JF, et al. Acute rupture of the diaphragm due to blunt trauma: diagnostic sensitivity and specificity of CT. AJR Am J Roentgenol 1996;166:1035–9.

[34] Shanmuganathan K, Mirvis SE, Chiu WC, et al. Penetrating torso trauma: triple-contrast helical CT in peritoneal violation and organ injury— a prospective study in 220 patients. Radiology 2004;231(3):775–84.

[35] Larici AR, Gotway MB, Litt HI, et al. Helical CT with sagittal and coronal reconstructions: accuracy for detection of diaphragmatic injury. AJR Am J Roentgenol 2002;179:451–7.

[36] Tresallet C, Menegaux F, Izzillo R, et al. Usefulness of CT reconstructed pictures for diaphragmatic rupture after blunt trauma. J Am Coll Surg 2004;198(4):666–7.

[37] Israel RS, Mayberry JC, Primack SL. Diaphragmatic rupture: use of helical CT scanning with multiplanar reformations. AJR Am J Roentgenol 1996;167:1201–3.

[38] Korolu M, Ernst RD, Oto A, et al. Traumatic diaphragmatic rupture: can oral contrast increase CT detectability? Emerg Radiol 2004;10:334–6.

[39] Rydberg J, Sandresegaran K, Tarver RD, et al. Routine isotropic scanning of the chest using a 40-channel CT scanner: value of reformatted coronal and sagittal images in showing anatomy and pathology. Presented at the 105th Annual Meeting of the American Roentgen Ray Society. New Orleans, Louisiana; May 15–20, 2005.

[40] Rydberg J, Sandresegaran K, Tann M, et al. Routine isotropic scanning of the abdomen and pelvis using a 40-channel CT scanner: value of reformatted coronal and sagittal images in showing pathology. Presented at the 105th Annual Meeting of the American Roentgen Ray Society. 2005.

[41] Worthy SA, Kang EY, Hartman TE, et al. Diaphragmatic rupture: CT findings in 11 patients. Radiology 1995;194(3):885–8.

[42] Nchimi A, Szapiro D, Ghaye B, et al. Helical CT of blunt diaphragmatic rupture. AJR Am J Roentgenol 2005;184:24–30.

[43] Bergin D, Ennis R, Keogh C, et al. The "dependent viscera" sign in CT diagnosis of blunt traumatic diaphragmatic rupture. AJR Am J Roentgenol 2001;177(5):1137–40.

[44] Leung JCM, Nance ML, Schwab CW, et al.

due to blunt trauma. Ann Emerg Med 1983; 12(6):351–7.

Thickening of the diaphragm: a new computed tomography sign of diaphragm injury. J Thorac Imaging 1999;14(2):126–9.

[45] Shanmuganathan K, Mirvis SE, White CS, et al. MR imaging evaluation of hemidiaphragms in acute blunt trauma: experience with 16 patients. AJR Am J Roentgenol 1996;167:397–402.

[46] Boulanger BR, Mirvis SE, Rodriquez A. Magnetic resonance imaging in traumatic diaphragmatic rupture: case reports. J Trauma 1992;32(1):89–93.

[47] Ammann AM, Brewer WH, Maull KI, et al. Traumatic rupture of the diaphragm: real-time sonography diagnosis. AJR Am J Roentgenol 1983;140:915–6.

[48] Kim HH, Shin YR, Kim KJ, et al. Blunt traumatic rupture of the diaphragm: sonography diagnosis. J Ultrasound Med 1997;16:593–8.

[49] Blaivas M, Brannam L, Hawkins M, et al. Bedside emergency ultrasonographic diagnosis of diaphragmatic rupture in blunt abdominal trauma. Am J Emerg Med 2004;22:601–4.

[50] McKenney KL. Ultrasound of blunt abdominal trauma. Radiol Clin North Am 1999;37(5): 879–93.

RADIOLOGIC
CLINICS
OF NORTH AMERICA

Radiol Clin N Am 44 (2006) 213–224

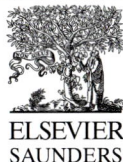

Chest Wall, Lung, and Pleural Space Trauma

Lisa A. Miller, MD*

- Pulmonary trauma
  Pulmonary contusion
  Pulmonary laceration
- Pleural trauma
  Pneumothorax
  Hemothorax
- Skeletal trauma
  Rib fractures

Sternal fracture
Sternoclavicular dislocation
Scapular fracture and scapulothoracic
  dissociation
- References

Thoracic injuries and related complications in the patient who has experienced blunt chest trauma have a mortality of 15.5% to 25% [1,2]. Once the hemodynamic stability of the patient is assured, a portable chest radiograph usually is obtained as the initial imaging evaluation. This examination is useful to screen for mediastinal hematoma, pneumothorax, pulmonary contusion, and osseous trauma. Chest radiographs frequently underestimate the severity and extent of chest trauma and, in some cases, fail to detect the presence of injury. CT is more sensitive than chest radiography in the detection of pulmonary, pleural, and osseous abnormalities in the patient who has chest trauma. With the advent of multidetector CT (MDCT), high-quality multiplanar reformations are obtained easily and add to the diagnostic capabilities of MDCT. This article reviews the radiographic and CT findings of chest wall, pleural, and pulmonary injuries that are seen in the patient who has blunt thoracic trauma.

Pulmonary trauma

Pulmonary contusion

Pulmonary contusions are the most common lung injury in blunt chest trauma, and occur in 17% to 75% of patients [3–7]. Injury to the walls of the alveoli and pulmonary vessels allows blood to leak into the alveolar and interstitial spaces [4,8]. Contusions can occur when the chest wall is compressed against the lung parenchyma at the time of impact, by shearing of the lung tissue across osseous structures, by rib fractures, or from previously formed pleural adhesions tearing the lung tissue [3]. The actual underlying mechanisms are complex: bursting effects at the gas–liquid interface of the alveolus, inertial effects of differential rates of acceleration between the low-density alveoli and heavier hilar structures, and implosion effects that are due to overexpansion of gas bubbles after passage of a pressure wave [9].

Department of Radiology, ShockTrauma Center, University of Maryland School of Medicine, Baltimore, MD, USA
* Department of Radiology, ShockTrauma Center, University of Maryland School of Medicine, 22 South Greene Street, Baltimore, MD 21201.
E-mail address: lmiller1@umm.edu

doi:10.1016/j.rcl.2005.10.006

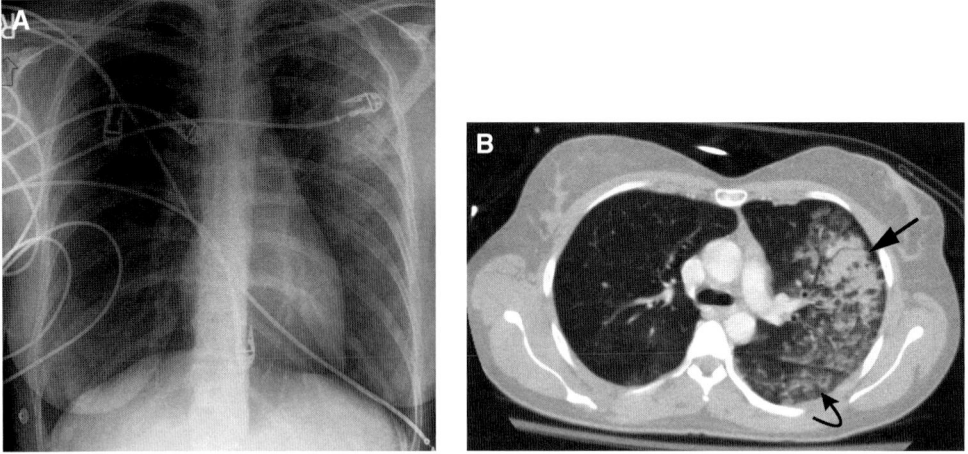

Fig. 1. Pulmonary contusion in a 26-year-old man who was involved in motor vehicle collision. (*A*) Admission chest radiograph demonstrates patchy air space disease throughout the lateral aspect of the left lung which represents pulmonary contusion. (*B*) Contrast-enhanced axial CT shows a moderate amount of pulmonary contusion throughout the lateral aspects of the left upper and lower lobes (*arrow*). A small amount of contusion, not visualized on the radiograph, is seen in the left lower lobe (*curved arrow*).

The complex pathophysiology of pulmonary contusion is reflected on the chest radiograph and CT as ill-defined, patchy, ground-glass density regions of opacification in mild contusion, to widespread areas of consolidation in more severe injury [Fig. 1]. Unlike other airspace diseases, such as pneumonia or aspiration pneumonitis, pulmonary contusions frequently are geographic or nonsegmental in location, and readily cross pleural fissures. Air bronchograms can be seen in pulmonary contusion, but may be absent if the bronchioles have filled with blood or fluid. On CT, sparing of 1 to 2 mm of subpleural lung may be present, especially in the pediatric population [10]. Typically, contusions are located adjacent to the osseous structures of the thoracic cage. An accompanying fracture often is absent, especially in the pediatric population in which there is greater musculoskeletal elasticity [11–13].

CT is clearly more sensitive in the detection of pulmonary injury compared with radiographs [Fig. 2] [5,14–18]. Radiographs may fail to detect the presence of pulmonary contusion for up to 6 hours after injury [13,19]. Using a canine model, Schild and colleagues [18] found that 38% of anesthetized dogs that sustained blunt chest trauma demonstrated a pulmonary contusion on chest radiograph, compared with 100% on CT. On radiography and CT, contusions may blossom in the first

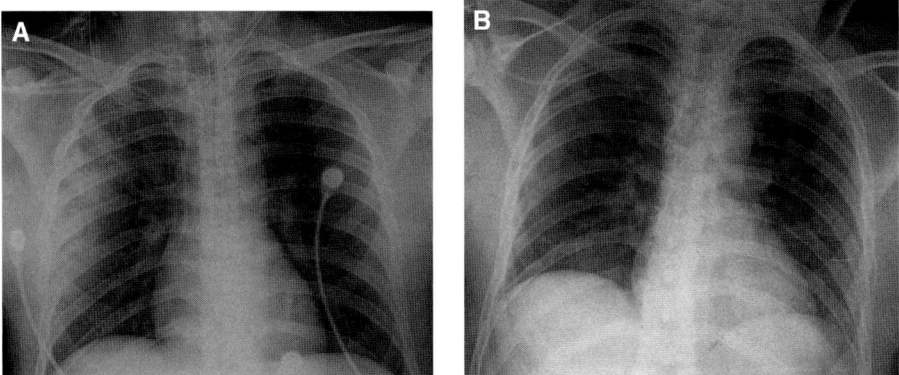

Fig. 2. Resolution of pulmonary contusion in a 19-year-old man who was involved in a motor vehicle collision. (*A*) Admission chest radiograph shows a moderate amount of pulmonary contusion seen throughout the lateral aspect of right lung. (*B*). Follow-up radiograph obtained 48 hours after admission shows complete resolution of right pulmonary contusion.

24 to 48 hours after injury as edema and hemorrhage accumulate in the parenchyma [8,20].

Clearance of contusions on radiographs typically is seen within 2 to 3 days, but complete resolution of severe contusion may take up to 14 days [13,21]. Persistence of airspace disease beyond this period suggests the development of pneumonia, aspiration, or adult respiratory distress syndrome (ARDS) [22].

Despite advances in diagnostic imaging and critical care medicine, pulmonary contusion carries a mortality of 10% to 25% [20,23], and is a predictor of the development of pneumonia and ARDS [20,24–26]. Recently, CT has been used to quantify the volume of contusion to predict clinical course and outcome. Miller and colleagues [20] used computer-generated measurements from three-dimensionally reconstructed admission chest CTs in 49 patients who had isolated pulmonary contusion from blunt trauma. They found that contusion volume was an independent predictor for the subsequent development of ARDS. In that study, patients who had greater than 20% contusion developed ARDS 82% of the time, compared with only 22% of patients who had less than 20% contusion.

Pulmonary laceration

A pulmonary laceration is formed when there is traumatic disruption of the lung architecture that results in formation of a cavity that is filled with air or blood [3]. Multiple mechanisms have been proposed to explain the formation of lacerations, including (1) rupture or shearing of lung tissue that is caused by sudden compression of the chest wall, (2) direct puncture of the lung by a fractured rib, (3) tearing of lung tissue adjacent to previously formed pleural adhesions, (4) rupture of alveoli due to high intra-alveolar pressures that are generated at time of trauma from closure of the glottis or sudden compression of a bronchus, and (5) compression of alveoli against the ribs or spine [3,7,13].

CT is superior to radiography in detecting lacerations [3,14,27]. On plain radiograph, pulmonary lacerations often are obscured initially because of the surrounding contusion, and become apparent over the next 48 to 72 hours as the contusion resolves. Lacerations are ovoid or round in shape because of the elastic recoil of the lung tissue, and have a thin 2- to 3-mm pseudomembrane of adjacent compressed lung parenchyma. The laceration may be lucent and filled with air, completely opacified as a result of blood accumulation within the cavity, or demonstrate an air–fluid level that is due to variable amounts of blood within the lumen [Fig. 3] [28]. The number and size of lacerations may range from a solitary laceration to numerous small lacerations that produce a "Swiss cheese" appearance [29].

Unlike pulmonary contusions, lacerations may take weeks to months to resolve. During this time, a laceration that is filled with clot may be misinterpreted as a lung nodule. Correlation with the history of recent trauma as well as serial chest radiographs that demonstrate the progressive decrease in size will help to make the correct diagnosis.

Complications of pulmonary lacerations are uncommon, and are evaluated best by CT. Potential complications include infection that leads to pulmonary abscess, enlargement of the laceration,

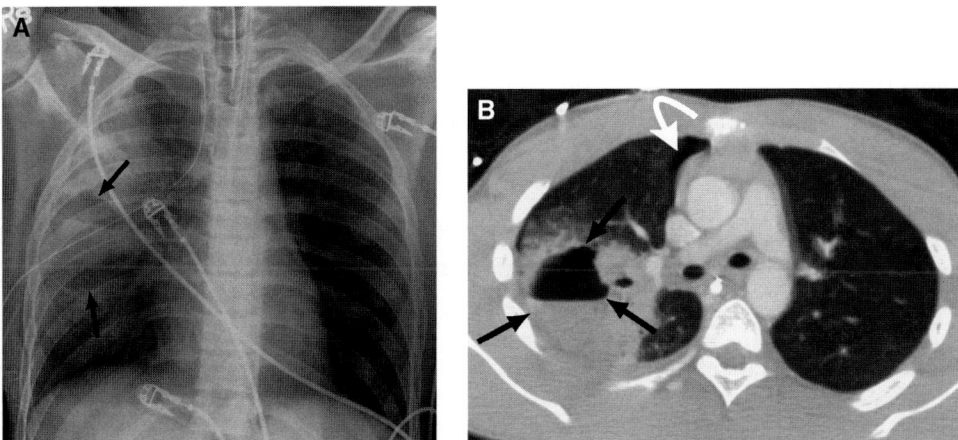

Fig. 3. Pulmonary laceration in a 24-year-old man who was admitted following a fall. (*A*) Chest radiograph demonstrates patchy contusion within the right upper lung. An ovoid lucency (*arrows*) within the area of contusion represents a pulmonary laceration. (*B*) CT image shows a large, right upper lobar pulmonary laceration (*arrows*) which is surrounded by extensive pulmonary contusion. An air–fluid level is seen within the laceration because of layering blood. A small right anterior pneumothorax also is seen (*curved arrow*).

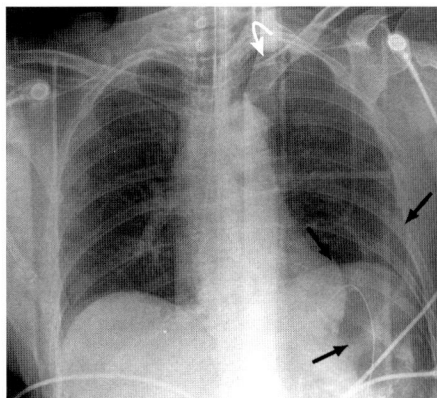

Fig. 4. Pneumothorax in a 30-year-old woman who was admitted following a fall. Supine chest radiograph demonstrates a moderate-sized left pneumothorax. The visceral pleura is visible at the lung apex (*curved arrow*). Hyperlucency (*arrows*) in the left lower chest is due to air within the nondependent portion of the anterior inferior pleural space.

or formation of a bronchopleural fistula. Superimposed infection with abscess formation within a pulmonary laceration is suggested clinically by fever and elevated white blood cell count. On CT, a pulmonary abscess appears as a thick-walled cavity with irregular inner margins, typically with an air–fluid level. Although most pulmonary abscesses respond to antibiotic therapy, CT-guided percutaneous drainage or endoscopic or surgical drainage may be required in as many as 11% to 21% of the patients who fail medical therapy [30,31].

Enlargement of a pulmonary laceration can occur if there is development of a ball–valve mechanism that allows expansion of the cavity from progressive influx of air [28]. The enlarging cavity can compress adjacent lung and cause impaired pulmonary function. The last complication, bronchopleural fistula, is formed when there is communication between a peripheral laceration, an adjacent bronchiole, and the pleural surface. This results in a persistent air leak that is unresponsive to chest tube placement.

Pleural trauma

Pneumothorax

Pneumothorax occurs in 30% to 40% of patients after blunt chest trauma. The most common cause is a rib fracture that lacerates the lung, but it also may be caused by rupture of a pre-existing bleb at the time of impact [32]. Clinical signs of pneumothorax can be subtle and difficult to elicit in a patient who has multisystem trauma. Detection of even a small, asymptomatic pneumothorax is important because up to one third can develop into a tension pneumothorax with potential cardio-

pulmonary decompensation [32–34]. A small pneumothorax also can enlarge during mechanical ventilation or general anesthesia [33,35].

CT is more sensitive than radiography for detecting pneumothorax. Ten to 50% of pneumothoraces that are seen on CT are not evident on the supine radiograph or detected clinically [3,14,33,36]. Radiographic signs of a pneumothorax can be subtle, and the appearance differs based on the patient position at the time that the radiograph was performed. In the supine position, air collects within the anterior costophrenic sulcus, which extends from the seventh costal cartilage to the eleventh rib at the midaxillary line [37,38]. This appears radiographically as abnormal lucency in the lower chest or upper abdomen, an abnormally wide and deep costophrenic sulcus (the "deep sulcus" sign), a sharply outlined cardiac or diaphragmatic border, depression of the hemidiaphragm, or as a "double diaphragm" sign that is seen when air outlines the dome and anterior insertion of the diaphragm [Fig. 4]. The tendency of air to collect in the anterior costophrenic sulcus in the supine position can be used to advantage in the detection of even a small pneumothorax when evaluating the abdominal CT, because this region typically is included on the upper abdominal images [32,33,36].

On the upright chest radiograph, a pneumothorax is seen as a thin, sharply defined line that represents the visceral pleura. No lung markings are seen beyond this line. Large bullae, skin folds, bedding, overlying tubes and catheters, and the medial scapular border can mimic the appearance of a pneumothorax. An upright expiratory chest radiograph or CT can assist in making the correct diagnosis in these cases.

Generally, patients who are symptomatic or who demonstrate a greater than 20% pneumothorax are

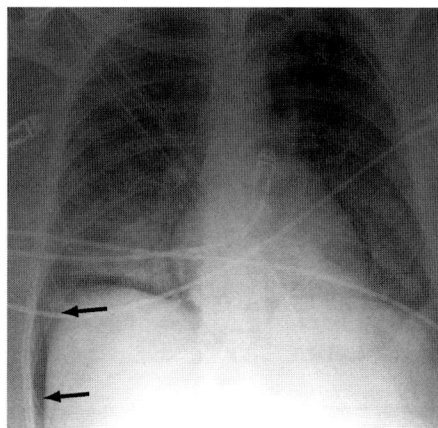

Fig. 5. Inferior pneumothorax. Supine chest radiograph shows a "deep sulcus" sign (*arrows*) within the right costophrenic angle from an inferior pneumothorax.

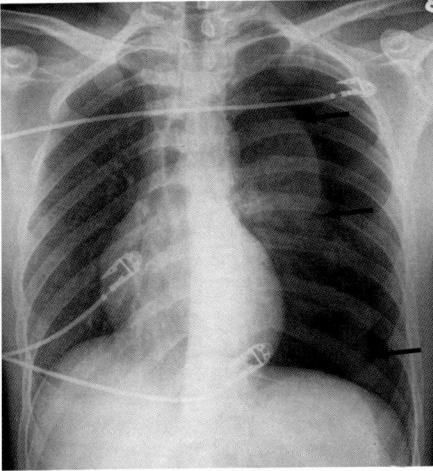

Fig. 6. Tension pneumothorax in a 22-year-old victim of assault. Chest radiograph demonstrates a left-sided tension pneumothorax. The left lung is compressed towards the hilum (*arrows*) and the mediastinum is shifted to the right. Widening of the intercostal spaces on the left and a sharply outlined, depressed left hemidiaphragm also is seen.

considered for chest tube placement [39,40]. Prophylactic insertion of a chest tube also may be considered in a patient who has a small, asymptomatic pneumothorax who will be placed on a mechanical ventilator or who will be undergoing a lengthy operative procedure.

A tension pneumothorax is a life-threatening condition in which air progressively accumulates in the pleural space as the result of a one-way valve mechanism, and causes high ipsilateral intrathoracic pressures. This can cause compression of the vena cava, which impairs venous return and decreases cardiac output. Radiographic signs of a ten-

sion pneumothorax include shift of the mediastinum to the contralateral side, abnormal lucency of the hemithorax with a collapsed lung in the hilar region, depression of the ipsilateral hemidiaphragm, and widening of the intercostal spaces [Figs. 5 and 6]. Prompt evacuation with needle aspiration or placement of a chest tube can be life saving. Tracheobronchial injury, bronchopleural fistula, or malpositioning of the chest tube should be considered if a pneumothorax does not respond completely to treatment [Fig. 7].

The phenomenon of re-expansion pulmonary edema can occur after placement of a chest tube. This syndrome develops almost immediately after resolution of the pneumothorax and is seen radiographically by unilateral or bilateral pulmonary edema [41–43]. The syndrome is more common in patients who are 20 to 50 years of age. A positive correlation exists between the development of this condition and the size of the pneumothorax as well as with the rapidity with which the pneumothorax is treated. The mortality rate of re-expansion pulmonary edema can be as high as 20%.

Hemothorax

Hemothorax is seen is approximately 50% of patients who sustain blunt chest trauma [44]. Bleeding into the pleural space can originate from injury to the pleura, chest wall, lung, diaphragm, or mediastinum. The appearance of hemothorax on a chest radiograph depends on the amount of blood that has collected in the pleural space and patient position. A small hemothorax may be undetected on a supine or upright chest radiograph, but a decubitus film can detect as little as 5 mL of fluid in the pleural space [45]. When the size of a hemothorax reaches approximately 200 mL, an upright chest radiograph demonstrates

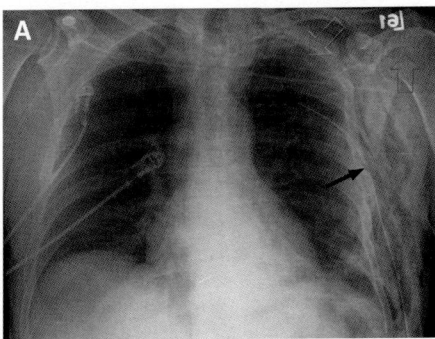

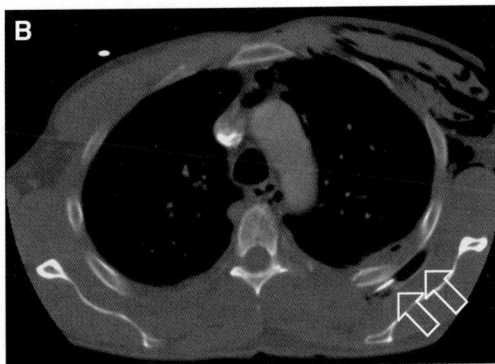

Fig. 7. Malpositioned chest tube. (*A*) Chest radiograph shows a small left pneumothorax (*large open arrows*), despite placement of a left-sided chest tube. The side hole of the chest tube lies within the chest wall (*black arrow*). (*B*) CT image shows placement of chest tube within the left thoracic wall (*arrows*). Left chest wall subcutaneous emphysema and a small amount of pneumomediastinum also are seen.

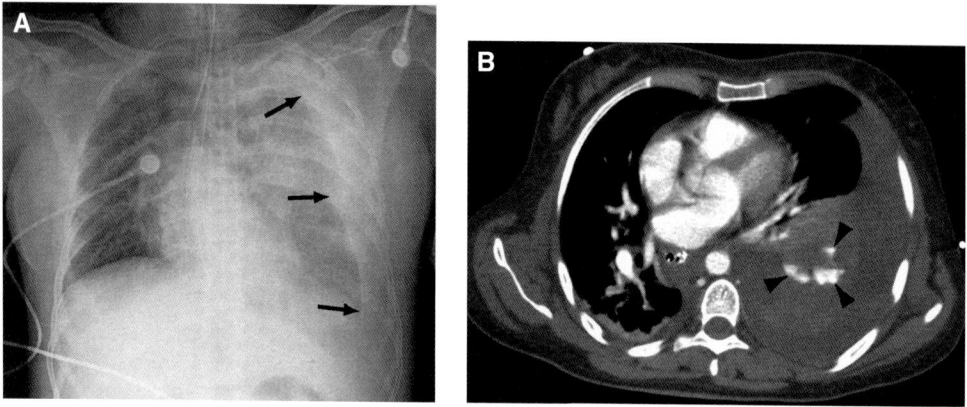

Fig. 8. Hemothorax in a 22-year-old patient who was involved in a motor vehicle collision. (*A*) Chest radiograph shows increased opacity of entire left hemithorax, a rim of increased density surrounding left lung (*arrows*), and shift of mediastinum to right as the result of a large left hemothorax. (*B*) CT image shows a large left hemothorax with shift of mediastinum to right. Multiple foci of high attenuation areas that are seen within compressed left lung indicate active bleeding (*arrowheads*) from the lung parenchyma. Transcatheter embolization controlled active bleeding.

blunting of the costophrenic angle. With progressive increase in size, a "meniscus" sign will be seen: a concave upward sloping of fluid in the costophrenic angle. In contrast, a straight air–fluid level on the upright chest radiograph indicates a hemopneumothorax. On a supine chest radiograph, a hemothorax layers in the dependent, posterior portion of the pleural space, and causes increased density of the entire hemithorax; this is appreciated best with a unilateral hemothorax. A hemothorax also may compress the lateral lung parenchyma, which is seen on the supine radiograph as a rim of density surrounding the lateral aspect and apex of the lung [Fig. 8]. A large hemothorax can opacify the hemithorax completely, and cause contralateral shift of the mediastinum as the result of mass effect.

CT is highly sensitivity in detecting a small hemothorax. In addition, the Hounsfield unit (HU) measurement of fluid in the pleural space can be used to identify the origin of the fluid. Hemothorax measures 35 to 70 HU, depending on the amount of clot present [28]. In contrast, a sympathetic serous pleural effusion, which can be seen in patients who have splenic, hepatic, or pancreatic injuries, typically measures less than 15 HU. Other causes of pleural effusion in the patient who has experienced trauma include chylothorax from injury to the thoracic duct [46]; the uncommon bilious effusion, which is caused by formation of a biliopleural fistula in the patient who has injury to the liver and the right hemidiaphragm [44,47]; and the rare urinothorax, which is caused by formation of a renopleural fistula or by way of lymphatic drainage across an intact diaphragm [48,49]. Differentiating among these last four entities is

difficult on CT, and usually requires thoracentesis for accurate diagnosis.

Clues to the source of the bleeding into the pleural space can be gleaned from the appearance on imaging studies. A hemothorax that is due to bleeding from venous origin typically is self-limiting because of the tamponade effect from the lung parenchyma and usually does not increase in size. Arterial bleeding, such as from an intercostal artery, can be inferred by progression of size on radiography or CT. CT also may demonstrate active bleeding within the hemothorax [Fig. 9]. This is seen as a focus of high density, typically within 10 HU of the nearest large artery. If delayed images

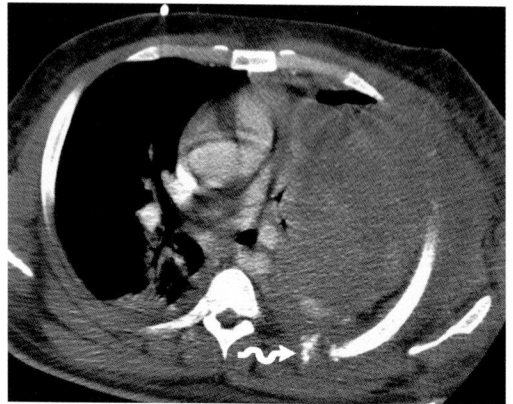

Fig. 9. Active bleeding from intercostal artery. CT shows a large left extrapleural hematoma displacing the heart to the right. Active bleeding (*arrow*) arises from the chest wall from torn intercostal artery.

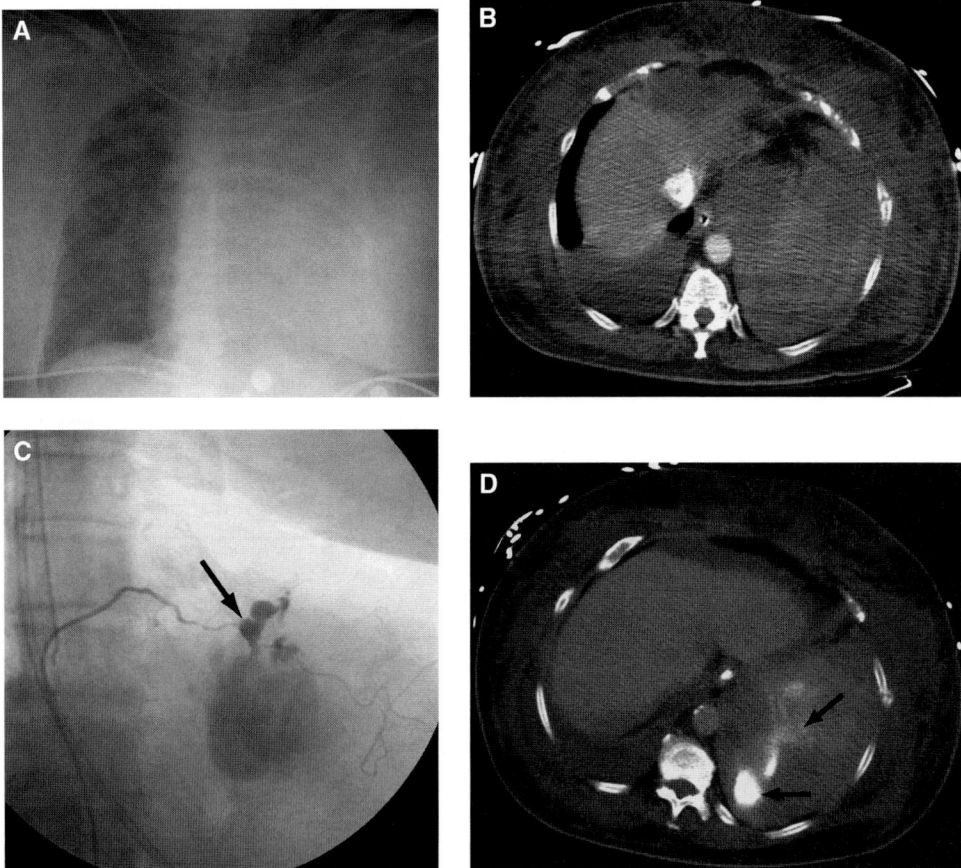

Fig. 10. Tension hemothorax in a 45-year-old woman who was involved in a motorcycle collision. (*A*) Chest radiograph shows a large left hemothorax with complete opacification of left hemithorax, mild shift of the mediastinum to right, and mild widening of intercostal spaces. Extensive pulmonary contusion is seen in the right lung. (*B*) CT image shows mixed attenuation hemothorax within left pleural space. (*C*) Arteriography of left intercostal artery demonstrates a large amount of active bleeding (*arrow*). Embolization was performed to control hemorrhage. (*D*) Axial CT image obtained 48 hours following angiography and embolization shows high attenuation area in pleural space representing extravasated intravenous contrast material (*arrows*) during recent angiography. Extravasated contrast material is much higher in attenuation compared with the attenuation of contrast material within the aorta.

are performed, the focus persists as a region of high density and may increase in size. Multiplanar CT reformatted images can be especially useful to demonstrate the site of active bleeding [Fig. 10].

Skeletal trauma

Rib fractures

Rib fractures are the most common skeletal injury in blunt chest trauma, and occur in approximately 50% of patients [50,51]. Fractures of the first through third ribs are a marker for high-velocity trauma because they are mostly protected by the clavicle, scapula, and upper chest wall musculature [52]. Although upper rib fractures are not asso-

ciated with an increased incidence of traumatic aortic injury [53,54], injury to the brachial plexus and subclavian vessels can be seen in 3% to 15% of patients who have upper rib fractures [52]. Fractures of the eighth to eleventh ribs should prompt careful evaluation for upper abdominal organ injuries. Patients who have right-sided rib fractures at these levels have a 19% to 56% probability of liver injury, whereas those who have left-sided fractures have a 22% to 28% probability of splenic injury [55,56]. In the elderly population, overall morbidity and mortality increases with an increasing number of ribs fractured [57–59].

A flail chest occurs when there are at least two fracture sites on each of three or more consecutive

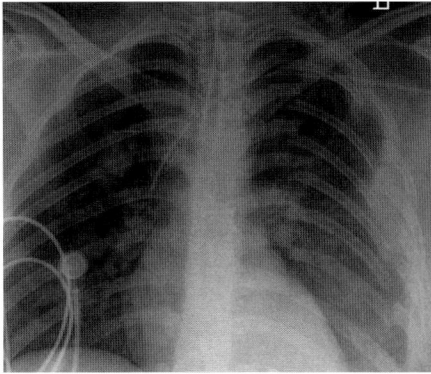

Fig. 11. Frontal chest radiograph of a 25-year-old woman who was involved in motor vehicle collision shows fractures at two locations in the left posterior third through to the eighth ribs. Patient required treatment for a flail chest.

ribs [Fig. 11]. This condition is seen in 5% to 13% of patients who have chest wall trauma [60]. In flail chest, a free-floating segment of ribs results, and causes focal chest wall instability. The paradoxic motion of the fracture segment alters normal pulmonary dynamics and promotes atelectasis, stasis of secretions, and pneumonia [28,61]; it may require early intubation for ventilatory support [62].

Traumatic pulmonary herniation can occur in patients who sustain severe blunt chest injury. In this rare entity, pleural-covered lung extrudes through a defect in the thoracic wall, which is caused by traumatic disruption of the ribs and chest wall musculature [Fig. 12] [63]. This injury usually involves the anterior chest wall of a patient who has sustained severe blunt chest injury [64], but also can be seen at sites of previous, percutaneously placed chest tubes [65]. The diagnosis is made readily by CT, which demonstrates the extent of chest wall injury and amount of herniated lung. Smaller herniations may be managed nonoperatively. Larger chest wall defects mandate urgent surgical repair to avoid ventilatory compromise and to prevent strangulation of lung parenchyma [64,65].

Sternal fracture

Sternal fractures occur in approximately 3% to 8% of patients who experience blunt chest trauma, and are seen most commonly in deceleration injuries or direct blows to the anterior chest wall [66].

Sternal fractures typically occur at the body or manubrium. Although a sternal fracture can be detected on a true lateral chest radiograph, in patients who have sustained trauma, the diagnosis is made more often on CT. A fracture that is oriented in the axial plane may be missed on standard CT images, and multiplanar reconstructed

images in the sagittal and coronal planes may be needed to detect the fracture.

Historically, a sternal fracture has been considered a marker for possible underlying cardiac injury, such as myocardial contusion. Recently, this view was challenged by several studies that showed essentially no correlation between a minimally displaced sternal fracture and cardiac injury [67,68]. A sternal fracture that is displaced significantly may warrant evaluation for potential cardiac trauma [69].

Varying amounts of anterior mediastinal hemorrhage are seen almost always with a sternal fracture. This isolated anterior mediastinal blood should not be confused with periaortic hemorrhage that is associated with traumatic aortic injury [66,70–73].

Sternoclavicular dislocation

Sternoclavicular dislocation accounts for 1% to 3% of all types of dislocations [74–76]. Anterior sternoclavicular dislocation is more common, and typically is evident on clinical examination by palpation and inspection. Although anterior dislocations typically have a benign course, they are a marker for high-energy trauma. Up to two thirds of patients have other chest injuries, such as pneumothorax, hemothorax, rib fractures, or pulmonary contusion [76–78]. Anterior dislocations usually are treated with conscious sedation and closed reduction.

A posterior sternoclavicular dislocation can be a cause of serious morbidity, but often it is clinically and radiographically occult. Often, it is detected initially on chest CT that is done for evaluation of other chest trauma. A posterior dislocation can result directly from anterior chest wall trauma or indirectly from force applied to the ipsilateral posterior shoulder, which drives the lateral

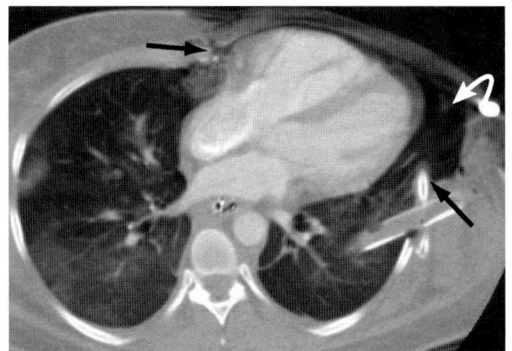

Fig. 12. Chest wall hernia in a 39-year-old woman who was involved in a motorcycle collision. There is a large soft tissue and bony defect (*arrows*) of the anterior left chest with herniation of heart and lung (*curved arrow*). Scattered areas of pulmonary contusion are present bilaterally. Thoracotomy was performed to repair chest wall hernia.

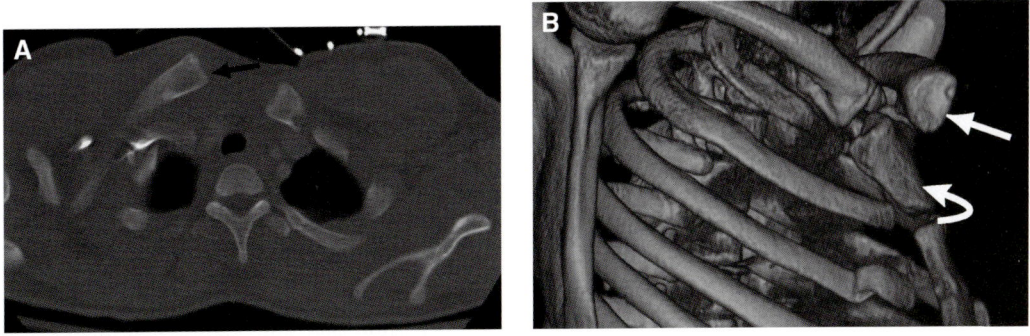

Fig. 13. Sternoclavicular joint dislocation in a 21-year-old man who was admitted following a motor vehicle collision. (*A*) CT image shows anterior subluxation of the right clavicular head (*arrow*) with associated soft tissue deformity of anterior chest wall. (*B*) Three-dimensional oblique image of sternoclavicular joints shows anterior subluxation of left clavicular head (*arrow*) in relation to manubrium (*curved arrow*).

end of the clavicle anteriorly and causes the medial clavicle to dislocate posteriorly [Fig. 13]. Impingement of the underlying mediastinal vessels; nerves, such as the brachial plexus and recurrent laryngeal nerve; esophagus; and trachea can occur by the dis-

placed clavicle, and may require additional evaluation with transcatheter angiography or endoscopy [78–82]. Open reduction by the orthopedic surgeon with assistance of a cardiothoracic surgeon may be required to treat this injury safely.

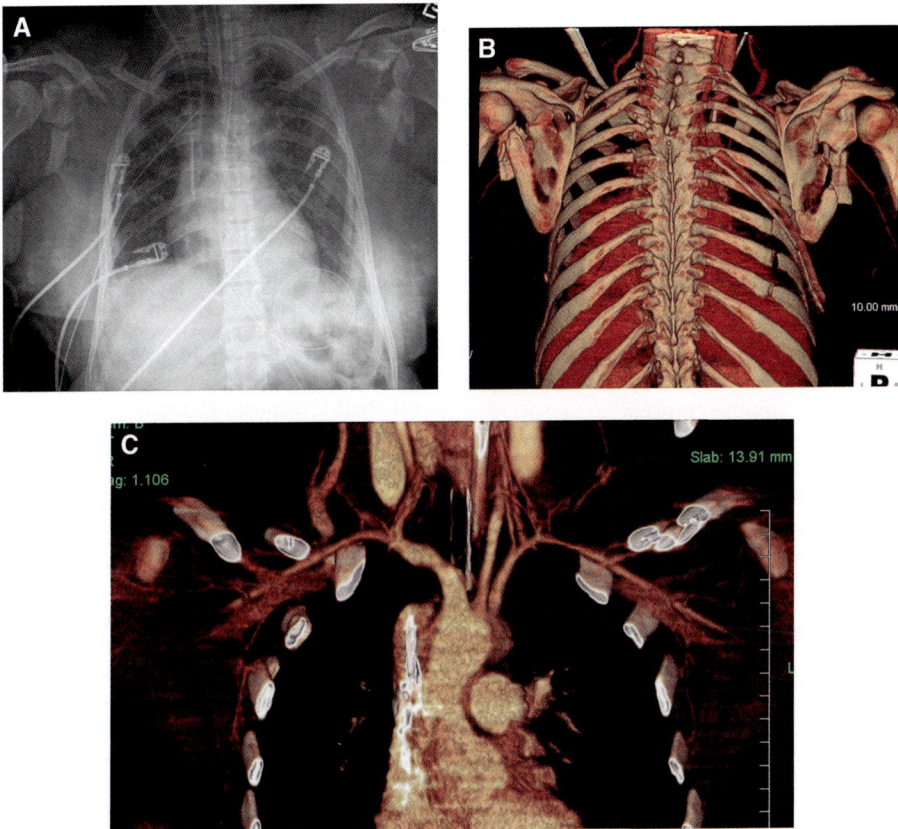

Fig. 14. Thoracoscapular dissociation. (*A*) Admission chest radiograph in a patient who sustained blunt trauma shows highly comminuted clavicle and scapular fractures with marked lateral displacement of both scapulae. (*B*) Three-dimensional rendering of injury from posterior view. (*C*) CT angiography showing occlusion of both axillary arteries.

Scapular fracture and scapulothoracic dissociation

Scapular fractures indicate high-force trauma, because the scapula is enveloped and protected by the large muscle masses of the posterior thorax. Isolated fractures are rare. Typically, scapular fractures are seen in a patient who has a severe chest trauma as the result of a motor vehicle accident or a fall [83–85]. Although most scapular fractures are treated nonoperatively, any fracture with involvement of the glenoid or scapular neck requires open reduction and internal fixation to allow normal scapulothoracic motion and stabilization of the shoulder girdle [86].

Scapulothoracic dissociation (STD) is a rare injury; only 62 cases have been described in the medical literature [87]. It was described originally by Oreck and colleagues [88] in 1984 as a "closed forequarter amputation with complete disruption of the musculotendinous attachments to the chest wall, with resultant lateral displacement of the scapula." This injury is seen most commonly in victims of a motorcycle collision in which there is violent distraction and rotation of the shoulder. Clinically, there is massive swelling in the region of the shoulder girdle. The upper extremity may be flaccid and pulseless as the result of associated subclavian or axillary artery and brachial plexus injury or avulsion [Fig. 14]. Radiographic signs of this injury include lateral scapular displacement in association with a clavicle fracture and acromioclavicular or sternoclavicular dissociation [88,89], presence of an apicolateral pleural cap, and axillary or superior mediastinal hematoma [90]. Multiple fractures of the upper extremity are common. STD can be difficult to detect on radiograph, and the scapulothoracic ratio was created to assist in the detection of this injury. The ratio is obtained by measuring the distance from the spinous process to a specific point on each scapula, such as the medial scapular border. Ratios that range from 1.07 [91] to 1.15 [90] have been described, and should raise suspicion of an STD in the patient who has sustained blunt chest trauma.

References

[1] Allen GS, Coates NE. Pulmonary contusion: a collective review. Am Surg 1996;62(11):895–900.

[2] Shorr RM, Crittenden M, Indeck M, et al. Blunt thoracic trauma. Analysis of 515 patients. Ann Surg 1987;206:200–5.

[3] Wagner RB, Crawford Jr WO, Schimpf PP. Classification of parenchymal injuries to the lung. Radiology 1988;167:77–82.

[4] Greene R. Lung alterations in thoracic trauma. J Thorac Imaging 1987;2:1–11.

[5] Toombs BD, Sandler CM, Lester RG. Computed tomography of chest trauma. Radiology 1981; 140:733–8.

[6] Webb WR. Thoracic trauma. Surg Clin North Am 1974;54:1179–92.

[7] Cohn SM. Pulmonary contusion: review of the clinical entity. J Trauma 1997;42:973–9.

[8] Fulton RL, Peter ET. The progressive nature of pulmonary contusion. Surgery 1970;67:499–506.

[9] Clemedson CJ. Blast injury. Physiol Rev 1956;36: 336–54.

[10] Donnelly LF, Klosterman LA. Subpleural sparing: a CT finding of lung contusion in children. Radiology 1997;204:385–7.

[11] Nakayama DK, Ramenofsky ML, Rowe MI. Chest injuries in childhood. Ann Surg 1989;210:770–5.

[12] Roux P, Fisher RM. Chest injuries in children: an analysis of 100 cases of blunt chest trauma from motor vehicle accidents. J Pediatr Surg 1992; 27:551–5.

[13] Goodman LR, Putman CE. The SICU chest radiograph after massive blunt trauma. Radiol Clin North Am 1981;19:111–23.

[14] Trupka A, Waydhas C, Hallfeldt KK, et al. Value of thoracic computed tomography in the first assessment of severely injured patients with blunt chest trauma: results of a prospective study. J Trauma 1997;43:405–11.

[15] Sivit CJ, Taylor GA, Eichelberger MR. Chest injury in children with blunt chest trauma: evaluation with CT. Radiology 1989;171:815–8.

[16] Karaaslan T, Meuli R, Androux R, et al. Traumatic chest lesions in patients with severe head trauma: a comparative study with computed tomography and conventional chest roentgenograms. J Trauma 1995;39:1081–6.

[17] Tocino I, Miller MH. Computed tomography in blunt chest trauma. J Thorac Imaging 1987;2: 45–9.

[18] Schild HH, Strunk H, Weber N, et al. Pulmonary contusion: CT vs plain radiograms. J Comput Assist Tomogr 1989;13:417–20.

[19] Blair E, Topuzlu C, Davis JH. Delayed or missed diagnosis in blunt chest trauma. J Trauma 1971; 11:129–45.

[20] Miller PR, Croce MA, Bec TK, et al. ARDS after pulmonary contusion: accurate measurement of contusion volume identifies high-risk patients. J Trauma 2001;51:223–30.

[21] Wiot JF. The radiologic manifestations of blunt chest trauma. JAMA 1975;231:500–3.

[22] Allen GS, Cox Jr CS. Pulmonary contusion in children: diagnosis and management. South Med J 1998;91:1099–106.

[23] Hoff SJ, Shotts SD, Eddy VA, et al. Outcome of isolated pulmonary contusion in blunt trauma patients. Am Surg 1994;60:138–42.

[24] Antonelli M, Moro ML, Capelli O, et al. Risk factors for early onset pneumonia in trauma patients. Chest 1994;105:224–8.

[25] Croce MA, Fabian TC, Davis KA, et al. Early and late acute respiratory distress syndrome:

two distinct clinical entities. J Trauma 1999;46:361–8.

[26] Ware LB, Matthay MA. The acute respiratory distress syndrome. N Engl J Med 2000;342:1334–49.

[27] Shin MS, Ho KJ. Computed tomography evaluation of posttraumatic pulmonary pseudocysts. Clin Imaging 1993;17:189–92.

[28] Shanmuganathan K, Mirvis SE. Imaging diagnosis of nonaortic thoracic trauma. Radiol Clin North Am 1999;37:533–51.

[29] Mirvis SE. Diagnostic imaging of acute thoracic injury. Semin Ultrasound CT MR 2004;25(2):156–79.

[30] Erasmus JJ, McAdams HP, Rossi S, et al. Percutaneous management of intrapulmonary air and fluid collections. Radiol Clin North Am 2000;38:385–93.

[31] Herth F, Ernst A, Becker HD. Endoscopic drainage of lung abscesses: technique and outcome. Chest 2005;127(4):1378–81.

[32] Tocino IM, Miller MH, Fairfax WR. Distribution of pneumothorax in the supine and semi recumbent critically ill adult. AJR Am J Roentgenol 1985;144:901–5.

[33] Wall SD, Federle MP, Jeffrey RB, et al. CT diagnosis of unsuspected pneumothorax after blunt trauma. AJR Am J Roentgenol 1983;141:919–21.

[34] Rhea JT, Novelline RA, Lawrason J, et al. The frequency and significance of thoracic injuries detected on abdominal CT scans in multiple trauma patients. J Trauma 1989;29:502–9.

[35] Enderson BL, Abdalla R, Frame SB, et al. Tube thoracostomy for occult pneumothorax: a prospective randomized study of its use. J Trauma 1993;35:726–9.

[36] Neff MA, Monk JS, Peters K, et al. Detection of occult pneumothoraces on abdominal computed tomographic scans in trauma patients. J Trauma 2000;49:281–5.

[37] Gordon R. The deep sulcus sign. Radiology 1980;136:25–7.

[38] Rhea JT, van Sonnenberg E, McLoud TC. Basilar pneumothorax in the supine adult. Radiology 1979;133:593–5.

[39] Weissberg D, Refaely Y. Pneumothorax: experience with 1,199 patients. Chest 2001;119(4):1292–3.

[40] Pacanowski JP, Waack ML, Daley BJ, et al. Is routine roentgenography needed after closed tube thoracostomy removal? J Trauma 2000;48(4):684–8.

[41] Gordon AH, Grant GP, Kaul SK. Reexpansion pulmonary edema after resolution of tension pneumothorax in the contralateral lung of a previously lung injured patient. J Clin Anesth 2004;16:289–92.

[42] Matsuura Y, Nomimura T, Murakami H, et al. Clinical analysis of reexpansion pulmonary edema. Chest 1991;100:1562–6.

[43] Smolle-Juettner FM, Prause G, Ratzenhofer B, et al. The importance of early detection and therapy of reexpansion pulmonary edema. Thorac Cardiovasc Surg 1991;39:162–6.

[44] Stark P. Pleura. In: Stark P, editor. Radiology of thoracic trauma. Boston: Andover Medical Publishers; 1993. p. 54–72.

[45] McLoud T. The pleura. In: Mcloud TC, editor. Thoracic radiology: the requisites. St. Louis (MO): Mosby, Inc.; 1998. p. 483–513.

[46] Ikonomidis JS, Boulanger BR, Brenneman FD. Chylothoax after blunt chest trauma: a report of 2 cases. Can J Surg 1997;40:135–8.

[47] Frankin DC, Mathai J. Biliary pleural fistula: a complication of hepatic trauma. J Trauma 1980;20:256–8.

[48] Parvathy U, Saldanha R, Balakrishnan K. Blunt abdominal trauma resulting in urinothorax from a missed ureteropelvic junction avulsion: case report. J Trauma 2003;54(1):187–9.

[49] Lahiry SK, Alkhafaji AH, Brown AL. Urinothorax following blunt trauma to the kidney. J Trauma 1978;18:608–10.

[50] Deluca SA, Rhea JT, O'Malley TO. Radiographic evaluation of rib fractures. AJR Am J Roentgenol 1982;138:91–2.

[51] Tocino I, Miller MH. Computed tomography in blunt chest trauma. J Thorac Imaging 1987;2:45–59.

[52] Fermanis GG, Deane SA, Fitzgerald PM. The significance of first and second rib fractures. Aust N Z J Surg 1985;55:383–6.

[53] Fisher RG, Ward BE, Ben-Menachem Y, et al. Arteriography and the fractured first rib: too much for too little? AJR Am J Roentgenol 1982;138:1059–62.

[54] Lee J, Harris Jr JH, Duke Jr JH, et al. Noncorrelation between thoracic skeletal injuries and acute traumatic aortic tear. J Trauma 1997;43:400–4.

[55] Shweiki E, Klena J, Wood GC, et al. Assessing the true risk of abdominal solid organ injury in hospitalized rib fracture patients. J Trauma 2001;50:684–8.

[56] Clark GC, Schecter WP, Trunkey DD. Variables affecting outcome in blunt chest trauma: flail chest vs pulmonary contusion. J Trauma 1998;28:298–304.

[57] Stawicki SP, Grossman MD, Hoey BA, et al. Rib fractures in the elderly: a marker of injury severity. J Am Geriatr Soc 2004;52:805–8.

[58] Sirmali M, Turut H, Topcu S, et al. A comprehensive analysis of traumatic rib fractures: morbidity, mortality and management. Eur J Cardiothorac Surg 2003;24:133–8.

[59] Bergeron E, Lavoie A, Clas D, et al. Elderly trauma patients with rib fractures are at greater risk of death and pneumonia. J Trauma 2003;54:478–85.

[60] LoCicero III J, Mattox KL. Epidemiology of chest trauma. Surg Clin North Am 1989;69(1):15–9.

[61] Wanek S, Mayberry JC. Blunt thoracic trauma: flail chest, pulmonary contusion, and blast injury. Crit Care Clin 2004;20:71–81.

[62] Velmahos GS, Vassiliu P, Chan LS, et al. Influence of flail chest on outcome among patients with severe thoracic cage trauma. Int Surg 2002;87:240–4.

[63] Taylor DA, Jacobson HG. Post-traumatic herniation of the lung. AJR Am J Roentgen 1962;87: 896–9.

[64] Lang-Lazdunski L, Bonnet PM, Pons F, et al. Traumatic extrathoracic lung herniation. Ann Thorac Surg 2002;74:927–9.

[65] Sadler MA, Sharpiro RS, Wagreich J, et al. CT diagnosis of acquired intercostal lung herniation. Clin Imag 1997;21:104–6.

[66] Athanassiadi K, Gerazounis M, Moustardas M, et al. Sternal fractures: retrospective analysis of 100 cases. World J Surg 2002;26:1243–6.

[67] Chiu WC, D'Amelio LF, Hammond JS. Sternal fractures in blunt chest trauma: a practical algorithm for management. Am J Emerg Med 1997; 15:252–5.

[68] Bu'Lock FA, Prothero A, Shaw C, et al. Cardiac involvement in seatbelt-related and direct sternal trauma: a prospective study and management implications. Eur Heart J 1994;15:1621–7.

[69] vonGarrel T, Ince A, Junge A, et al. The sternal fracture: radiographic analysis of 200 fractures with special reference to concomitant injuries. J Trauma 2004;57:837–44.

[70] Sturm JT, Luxenberg MG, Moudry BM, et al. Does sternal fracture increase the risk for aortic rupture? Ann Thorac Surg 1989;48:697–8.

[71] Hills MW, Delprado AM, Deane SA. Sternal fractures: associated injuries and management. J Trauma 1993;35:55–60.

[72] Brookes JG, Dunn RJ, Rogers IR. Sternal fractures: a retrospective analysis of 272 cases. J Trauma 1993;35:46–54.

[73] Harley DP, Mena I. Cardiac and vascular sequelae of sternal fractures. J Trauma 1986;26: 553–5.

[74] Nettles JL, Linscheid RL. Sternoclavicular dislocations. J Trauma 1968;8:158–64.

[75] Cope R. Dislocations of the sternoclavicular joint. Skeletal Radiol 1993;22:233–8.

[76] Stark P, editor. Chest cage injuries. Radiology of thoracic trauma. Boston: Andover Medical Publishers; 1993. p. 7–16.

[77] deJong KP, Sukul DM. Anterior sternoclavicular dislocation: a long term follow-up study. J Orthop Trauma 1990;4:420–3.

[78] Rockwood CA, Wirth MA. Injuries to the sternoclavicular joints. In: Rockwood CA, Green DP, Bucholtz RW, editors. Fractures in adults. 5th edition. Philadelphia: Lippincott-Raven; 2001. p. 1245–92.

[79] Ono K, Inagawa H, Kiyota K, et al. Posterior dislocation of the sternoclavicular joint with obstruction of the innominate vein: case report. J Trauma 1998;44(2):381–3.

[80] Mirza AH, Alam K, Ali A. Posterior sternoclavicular dislocation in a rugby player as a cause of silent vascular compromise: a case report. Br J Sports Med 2005;39(5):28.

[81] Buckerfield CT, Castle ME. Acute traumatic retrosternal dislocation of the clavicle. J Bone Joint Surg Am 1984;66:379–85.

[82] Jougon JB, Lepront DJ, Dromer CEH. Posterior dislocation of the sternoclavicular joint leading to mediastinal compression. Ann Thorac Surg 1996;61:711–3.

[83] Imatani RJ. Fractures of the scapula: a review of 53 fractures. J Trauma 1975;15:473–8.

[84] Veysi VT, Mittal R, Agarwal S, et al. Multiple trauma and scapular fractures: so what? J Trauma 2003;55(6):1145–7.

[85] Rowe CR. Fractures of the scapula. Surg Clin North Am 1963;43:1565–71.

[86] McGahan JP, Rab GT, Dublin A. Fractures of the scapula. J Trauma 1980;20:880–3.

[87] Zelle BA, Pape HC, Gerich TG, et al. Functional outcome following scapulothoracic dissociation. J Bone Joint Surg Am 2004;86(1):2–8.

[88] Oreck SL, Burgess A, Levine AM. Traumatic lateral displacement of the scapula: a radiographic sign of neurovascular disruption. J Bone Joint Surg Am 1984;66:758–63.

[89] Ebraheim NA, Pearlstein SR, Savolaine ER, et al. Scapulothoracic dissociation (closed avulsion of the scapula, subclavian artery, and brachial plexus): a newly recognized variant, a new classification, and a review of the literature and treatment options. J Orthoped Trauma 1987;1: 18–23.

[90] Ridpath CA, Nork S, Linnau K, et al. Scapulothoracic dissociation: are there reliable chest radiographic findings? Emerg Rad 2001;8:304–7.

[91] Kelbel JM, Jardon OM, Huurman WW. Scapulothoracic dissociation. A case report. Clin Orthop Relat Res 1986;209:210–4.

RADIOLOGIC
CLINICS
OF NORTH AMERICA

Radiol Clin N Am 44 (2006) 225–238

ELSEVIER
SAUNDERS

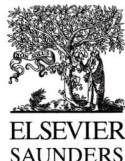

Imaging of Penetrating Chest Trauma

Kathirkamanathan Shanmuganathan, MD[a],*,
Junichi Matsumoto, MD[b]

- Basic ballistics
- Imaging of penetrating chest trauma
  Wound tracks
  Injury to chest wall, pleura, and lung
  Hemothorax and pleural effusions
  Pulmonary contusion
  Pulmonary lacerations
- *Transmediastinal gunshot wounds*
  Cardiac and pericardial injuries
  Tracheobronchial injuries
  Esophageal injury
- Summary
- References

Firearm-related injuries have become a public health problem that has a devastating impact on American society; as a result of their frequency and lethality, they inflict substantial emotional and financial costs. For every firearm death it is estimated that there are three to five other nonfatal firearm injuries [1]. There has been a steady increase in the number of patients who are admitted with penetrating injuries to urban trauma centers throughout the United States [2,3].

Basic ballistics

Penetrating injuries to the chest can result from stabbing or gunshot wounds. All stab wounds are considered low-energy injuries. Gunshot wounds can be divided into high- and low-energy injuries. High-energy gunshot wounds have a muzzle velocity greater than 1000 to 2500 feet per second. Most penetrating chest injuries that are seen in the civilian environment are the result of knife or low-energy handgun wounding.

The extent of tissue damage that is caused by a projectile is more severe for high-energy missiles [4,5]. Permanent and temporary cavities form from high-energy injuries that result in substantial tissue damage along the wound tract and in surrounding tissues. The temporary cavity formed is insignificant and does not contribute to the amount of tissue damage in long- or intermediate-range civilian gunshot wounds. Low-energy weapons, such as a knife or ice pick, which are hand driven, damage tissue only from the sharp cutting edge or point.

Imaging of penetrating chest trauma

Approximately 4% to 15% of admissions to major trauma centers are attributable to penetrating thoracic injuries [6]. Most penetrating injuries to the chest are caused by knives or handgun bullets [7,8]. Unlike injury to the chest wall, pleura, and lung, transmediastinal knife and gunshot wounds that enter within the tight confines of the mediastinum are associated with injuries to vital structures,

[a] Department of Diagnostic Radiology, University of Maryland School of Medicine, Baltimore, MD, USA
[b] Department of Emergency and Critical Care Medicine, St. Marianna University School of Medicine, Kanagawa, Japan
* Corresponding author. Department of Diagnostic Radiology, University of Maryland School of Medicine, 22 South Greene Street, Baltimore, MD 21201.
E-mail address: kshanmuganathan@umm.edu (K. Shanmuganathan).

doi:10.1016/j.rcl.2005.10.002

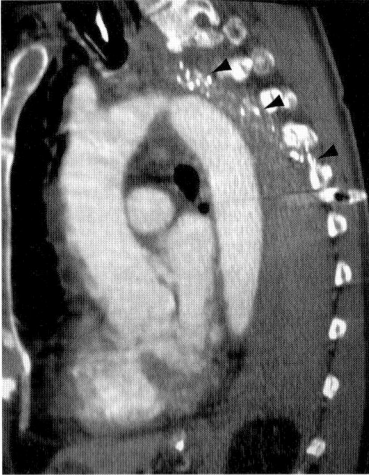

Fig. 1. Wound track outlined by bullet fragments in a patient who has transmediastinal gunshot wound. Sagittal multiplanar reformatted MDCT image shows a bullet track extending from posterior mediastinum adjacent to the thoracic spine into the middle mediastinum, outlined by bullet fragments (*arrowheads*). Note proximity of bullet track to the posterior arch of the thoracic aorta.

Wound tracks

The presence of air, hemorrhage, and bone or bullet fragments along the wound track allows identification of the course of the bullet or knife on multidetector row CT (MDCT). Usually, as compared with low-energy stab wounds, gunshot tracks create larger amounts of hemorrhage, air, bone, and metal fragments [Fig. 1] that enable the bullet's course to be demonstrated more clearly by MDCT. Even low-energy knife wound tracks through the lung may be well demonstrated by MDCT because of hemorrhagic cavitation that occurs from the elastic recoil property of lung parenchyma; however, detecting the extension of knife wound tracks to the mediastinum and their precise relationship to the vital mediastinal structures may be challenging [Fig. 2]. It is important to know the wound entry site and use optimal MDCT windows and levels (window = 550, level = 75) to improve identification of wounds that may reach the mediastinum. Images also should be reviewed in bone and lung window settings to aid in determining the precise extent of the wound and its relationship to the mediastinum.

including the heart, great vessels, esophagus, and trachea [6,9,10]. Injuries to vital vascular structures, such as the heart, aorta and its major branches, and the pulmonary artery and veins, are likely to cause rapidly fatal injures. Chest radiographs are the most common imaging study performed to evaluate these patients.

Injury to chest wall, pleura, and lung

From 88% to 97% of patients who are admitted with penetrating injuries to the chest have involvement of the chest wall, pleura, or lung [6,11]. Up to 62% of patients who are admitted following civilian penetrating injuries to the chest are asymptomatic and have normal chest radiographs

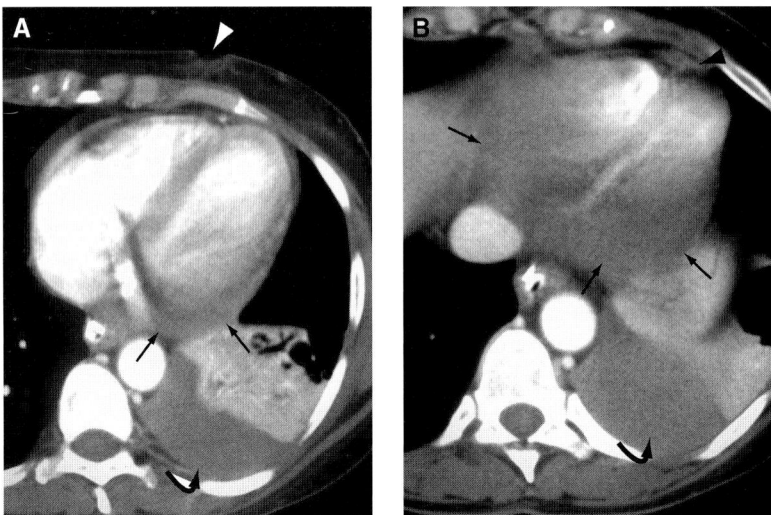

Fig. 2. Subtle wound tract in a 47-year-old woman who was stabbed in the juxtacardiac region of the left chest. (*A* and *B*) Axial MDCT images show entry site (*white arrowhead*) with a small amount of anterior mediastinal hemorrhage (*black arrowhead*) along subtle knife track. The presence of hemopericardium (*arrows*) and hemothorax (*curved arrow*) indicate violation of pleura and pericardium by the knife.

[12]. A hemopneumothorax occurs in 41% to 45% of symptomatic patients, and most of these patients require immediate intercostal tube drainage [13,14]. Patients who have isolated pneumothorax or hemothorax diagnosed on admission chest radiographs are less likely to need intercostal tube drainage, and usually do not deteriorate clinically compared with patients who have hemopneumothorax.

Delayed complications from chest stab wounds are well recognized and occur in from 8% to 12% of asymptomatic patients with normal chest radiographs, usually from 2 to 5 days after injury [6,13,14]. The appropriate in-hospital observation time to detect potential delayed complications is controversial. Ordog and colleagues [8] reported the initial chest radiograph was 92.5% sensitive and had a negative predictive value of only 87% in detecting injuries. The negative predictive value of chest radiographs for thoracic injury increased

to 99.9% at 6 hours after injury and allowed subsequent outpatient management. Follow-up chest radiographs are obtained after a 4- to 6-hour period of observation at our institution to detect delayed complications.

Pneumothorax is a common complication of penetrating thoracic trauma. The location of the pneumothorax depends on patient position, the amount of pleural space air, the presence of pleural adhesions, and regions of atelectasis. Typically, air in the pleural space collects in the apicolateral aspect of the hemithorax in the erect or semierect patient. Air within the pleural space is diagnosed by visualizing the visceral pleura as a thin sharp line with the absence of lung markings peripheral to this line. In the supine position, the most nondependent part of the hemithorax is the anterior costophrenic sulcus, which extends from the seventh costal cartilage laterally to the eleventh rib in the midaxillary line [Fig. 3] [15,16]. Prompt diagno-

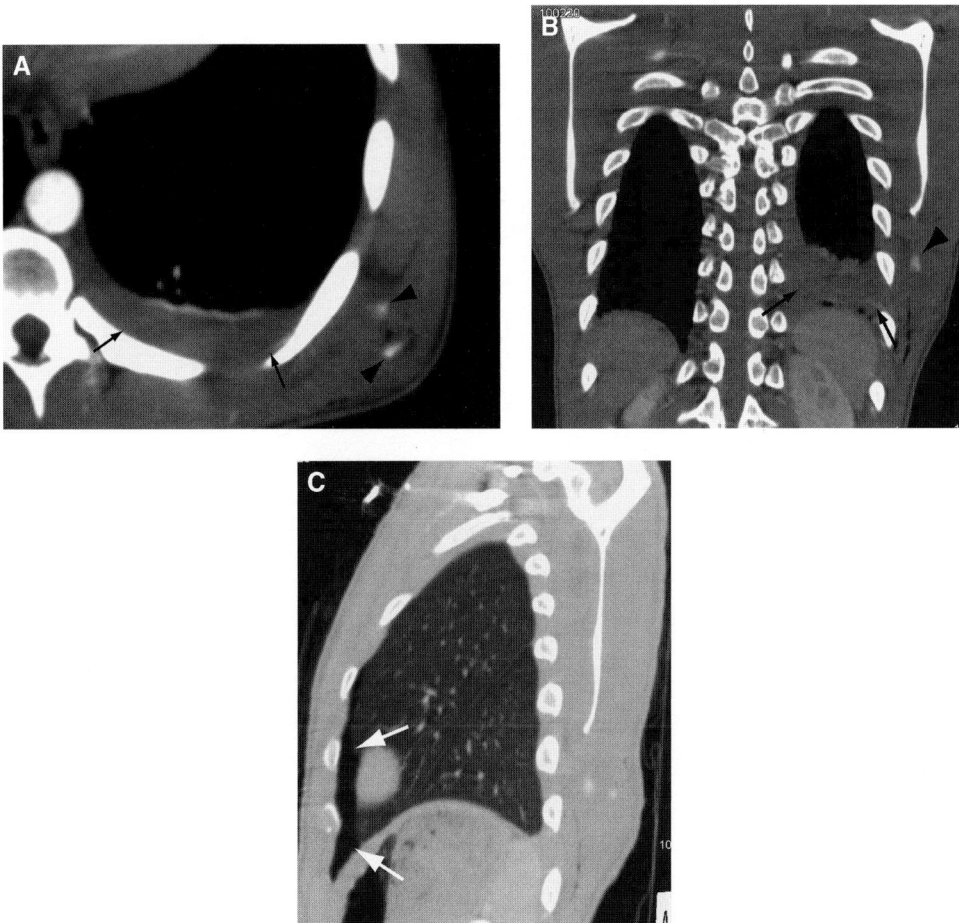

Fig. 3. Stab wound to left thoracoabdominal region with active bleeding in chest wall. Axial (*A*), coronal (*B*), and sagittal (*C*) multiplanar reformatted MDCT images show active bleeding (*arrowheads*) within the left lower chest wall along wound track with a small hemothorax (*black arrows*) and anterior inferior pneumothorax (*white arrows*).

sis, even of a small pneumothorax, is important, because significant respiratory and cardiovascular embarrassment may develop, especially for patients who have impaired pulmonary function or are receiving mechanical ventilation. The literature indicates that small pneumothoraces are not recognized initially by clinical examination or by admission chest radiography in 30% to 50% of trauma patients, and are only diagnosed after thoracic CT [17,18].

Hemothorax and pleural effusions

Hemothorax is a common occurrence in penetrating trauma [see Fig. 3]. It may be the result of a laceration/contusion of lung parenchyma, or injury to the visceral pleura, diaphragm, internal mammary, intercostal arteries [Fig. 4], heart, or great vessels [Figs. 5 and 6]. When more than 1500 mL of blood accumulates in the pleural space it is called a massive hemothorax [see Fig. 4]. Indications for thoracotomy include the immediate drainage of 1000 mL of blood from the pleural cavity, on-going hemorrhage that results in thoracostomy tube output of 200 mL/h or greater for 4 hours, or the presence of a large amount of clotted blood in the pleural space that prevents complete evacuation of blood. Clotted blood provides an ideal nidus for secondary infection and later development of empyema. Residual blood in the pleural cavity may entrap a significant portion of normal lung with subsequent loss of function from the ensuing fibrothorax and adhesions. To prevent or minimize these complications, surgeons have started using

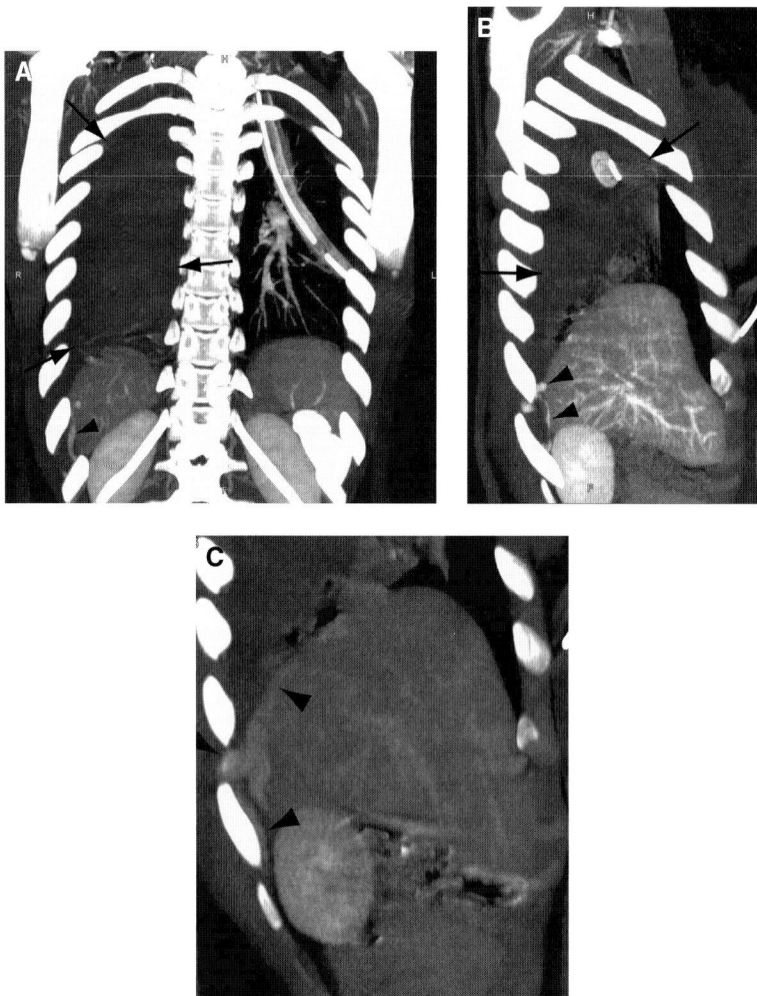

Fig. 4. Massive hemothorax in a young woman who was stabbed bilaterally in the lower chest. Coronal (*A*) and sagittal (*B*) three-dimensional images show a massive hemothorax (*arrows*) with active bleeding (*arrowheads*) from the tenth right intercostal artery. (*C*) Delayed three-dimensional sagittal image shows increase in area of active bleeding. Right thoracotomy was performed to control hemorrhage and evacuate the hemothorax.

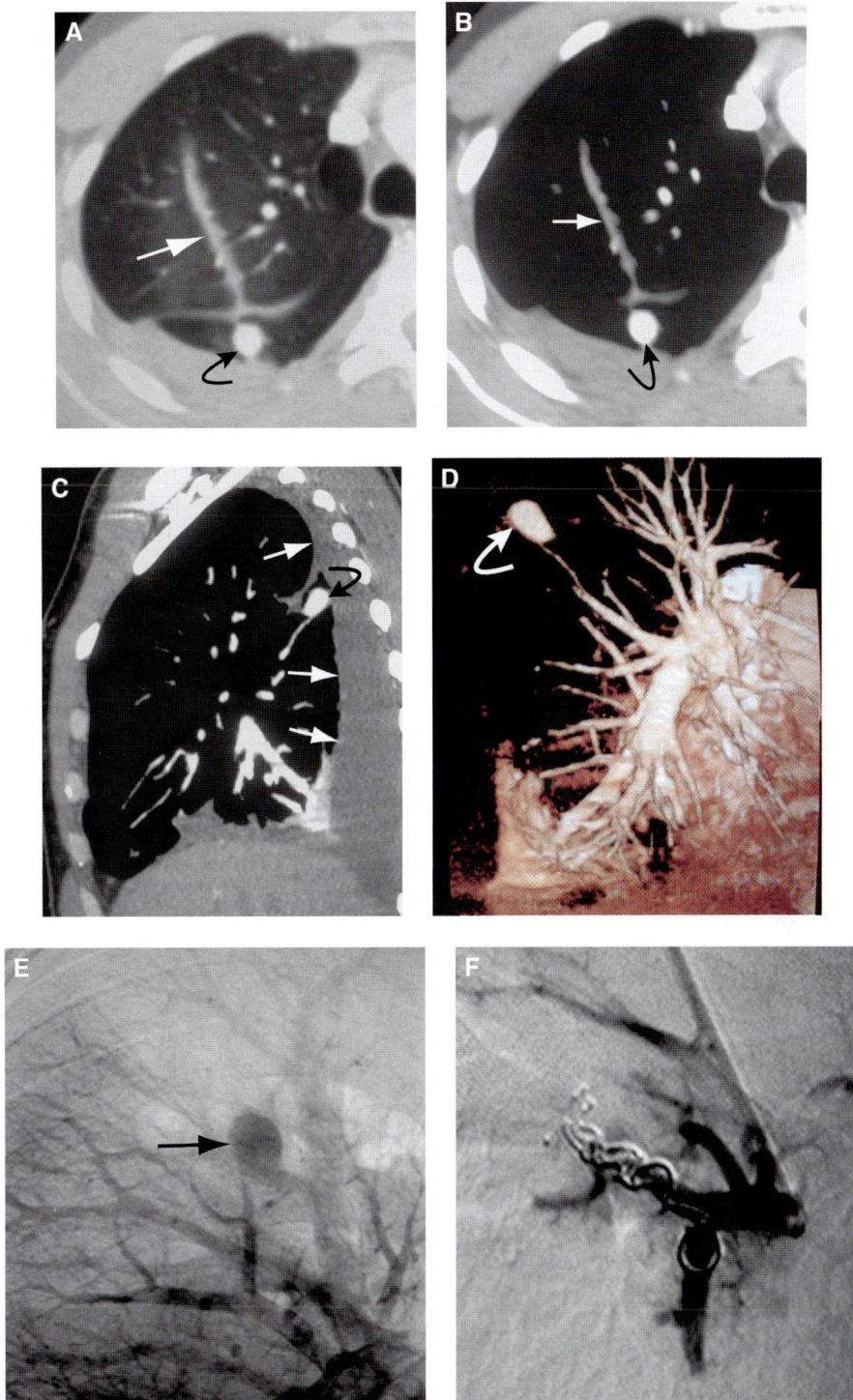

Fig. 5. Pulmonary artery branch pseudoaneurysm in a 37-year-old man who was stabbed in the right chest. Follow-up MDCT. (*A* and *B*) Axial images show a high attenuation rounded lesion (*curved arrow*) in the posterior superior segment of the lower lobe and end of the wound track (*arrow*). Sagittal multiplanar reformatted (*C*) and three-dimensional coronal oblique (*D*) images show a pseudoaneurysm arising from a peripheral posterior branch of the right superior pulmonary artery. A moderate amount of hemothorax (*arrows*) is seen in the posterior right thorax. (*E*) Pulmonary angiogram confirms the pseudoaneurysm (*arrow*). (*F*) Posttranscatheter embolization images confirm successful treatment of pulmonary artery branch pseudoaneurysm.

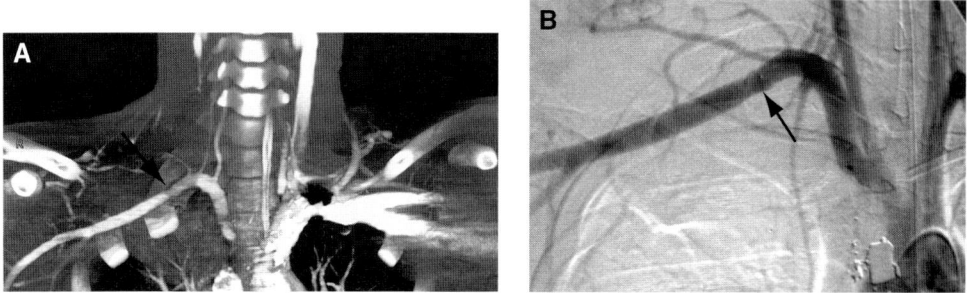

Fig. 6. Subclavian artery injury following a gunshot wound to the right thoracic inlet in an 18-year-old man. Three-dimensional coronal MDCT (*A*) and arch aortogram (*B*) images show an injury (*arrow*) to the subclavian artery posterior to the first rib.

minimally invasive surgical techniques, including video-assisted thoracoscopy, to evacuate retained hemothorax [6,19].

MDCT attenuation values help to distinguish serous effusion (low attenuation) from hemothorax, which has an MDCT attenuation of 35 to 70 Hounesfield units, depending upon the degree of clot retraction. Also, active hemorrhage [see Figs. 3 and 4] into the pleural space can be delineated directly by MDCT by use of power-injected intravenous contrast and contrast bolus timing techniques. The optimum window for thoracoscopy is between days 2 and 5 after injury (ie, before clot organization and adhesion formation) [20]. Although chest radiographs are the most frequently obtained imaging study that is used to follow hemothoraces, they are unreliable in diagnosing and precisely determining the amount of retained blood clot in the thoracic cavity [19]. A prospective study by Velmahos and colleagues [19] that evaluated the accuracy of chest radiographs for judging the amount of residual hemothorax, found that radiography was misleading in 48% of patients. In this study, chest radiographs identified only 10 of the 20 patients who were diagnosed initially by CT as having residual hemothorax of more than 300 mL. Seven patients who were believed to have intraparenchymal injury by chest radiography actually had retained hemothorax on CT. CT was required to select appropriate patients for thoracoscopy.

Bilious pleural effusion is rare and results from concomitant laceration of the right lung, right hemidiaphragm, and liver which permits formation of a biliary–pleural fistula [21]. Another etiology of pleural fluid that should be considered in the setting of penetrating chest trauma is chylothorax secondary to interruption of the thoracic duct, which is suggested by low or negative fluid attenuation values. Most thoracic duct injuries (88%) occur from superior mediastinal wounds

at the junction on the thoracic duct and left subclavian vein (Porier's triangle) and require early surgical intervention [6].

Pulmonary contusion

Pulmonary contusion is a common primary lung injury after penetrating chest trauma [22,23]. Direct injury to the interstitium and alveoli occurs along the wound track and temporary cavity. Disruption of small blood vessels and damage to the alveolar capillary membrane lead to hemorrhage into the parenchyma at the time of trauma, followed in 1 to 2 hours by interstitial edema, which peaks 24 hours after injury [22,24]. The extent of parenchymal damage depends on the energy of the projectile. The lung injury creates ventilation/perfusion mismatch, intrapulmonary shunts, decreased lung compliance, and increased lung water [25].

MDCT is superior to supine chest radiographs in diagnosing pulmonary contusion [26,27]. On MDCT, pulmonary contusions appear as unilateral or bilateral, patchy or diffuse air space filling that tends to be peripheral, nonsegmental, and geographic in distribution [Fig. 7]. Air-bronchograms frequently are not seen within contusion because of blood filling the adjacent small airways. Multiplanar reformatted (MPR) and minimum–maxiumum intensity images (MiniMIP) in the sagittal and coronal planes are optimal to display the extent and distribution of injury and the relationship between the lung injury and airways [see Fig. 7].

Pulmonary contusion usually is seen on admission MDCT or those that are performed within 6 hours after admission. Typically, pulmonary contusions begin to resolve on chest radiographs within 48 to 72 hours, but may not appear to be clearing for 5 to 7 days. Complete clearing of contusions usually occurs by 10 to 14 days after injury [28]. Superimposed pathologic processes, including infection, aspiration, atelectasis, or adult respiratory distress syndrome (ARDS), may result

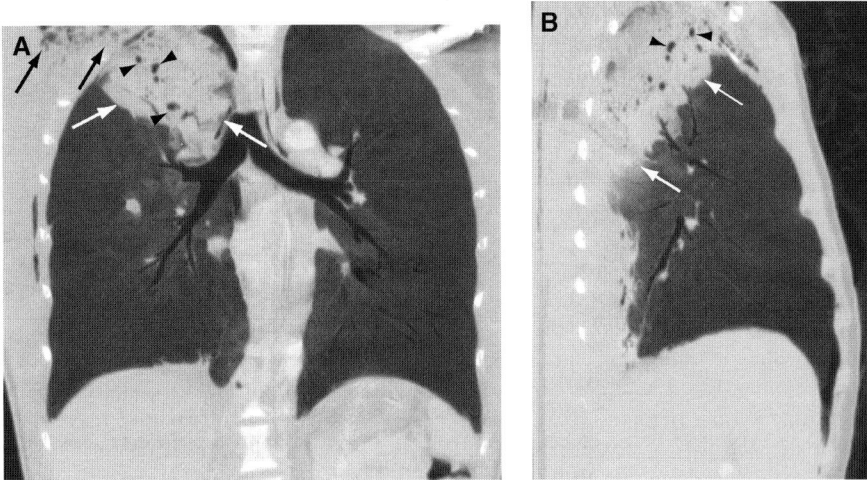

Fig. 7. Pulmonary contusion and laceration following gunshot wound to right anterior thoracic inlet in an 18-year-old man. Coronal (*A*) and sagittal (*B*) miniMIP images show an area of pulmonary contusion (*white arrows*) in right upper lobe. Small pulmonary lacerations (*arrowheads*) are seen within the area of contusion. Bullet track (*black arrows*) is outlined by air.

in failure of the lung density to resolve in this time period [26].

Pulmonary lacerations

Lung laceration is a common injury after penetrating chest trauma [23,26,29]. Because lung lacerations are surrounded by pulmonary contusions [see Fig. 7], they frequently are overlooked on initial chest radiographs, and in the past, were considered to be an uncommon result of blunt chest trauma. MDCT is far more sensitive than chest radiography in detecting lung laceration and any associated complications [29,30]. Because of the elastic recoil of the lung, lacerations typically are ovoid or elliptical in shape and are seen along, or adjacent, to wound tracts [Fig. 8]. An air–fluid level may be seen with hemorrhage into the cavity, or hemorrhage may fill the cavity completely and create a mass-like uniform density. A crescent of air may occur when a clot forms within the laceration, and result in an "air-meniscus" sign. Unlike pulmonary contusions, lung lacerations resolve slowly over a period of 3 to 5 weeks. Patients who have ARDS or who receive positive pressure ventilatory support may have lacerations that persist for months [31]. Usually, posttraumatic pneumatoceles resolve without prophylactic antibiotics or surgical intervention [32].

Lacerations of the lung generally are benign lesions, but occasionally, complications can occur. The presence of secretions or blood within the posttraumatic pneumatocele and endotracheal intubation provide a nidus and route for infection and abscess formation. A bronchopleural fistula may result from communication of a pulmonary laceration with a bronchus and the pleural surface.

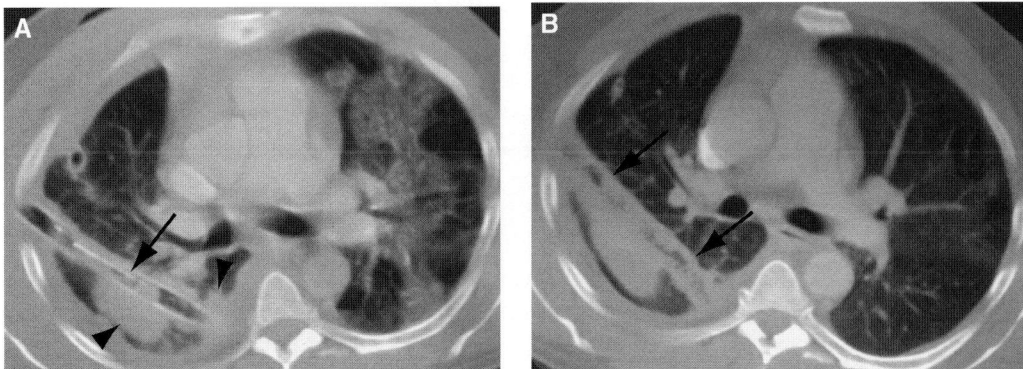

Fig. 8. Iatrogenic lung laceration. (*A*) Axial MDCT image shows a right intraparenchymal chest tube (*arrow*) surrounded by pulmonary contusion (*arrowheads*). (*B*) Axial MDCT image obtained following removal of right chest tube shows lung laceration (*arrows*) with hemorrhage within chest tube track.

A persistent air leak into the pleural space may not respond to chest tube placement, and may require pulmonary surgical resection to close the fistula. A ball-valve mechanism also may develop in posttraumatic pneumatoceles, which permit elevated pressure and expansion of the cavity with compression of adjacent normal lung. Such a development creates a large ventilatory dead-space with the potential for significant impairment of pulmonary function.

Transmediastinal gunshot wounds

Civilian patients who are admitted with potential transmediastinal gunshot wounds and who maintain a systolic blood pressure greater than 100 mm Hg in the absence of obvious bleeding do not warrant immediate surgery [9,10,33]. Pre-

hospital mortality from transmediastinal penetrating injury may be as high as 86% for cardiac injuries, 92% for thoracic vascular injuries, and 11% for pulmonary injuries [6,7]. Most patients (60%) who have transmediastinal gunshot wounds, who do not require immediate surgery will need imaging studies to diagnose injuries and plan treatment [6–10,34,35]. Occult injuries to mediastinal structures are not uncommon, and any possible transmediastinal trajectory must be assumed to have created life-threatening injuries [Figs. 1 and 9–14] [9,10,33]. A significant increase in morbidity and mortality is associated with delayed recognition of such injuries [35].

MDCT is optimally suited to visualize wounds that penetrate the great vessels see [Figs. 6, 9, and 10] pericardium [see Fig. 11], thoracic esophagus

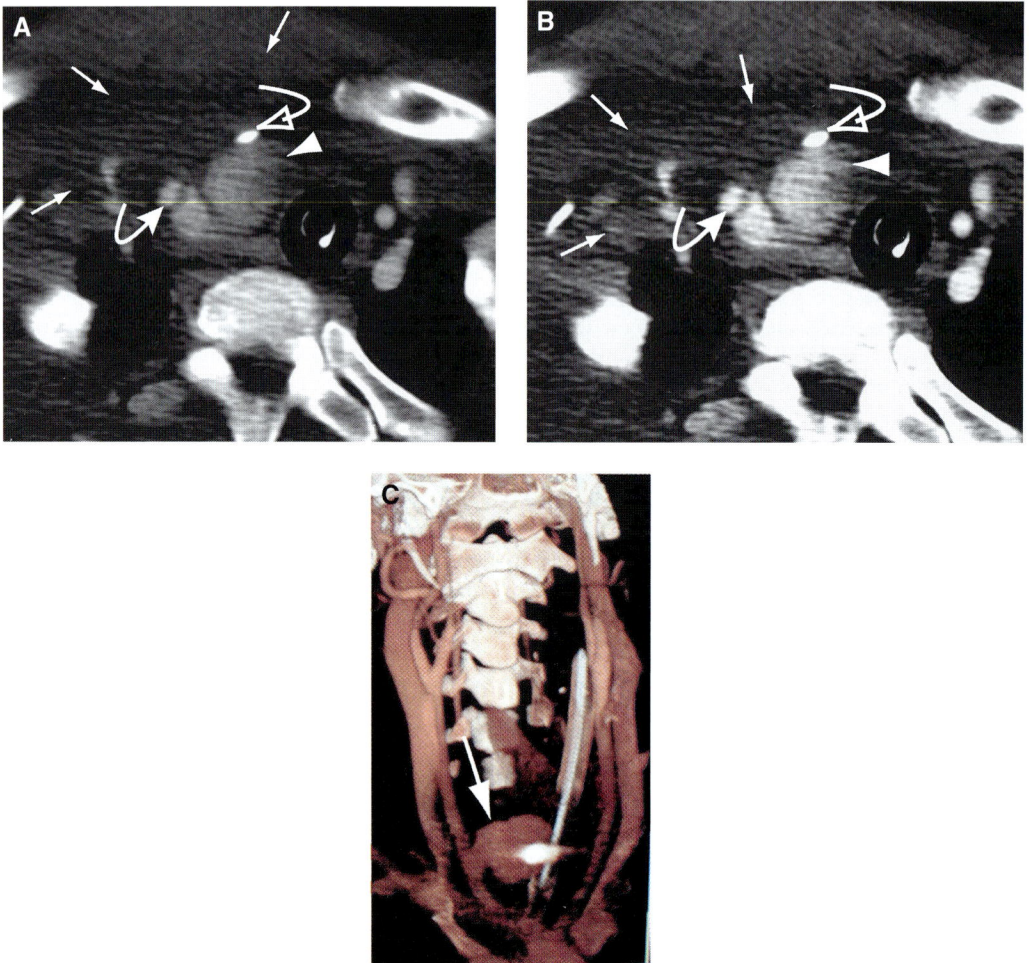

Fig. 9. Transmediastinal gunshot wound with major vascular injury. (*A* and *B*) Axial MDCT images show a right upper mediastinal hematoma (*arrows*) displacing the trachea to the left side. A large pseudoaneurysm (*arrowhead*) is seen arising from the right common carotid artery (*solid curved arrow*). A bullet fragment (*open curved arrow*) is seen anterior to the pseudoaneurysm. (*C*) Three-dimensional image shows a pseudoaneurysm (*arrow*) arising from the proximal right common carotid artery. Based on MDCT findings, surgery was performed to treat the pseudoaneurysm.

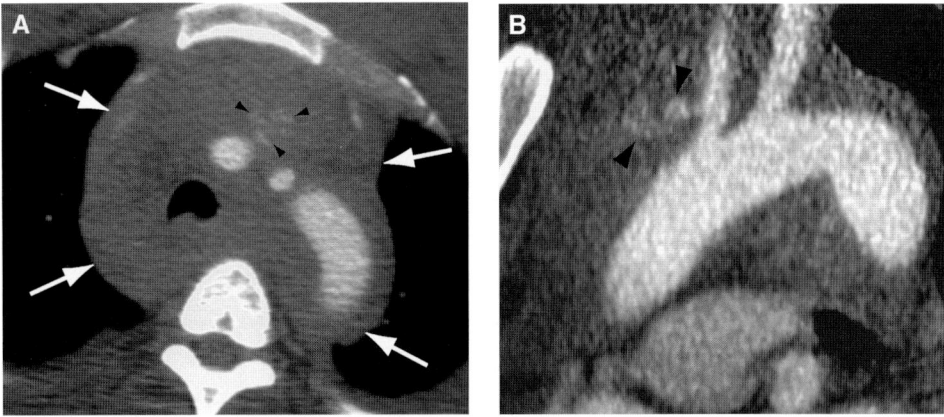

Fig. 10. Transmediastinal stab wound with major vascular injury in a 58-year-old man. Axial (*A*) and MPR (*B*) MDCT images show a large mediastinal hematoma (*arrows*) with active bleeding (*arrowheads*) from the right common carotid artery. At thoracotomy following MDCT, the right common carotid artery was found to be transected.

[see Fig. 14], trachea [see Figs. 13 and 14], and thoracic spine. This capability arises from the capacity to obtain volumetric data at peak contrast enhancement and with minimal misregistration and motion artifact. MDCT is readily available in most institutions in the United States, and is less expensive, time-consuming, and invasive than angiography or endoscopy. Traditionally, radiography, echocardiography, angiography, esophagoscopy, brochoscopy, and contrast barium swallow have been considered the required studies to evaluate the mediastinal for vascular and aerodigestive injuries. These investigations often remove the patient from an environment of ideal clinical support and monitoring. If, by MDCT, the wound track does not traverse the mediastinum or is demonstrated not to be in close proximity to vital struc-

tures, the traditional work-up of these patients is unnecessary [10]. A prospective study by Hanpeter and colleagues [10] evaluated 25 gunshot wounds to the chest with potential violation of the mediastinum as determined by chest radiographs and the entry and exit sites of bullet wounds using single-slice helical CT. Routine work-up of these patients would have required angiography, endoscopy, and contrast swallow. Proximity injuries to the mediastinum required further diagnostic studies, including angiography (n = 8) and contrast swallow (n = 9) in 12 patients. Thoracotomy was performed based on CT findings in one patient to remove a bullet that was lodged within the myocardium. Eleven patients did not need further diagnostic studies, because CT demonstrated the wound tract was well away from any vital mediastinal structure.

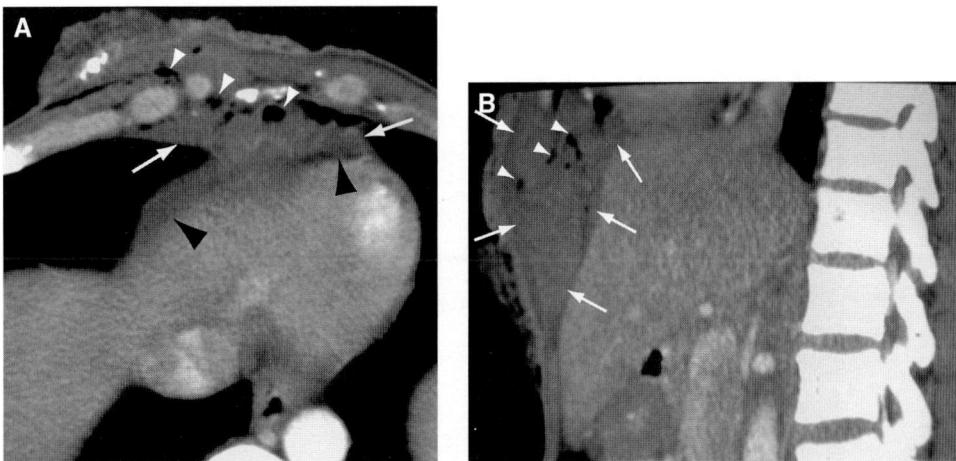

Fig. 11. Pericardial stab wound. Axial (*A*) and MPR (*B*) MDCT images show a stab wound track outlined by air (*white arrowheads*). A moderate-sized anterior mediastinal and extraperitoneal anterior abdominal hematoma (*arrows*) also is seen. The presence of a small amount of hemopericardium (*black arrowheads*) indicates an injury to the pericardium.

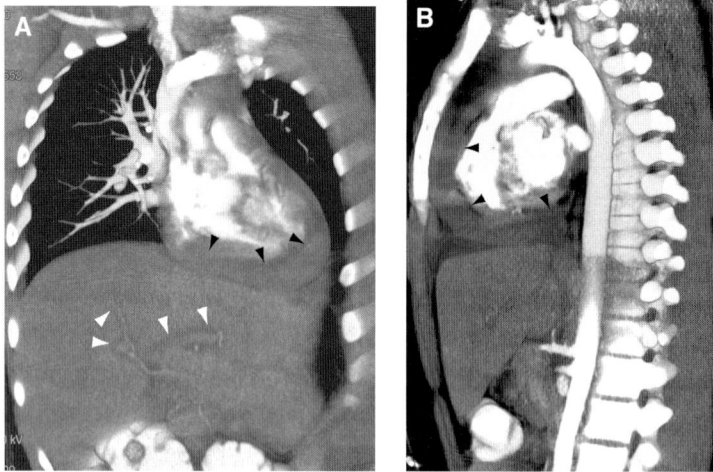

Fig. 12. Pericardial tamponade in an 18-year-old man who was stabbed in the precordium. Coronal (*A*) and sagittal (*B*) three-dimensional MDCT images show a large amount of hemopericardium (*black arrowheads*). Periportal lymphedema (*white arrowheads*) resulting from cardiac tamponade is seen.

MDCT provided valuable and accurate information to plan further work-up and therapy. At our institution, MDCT also helps to reduce the number of routine, invasive time-consuming angiographic and endoscopic studies [see Figs. 9 and 10] in patients who have penetrating chest injury. Further studies with larger numbers of patients are needed to define further the accuracy of MDCT for mediastinal violation as well as injury to particular mediastinal structures.

Cardiac and pericardial injuries

Injuries to intrapericardial structures have a mortality of approximately 60% to 80% [9,10,33,36,37]. Patients who have entrance wounds in a juxtacar-

diac location—defined by the area between the midcalvicular lines laterally, the clavicles superiorly, and the costal margin inferiorly—are likely to have injuries to the heart, intrapericardial aorta, pulmonary arteries, or veins [see Figs. 2 and 11] [36]. Demetriades and Van Der Veen [37] reviewed 532 penetrating cardiac injuries, including 125 patients who were admitted to the hospital with vital signs and 407 who died before hospital arrival. The distribution of injuries involved a ventricle (right, 35%; left, 25%), atrium (right, 33%; left, 14%), or aorta (14%).

The clinical presentation of patients who have penetrating cardiac wounds is determined by the location of any cardiac injury, the rate of bleeding

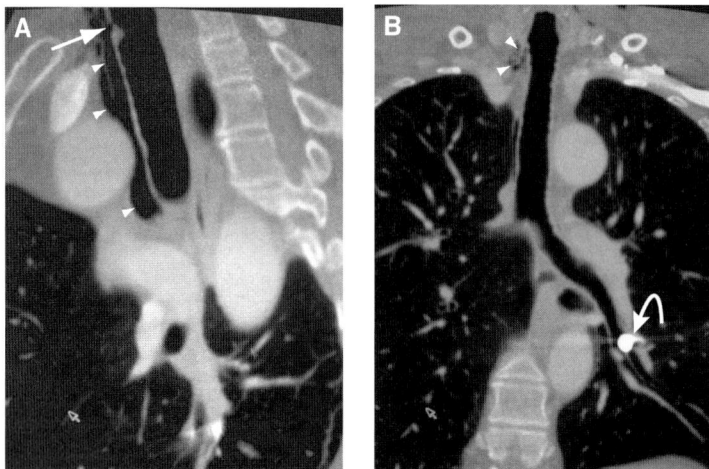

Fig. 13. Tracheal injury following a gunshot wound in a 54-year-old man. Entry wound was at the anterior sternal notch. Sagittal (*A*) and coronal (*B*) MDCT MPR images show paratracheal air (*arrowheads*) tracking anterior and lateral to trachea with a defect (*arrow*) in the anterior wall of trachea. The bullet (*curved arrow*) has fallen down the airway and is lodged in a branch of left lower lobe bronchus. Bronchoscopy was used to retrieve the bullet.

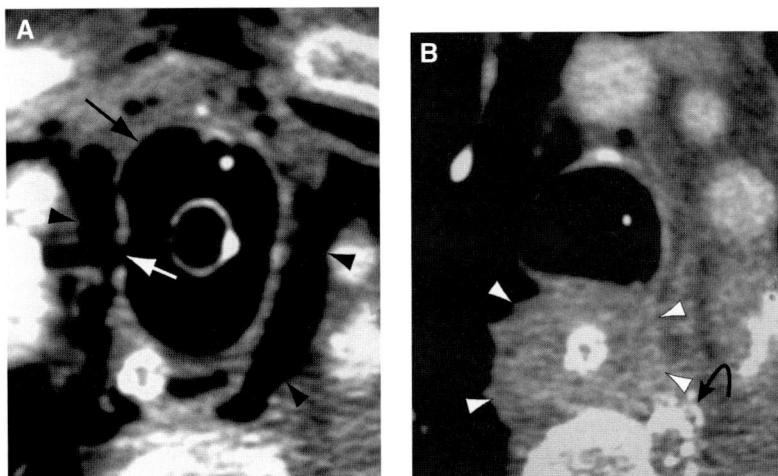

Fig. 14. Transmediastinal gunshot wound with tracheal and esophageal injury. (*A* and *B*) Axial MDCT images show an abnormal contour and an anteroposterior diameter of the tracheal balloon (*black arrow*), a defect in the right tracheal wall (*white arrow*), and paratracheal air (*black arrowheads*) indicating a tracheal injury. On inferior images, the esophageal wall is thickened (*white arrowheads*) and bullet fragments are seen adjacent to the esophagus. At surgery, tracheal and esophageal injuries were confirmed.

from the cardiac wound, and the size of the pericardial rent [38]. Most patients who have penetrating cardiac injuries present with unstable vital signs. Up to 80% of patients who have cardiac stab wounds present with tamponade [see Fig. 12] [38]. A small group of patients is relatively asymptomatic and maintains stable vital signs.

Echocardiography is the preferred method of diagnosing cardiac injuries in stable patients who have proximity injuries to the heart [38–41]. Nagy and colleagues [42] substituted conventional chest CT when echocardiography was not available to diagnose hemopericardium. The study included 45 patients who had precordial stab wounds and 15 patients who had transmediastinal gunshot wounds. None of the 56 patients who did not have evidence of pericardial fluid by CT had cardiac injury. This group of patients was observed in-hospital for a minimum of 24 hours. Three patients had pericardial fluid and one patient had an indeterminate CT for pericardial fluid. A subxiphoid pericardial window was performed in all four patients and was positive in two; both had cardiac injury. The other two patients had a negative subxiphoid pericardial window and required no further studies.

MDCT findings of cardiac and pericardial injuries include wound tracks that extend to the pericardium, a defect in the pericardium or myocardium, hemopericardium or pneumopericardium, herniation of the heart or a portion thereof through a pericardial rent, and intrapericardial or intracardiac bullets [see Figs. 2, 11, and 12] [43]. Faster MDCT scanners with the capability of obtaining 40 or 64 slices per subsecond rotation using cardiac gat-

ing techniques will reduce cardiac and respiration motion significantly, and produce consistently high-resolution images of the heart and intrapericardial vascular structures. Use of these scanners with gating techniques for penetrating trauma near the heart will permit diagnosis of the exact location and extent of injury and provide valuable information about cardiac function.

Tracheobronchial injuries

Tracheobronchial injury (TBI) has been reported in 2.8% to 5.4% of autopsy series of trauma victims [44–46]. Isolated tracheal injury accounts for 25% of all TBIs [44]. Penetrating trauma is less likely to injure the trachea (incidence of blunt trauma:penetrating trauma, 8:5) and generally involves the cervical trachea [46]. These injuries are uncommon and often go unrecognized because of a lack of visible external signs of injury. Early symptoms may be nonspecific and minimal and result in diagnosis only when late symptoms develop that suggest TBI, or the diagnosis may be established only at surgery or autopsy. TBI should be suspected in all patents who have penetrating wounds that enter the chest or neck [47]. A retrospective review of tracheal injuries over a 5-year period by Chen and colleagues [46] revealed that penetrating injuries most commonly involved the anterior aspect of the cervical trachea, with injuries to the rings and the ligamentous portion between the tracheal cartilages. A high incidence (31%) of concurrent esophageal and major vascular injuries is seen with penetrating TBI [46].

CT has an overall sensitivity of 85% in detecting tracheal injury [46]. MDCT volumetric data, with less partial volume averaging and motion artifact, produce high-resolution MPR and Mini MIP coronal and sagittal images of the trachea and mainstem bronchi [see Figs. 7 and 13] [48] that might help to delineate airway injury in cases of delayed presentation of subacute or chronic airway injury. Compared with chest radiography, MDCT is sensitive to less pneumomediastinum, and this may be the only sign of TBI. On MDCT, extrapulmonary air in direct contact with the trachea (paratracheal air) [see Figs. 13 and 14] and pneumomediastinum are not significant or pathognomonic findings of TBI [46]. Direct MDCT signs of airway injury include an overdistended endotracheal tube balloon with a transverse diameter measuring more than 2.8 cm [see Fig. 14], herniation of the endotracheal balloon outside of the walls of the airway [see Fig. 14], an endotracheal tube projecting outside of the airway, fracture or deformity of the cartilaginous rings of the airway, and airway wall discontinuity [Figs. 13 and 14] [46,49].

Bronchoscopy is the diagnostic modality of choice to confirm TBI, and early diagnosis is essential to obtain successful primary reanastamosis and optimal long-term results [50]. Although complete transection of the trachea usually is diagnosed during the initial admission, partial tears of the trachea and complete or partial tears of the bronchi may be detected only as a late sequela of TBI, including tracheal stenosis, tracheoesophageal fistula, empyema, mediastinitis, or bronchiectasis.

Esophageal injury

All forms of trauma account for only 10% to 19% of esophageal perforations [51,52]. Any case of penetrating trauma that traverses the mediastinum with the wound tract extending in proximity to the esophagus on MDCT requires definitive exclusion of esophageal injury [see Fig. 14]. In a review of 77 patients who had penetrating esophageal injuries, physical findings were present in only 34%. A multicentric retrospective study by Asensio and colleagues [53] on 405 patients who had penetrating esophageal injury reported a statistically significant, high incidence of morbidity and mortality when surgical repair was delayed. The uncommon nature of this injury, lack of specific clinical signs or chest radiographic findings, and the necessity for early diagnosis to avoid complications warrant a high index of clinical suspicion.

Most penetrating injuries involve the cervical esophagus and are associated with injuries to the respiratory tract (81%) [see Fig. 14], central nervous system (23%), and vascular system (21%) [53]. The most common presenting symptom is chest pain, followed by fever, dyspnea, and chest wall crepitus [54]. Other signs and symptoms include dysphagia, odynophagia, hematemesis, stridor, abdominal tenderness, and a mediastinal crushing sound (Hamman's sign). The most common chest radiographic signs are cervical and mediastinal emphysema (60%) and left pleural effusion (66%) [55]. Other radiologic signs of esophageal disruption include alteration of the mediastinal contour that is due to leakage of fluid, associated mediastinal hemorrhage, or inflammatory reaction.

In the authors' practice, esophagography is the initial study that is used to evaluate suspected esophageal injury in patients who have transmediastinal penetrating injuries. Contrast esophagogram is performed first with water-soluble contrast, and, if negative, it is performed with barium sulfate contrast. Fluoroscopic guidance is ideal, but if it is not possible because of the patient's condition, contrast can be instilled into the upper esophagus with chest radiographs performed during injection of water-soluble contrast after the position of the nasogastric tube is verified as appropriate.

The role of MDCT scanning in the diagnosis of traumatic esophageal perforation is not established. The demonstration of air bubbles, bone, or bullet fragments [see Fig. 14] in the mediastinum which are localized adjacent to the esophagus suggests esophageal perforation. Direct MDCT findings of esophageal injury include wall thickening [see Fig. 14], a defect in the esophageal wall adjacent to the wound tract, and extravasation of oral contrast material into the mediastinum. MDCT of the chest is used to verify the presence or absence of mediastinal involvement [10,56]. Demonstration of a ballistic tract that unequivocally does not involve the mediastinum avoids the need to evaluate the esophagus, aorta, and mainstem bronchi. Knife wounds to the chest tend to have a less predictable course because of minimal hemorrhage and air along the wound tract, and thus, are likely to require more extensive imaging assessment if there is any doubt regarding the course of penetrating trauma.

Summary

Chest radiograph is the most common imaging study that is performed in patients who have penetrating thoracic injury. With the introduction of MDCT technology, significant advances have been made in the ability to obtain high-resolution volumetric data during peak vascular contrast enhancement in patients who have penetrating chest injuries. This development has resulted in a marked increase in the number of hemodynamically stable sustaining penetrating chest traumas that are imaged with MDCT. The volumetric data that are acquired can be used to perform high-resolution axial, MPR,

MIP, and three-dimensional color images. Improved image quality and manipulation of volumetric data allow a more accurate diagnosis of the extent and course of penetrating injury, and often allow delineation of the precise injuries that have been sustained. The need for further diagnostic work-up or intervention frequently can be determined from the MDCT results.

References

[1] Annest JL, Mercy JA, Gibson DR, et al. National estimate of nonfatal firearm-related injuries: beyond the tip of the iceberg. JAMA 1995;273: 1749–54.

[2] Schwab CW. Violence: American uncivil war. Presidential address, Sixth Scientific Assembly of the Eastern Association for the Surgery of Trauma. J Trauma 1993;35:657–65.

[3] The Violence Prevention Task Force of the Eastern Association for the Surgery of Trauma. Violence in America: a public health crisis–the role of firearms. J Trauma 1995;38:163–8.

[4] Hollerman JJ, Fackler ML, Coldwell DM, et al. Gunshot wounds: 1. Bullet, ballistics, and mechanism of injury. AJR Am J Roentgenol 1990;155: 685–90.

[5] Ledgerwood AM. The wandering bullet. Surg Clin North Am 1997;57:97–109.

[6] Von Oppell UO, De Groot M. Penetrating thoracic injuries: what have we learned? Thorac Cardiov Surg 2000;48:55–61.

[7] Richardson JD, Spain DA. Injury to lung and pleura. In: Mattox KL, Feliciano DV, Moore EE, editors. Trauma. 4th edition. New York: McGraw-Hill Companies Inc.; 2000. p. 523–43.

[8] Ordog GJ, Wasserberger J, Balasubramanium S, et al. Asymptomatic stab wounds of the chest. J Trauma 1994;36:680–4.

[9] Renz BM, Cava RA, Feliciano DV, et al. Transmediastinal gunshot wounds: a prospective study. J Trauma 2000;48:416–22.

[10] Hanpeter DE, Demetriades D, Asensio JA, et al. Helical computed tomographic scan in the evaluation of mediastinal gunshot wounds. J Trauma 2000;49:689–95.

[11] Oparah SS, Mandal AK. Penetrating stab wounds to the chest: experience with 200 consecutive cases. J Trauma 1976;16:868–72.

[12] Kerr TM, Sood R, Buckman RF, et al. Prospective trial of the six hour rule in stab wounds of the chest. Surg Gynecol Obstet 1989;169:223–5.

[13] Muckart DJJ, Luvuno FM, Baker LW. Penetrating injuries of the pleural cavity. Thorax 1984;39: 789–93.

[14] Shatz DV, Pedraja J, Erbella J, et al. Efficacy of follow-up evaluation in penetrating thoracic injuries: 3- vs 6-hour radiographs of the chest. J Emerg Med 2000;20:281–4.

[15] Gordon R. Deep sulcus sign. Radiology 1980; 136:25–7.

[16] Ziter FM, Westcott JL. Supine subpulmonary pneumothorax. AJR Am J Roentgenol 1981;137: 699–701.

[17] Rhea JT, Novelline RA, Lawrason J, et al. The frequency and significance of thoracic injuries detected on abdominal CT scans in multiple trauma patients. J Trauma 1989;29:502–9.

[18] Rhea JT, van Sonnenburg E, McLoud TC. Basilar pneumothorax in the supine adult. Radiology 1979;133:593–5.

[19] Velmahos GC, Demetriades D, Chang L, et al. Predicting need for thoracoscopic evacuation of residual traumatic hemothorax: chest radiograph is insufficient. J Trauma 1999;46:65–70.

[20] Meyer DM, Jessen ME, Wait MA, et al. Early evacuation of traumatic retained hemothoraces using thoracoscopy: a prospective randomized trial. Ann Thorac Surg 1997;64:1396–401.

[21] Stark P. Pleura. In: Radiology of thoracic trauma. Boston: Andover Medical Publishers; 1993. p. 54–72.

[22] Greene R. Lung alterations in thoracic trauma. J Thorac Imaging 1987;2(3):1–11.

[23] Cohen MC. Pulmonary contusion: review of the clinical entity. J Trauma 1997;42(5):973–9.

[24] Fluton RL, Peter ET. The progressive nature of pulmonary contusion. Surgery 1970;67: 499–502.

[25] Oppenheimer L, Craven KD, Forkert L, et al. Pathophysiology of pulmonary contusion in dogs. Am J Physiol 1979;47:718–28.

[26] Mirvis SE, Tobin KD, Kostrubiak I, et al. Thoracic CT in detecting occult disease in critically ill patients. AJR Am J Roentgenol 1987;148:685–9.

[27] Sivit CJ, Taylor GA, Eichelberger MR. Chest injury in children with blunt abdominal trauma: evaluation with CT. Radiology 1989;171:815–8.

[28] Goodman LR, Putman CE. The SICU chest radiograph after massive blunt trauma. Radiol Clin North Am 1981;19(1):111–23.

[29] Wagner RB, Crawford WO, Schimpf PP. Classification of parenchymal lung injuries of the lung. Radiology 1988;167:77–82.

[30] Myung SS, Kang J. Computed tomography evaluation of posttraumatic pulmonary pseudocysts. Clin Imaging 1993;17:189–92.

[31] Kato R, Horinouchi H, Maennaka Y. Traumatic pulmonary pseudocyst. J Thorac Cardivas Surg 1989;97:309–12.

[32] Ulstad DR, Bjelland JC, Quan SF. Bilateral paramediastinal posttraumatic lung cyst. Chest 1990; 97:242–4.

[33] Richardson JD, Flint LM, Snow NJ, et al. Management of transmediastinal gunshot wound. Surgery 1981;90:671–6.

[34] Cornwell III EE, Kennedy F, Ayad IA, et al. Transmediastinal gunshot wounds: reconsideration of the role of aortography. Arch Surg 1996;131: 949–52 [discussion 952–3].

[35] Gasparri MG, Lorelli DR, Karlovich KA, et al. Physical examination plus chest radiography in penetrating periclavicular trauma: the appropri-

ate trigger for angiography. J Trauma 2000;49: 1029–33.

[36] Duncan OA, Scalea TM, Sclafani SJA, et al. Evaluation of occult cardiac injuries using sub-xiphoid pericardial windows. J Trauma 1989; 29(7):955–60.

[37] Demetriades D, Van Der Veen BW. Penetrating injuries of the heart: experience over two years in South Africa. J Trauma 1983;23(12):1034–41.

[38] Ivatury RR. Injured heart. In: Mattox KL, Feliciano DV, Moore EE, editors. Trauma. 4th edition. New York: McGraw-Hill Companies Inc.; 2000. p. 545–58.

[39] Harris DG, Papagiannopoulus KA, Pretorius J, et al. Current evaluation of stab wounds. Ann Thorac Surg 1999;68:2119–222.

[40] Rozycki GS, Feliciano DV, Ochsner MG, et al. The role of ultrasound in patients with possible penetrating cardiac wounds: a prospective multi-center study. J Trauma 1999;469(4):543–51.

[41] Bllaivas M, DeBehnke D, Phelen MB. Potential errors in the diagnosis of pericardial effusion on trauma ultrasound for penetrating injuries. Acad Emerg Med 2000;7(11):1261–6.

[42] Nagy KK, Gilkey SH, Roberts RR, et al. Computed tomography screens stable patients at risk for penetrating cardiac injury. Acad Emerg Med 1996; 3(11):1024–7.

[43] Killeen KL, Poletti PA, Shanmuganathan K, et al. CT diagnosis of cardiac and pericardial injuries. Emerg Radiol 1999;6:339–44.

[44] Mason AC, Mirvis SE, Templeton PA. Imaging of acute tracheobrochial injury: review of the literature. Emerg Radiol 1994;1:250–60.

[45] Lee RB. Traumatic injury of cervicothoracic trachea and major bronchi. Chest Surg Clin N Am 1997;7(2):285–304.

[46] Chen J, Shanmuganathan K, Mirvis SE, et al. Using CT to diagnose tracheal rupture. AJR Am J Roentgenol 2001;176:1273–80.

[47] Rossbach MM, Johnson SB, Gomez MA, et al. Management of major tracheobronchial injuries: a 28-year experience. Ann Thorac Surg 1998; 65:182–6.

[48] Wan YL, Tasi KT, Yeow KM, et al. CT findings of bronchial transection. Am J Emerg Med 1997; 15:176–7.

[49] Rollings RJ, Tocino I. Early radiographic signs of tracheal rupture. AJR 1987;148:695–8.

[50] Balci AE, Eren N, Erne S, et al. Surgical treatment of post-traumatic tracheobrochial injuries: 14 year experience. Eur J Cardiothorac Surg 2002; 22(6):984–9.

[51] Bladergroen MR, Lowe JE, Postlethwait RW. Diagnosis and recommended management of esophageal perforation and rupture. Ann Thorac Surg 1986;42:235–9.

[52] Jones II WG, Ginsberg RJ. Esophageal perforation: a continuing challenge. Ann Thorac Surg 1992;53:534–43.

[53] Asensio JA, Chahwan S, Forno W, et al. Penetrating esophageal injuries: multicentric study of the American Association for the Surgery of Trauma. J Trauma 2001;50:289–96.

[54] Nesbitt JC, Sawyer JL. Surgical management of esophageal perforation. Am Surg 1987;53: 183–91.

[55] Van Moore A, Ravin CE, Putman CE. Radiologic evaluation of acute chest trauma. CRC Crit Rev Diagn Imaging 1983;19:89–110.

[56] LeBlang SD, Dolich MO. Imaging of penetrating thoracic trauma. J Thorac Imaging 2000;15: 128–35.

RADIOLOGIC
CLINICS
OF NORTH AMERICA

Radiol Clin N Am 44 (2006) 239–249

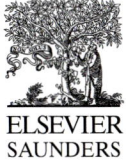

Thoracic Angiography and Intervention in Trauma

Patrick C. Malloy, MD*, Howard Marks Richard III, MD

- Mechanism of arterial injury in thoracic aortic trauma
- Thoracic angiography in trauma
  Technique
  Thoracic aortography
  Selective arteriography
  Radiation protection
- Vascular anatomy and findings
  Traumatic pseudoaneurysm in blunt chest injury
  Traumatic dissection
- Penetrating trauma to the aorta
- Thoracic anomalies and normal variants
- Aortic branches
- Thoracic venous injuries
- Interventions
- Summary
- References
- Further reading

Angiography and intervention in patients who have sustained thoracic trauma has evolved significantly in the past decade. The widespread availability of multidetector-row CT (MDCT) and the continuing development of minimally invasive techniques for the treatment of patients who have thoracic vascular injury have changed patient care and physician practice significantly. In the late 1980s, for example, thoracic angiography was a first-line modality for the diagnosis of thoracic aortic injury (TAI), and was performed based on mechanism of injury, clinical signs, and chest radiographic findings.

TAI most often required emergent surgery, which carried significant morbidity and mortality, particularly in older patients. By the mid-1990s, advances in technology allowed spiral CT to act as the first-line diagnostic modality in thoracic trauma. Controversy ensued over the validity of a "negative" CT scan; however, within a short time in the late 1990s, the weight of clinical experience—together with rapid, continued improvements in technology —allowed CT to take the initial, and the definitive, role in the evaluation of the patient who had sustained trauma [1–5]. Aortography, at this time, was used only as a problem solver when the results of MDCT were ambiguous because of technical factors or the lack of dynamic flow information. Current trauma practice using multichannel scanners often allows for rapid, isotropic imaging during peak aortic enhancement, which permits accurate three-dimensional reconstruction and definitive diagnosis. These advancements in imaging have effected a significant shift in clinical practice.

Mechanism of arterial injury in thoracic aortic trauma

The mechanisms of injury in chest trauma are divided into two main categories: penetrating and

Department of Diagnostic Radiology, University of Maryland Medical System, Baltimore, MD, USA
* Corresponding author. Department of Diagnostic Radiology, University of Maryland Medical System, 22 South Greene Street, Baltimore, MD 21201.
E-mail address: pmalloy@umm.edu (P.C. Malloy).

0033-8389/06/$ – see front matter. Published by Elsevier Inc.
radiologic.theclinics.com
doi:10.1016/j.rcl.2005.11.001

blunt chest trauma. Most patients who present with thoracic great vessel injury have sustained penetrating trauma and have a dire prognosis; most die before they reach medical care [6,7].

Aortic injuries that are due to blunt trauma are increasing in incidence [8]. Aortic injury that results from blunt trauma may range from intimal injury to medial disruption and contained extravasation. TAI from blunt chest trauma occurs most frequently as the result of motor vehicle collisions, and is estimated to account for as many as 10% to 15% of vehicular collision–related deaths. Approximately 70% to 90% of patients who sustain this injury die at the accident scene. Of the 10% to 30% of patients who survive, the prognosis is dismal in the absence of definitive repair; up to 50% succumb within 24 hours and 90% die within 4 months. More than 90% of patients have associated injuries that require a major operation that may impact the timing of definitive aortic repair [8].

The mechanism of injury in blunt traumatic aortic injury involves high-speed deceleration. In motor vehicle collisions, the typical injury occurs as the chest strikes the steering wheel, which transmits decelerating forces across the mediastinum. In addition, the sudden deceleration may induce injury from vascular compression between the sternum and thoracic spine, and by the sudden induction of severe intraluminal hypertension [9,10]. The area of the aorta that is most susceptible to injury is the transition point from the transverse arch—which is stabilized by the arch great vessels—to the descending thoracic aorta—which is fixed by the ligamentum arteriosum and intercostal arteries. At this point, the aorta is mobile and continues to move forward as the tethered portions decelerate with the remainder of the chest, and results in aortic injury.

Thoracic angiography in trauma

Technique

The technique that is used in thoracic aortography and selective angiography often is dictated by clinical history, including mechanism of injury, physical findings, and findings on contrast-enhanced MDCT. Arterial access is obtained most often from the common femoral arteries, although the brachial or axial approach may be used. Generally, femoral approaches are preferred because of a slightly lower incidence of puncture site complications and wider experience with closure devices in femoral access sites. These devices may play an important role in the patient who has sustained trauma, particularly in the acute setting; rapid blood loss and hemodilution may lead to a sig-

nificant acute coagulopathy, and increase the risk of arterial puncture site complications.

Thoracic aortography

Thoracic aortography requires the rapid delivery of contrast to nearly completely replace the volume of flowing blood with rapid, high-detail imaging. This requires the use of high-pressure injectors that are capable of injecting at 1050 psi or greater, and digital angiography systems that are capable of imaging a 15-inch or greater field-of-view at up to 15 frames per second, using a 1024 × 1024 image capture device, with appropriate postprocessing capabilities. After thoracic trauma, patients often exhibit hyperdynamic flow in the thoracic aorta. Absence of proper technique and equipment may lead to ambiguous imaging or excessively high amounts of iodinated contrast.

A 5- or 6-French pigtail catheter is inserted into the ascending thoracic aorta under fluoroscopic guidance. The use of endhole catheters or the injection of large-caliber sheaths for thoracic angiography is inadvisable. The lack of ability to achieve sufficient injection volumes and propensity for catheter "whip" at high flow rates in a large vessel can lead to vessel trauma and inadvertent injections of high contrast volumes into branch vessels. A test injection confirms placement of the catheter, and allows for assessment of flow within the aorta. This is particularly essential in cases of traumatic dissection (see elsewhere in this issue) where flow characteristics in the aorta may be altered significantly. In aortic root injections, contrast generally is injected at a rate of 25 to 30 mL/s, for a total of 50 to 60 mL of contrast. For imaging of the descending thoracic aorta, the pigtail catheter is placed with its tip just caudal to the origin of the left subclavian artery. Contrast is injected at a rate of 15 to 20 mL/s, for a total of 30 to 40 mL of contrast. Images may be acquired at rates that range from 5 to 15 frames per second. Generally, the higher rates are required for the acutely injured patient in whom it may be inadvisable to attempt, or impossible to achieve, success using motion suppression and suspended respiration. It is essential to obtain two or more views of the aorta at orthogonal angles that are separated by at least 30°. For thoracic arch imaging, the left anterior oblique (LAO) projection is used most widely, because this view "unfolds" the arch and profiles the expected position of insertion of the ligamentum arteriosum, the most common site of injury in initial survivors of blunt chest trauma. In blunt chest trauma, two orthogonal views may be sufficient to exclude significant aortic injury. At least three views are required in penetrating trauma, because a small pseudoaneurysm may be missed as a result of overlap with the aortic lumen. Although in most cases the initial diagnosis will be made by earlier CT, familiarity with these principles guides the proper depiction of arterial pathology during endovascular interventions, and helps to improve procedural success and outcomes.

Selective arteriography

In the clinical situation of suspected or confirmed thoracic aortic branch vessel injury, selective angiography may be required to evaluate the flow characteristics of the injury and to treat the injury primarily. A variety of catheter shapes is available that can be divided into curved tip and reverse curve types. Although the selection of any individual catheter may be dependent on the individual operator's experience and preference, several general points are worthy of mention. Use of catheters with inner diameters of 0.038 inches allows coaxial placement of a 3-French microcatheter, which may be useful later for superselective coil or particulate embolization, as in the case of acute intercostal, internal mammary, or other thoracic aortic branch vessel injury. In addition, the use of reverse curve catheters may be particularly helpful in selective catheterization of the middle to lower thoracic intercostal arteries, particularly if they are of narrow caliber. Care should be taken in reforming the reverse curve catheter, because older individuals who have preexistent atherosclerotic disease of the proximal aorta are at risk for embolic stroke from catheter manipulations.

Radiation protection

The opportunity to treat an arterial injury primarily through a small skin nick in the groin is compelling, but carries the risk for excessive radiation exposure to the patient and operator. As endovascular techniques evolve, the opportunity to treat these lesions and the attractiveness of the approach will continue to increase. With greater technical complexity, however, comes the potential for exposure issues that result from prolonged fluoroscopy times. To mitigate this risk, interventionalists are advised to follow the following techniques: (1) maintain and inspect fluoroscopic equipment regularly to ensure that the equipment stays within the U.S. Food and Drug Administration maximum fluoroscopic output of 10 R/min; (2) minimize the use of electronic magnification whenever possible; (3) avoid fluoroscopy of the same anatomic area in the same projection for prolonged periods (ie, rotate tube to different obliquities if possible to vary peak skin entrance site); (4) keep image intensifier as close to the patient as possible· (5) use operator barriers properly, including regularly inspected aprons, proper eye protection, and under and over table shields; and (6) minimize angiographic acquisition with the operator and staff at tableside.

Vascular anatomy and findings

Traumatic pseudoaneurysm in blunt chest injury

The typical site of injury is the proximal descending thoracic aorta at the insertion of the ligamentum arteriosum just distal to the left subclavian artery. This region represents a mobile segment of aorta interposed between the fixed transverse arch and descending thoracic aorta. Upon impact, the transverse and descending aorta decelerate with the chest, whereas the interposing segment continues to move forward which causes the injury. Inju-

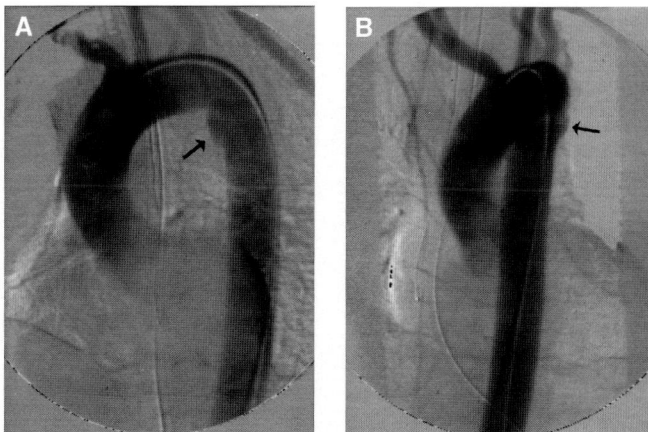

Fig. 1. AP (*A*) and LAO (*B*) aortograms demonstrate an aortic pseudoaneurysm (*arrows*). Note the contour defect in both views.

ries may range in severity from focal intimal disruption, partial rupture that involves the intima and media, to transection involving full-thickness aortic injury, which may be partial or circumferential [11,12].

Pseudoaneurysm with an epicenter at or near the expected site of insertion of the ligamentum arteriosum is the classic aortographic finding of TAI that is due to blunt chest trauma [Fig. 1]. The pseudoaneurysm appears as a double-density outpouching that typically is seen best in the LAO view. Although small pseudoaneurysms only may be seen as a double density on views that do not profile the contour of the injury [Fig. 2], most traumatic pseudoaneurysms are of sufficient size to be visualized readily on standard anteroposterior (AP), LAO, and right anterior oblique (RAO) views. Typically, the pseudoaneurysm has acute margins with the aortic wall on at least one view, demonstrates a double density with respect to the aortic lumen, and may display delayed washout. The pseudoaneurysm may be confined to the anteromedial region of the thoracic aorta at the level of the ligamentum arteriosum or it may extend circumferentially. Active extravasation of contrast typically is not seen because the patient likely would have impending cardiovascular collapse and would be too unstable to undergo angiography. Less typical findings at angiography include a focal irregularity or filling defect along the anteromedial surface of the aortic lumen that is due to intimal disruption and a partial thickness tear.

Traumatic dissection

A focal intimal injury may appear as a linear mobile filling defect at the site of trauma. Other findings include a focal globular filling defect that presumably is caused by focal clot that is due to localized intimal injury. True traumatic aortic dissection, which represents a longitudinal separation of the media along the long axis of the thoracic aorta, is rare [12].

Penetrating trauma to the aorta

Penetrating aortic trauma represents a special challenge to traditional aortography. Most survivors of penetrating aortic trauma show contained pseudoaneurysms angiographically that may vary widely in size. Small pseudoaneurysms may not be detected using the standard two orthogonal view–angiogram. Simple geometric modeling demonstrates the fallibility of conventional aortography in the detection of subtle traumatic injury. For example, in a patient who has a thoracic aortic cross-sectional diameter of 2.5 cm, a pseudoaneurysm of up to 10 mm may appear only as a subtle double density, rather than a contour abnormality. Therefore, three or more views with a total angular separation of at least 120° should be obtained to avoid missing subtle findings [Fig. 3].

A typical finding on thoracic aortography, in the setting of penetrating injury, is a small pseudoaneurysm at the site of vessel injury (also see elsewhere in this issue). Unlike blunt chest trauma, where the mechanism of injury makes the site of injury more predictable, findings in penetrating trauma may be highly variable, and dependent on the trajectory of the bullet, knife, or other object that caused the injury. The epicenter of the pseudoaneurysm may be seen at any point along the circumference of the aorta at any level in the chest. MDCT with optimal contrast bolus timing is superior to angiography in this setting, and avoids the above limitations. MDCT further offers the option for multiplanar reconstruction, which may enhance

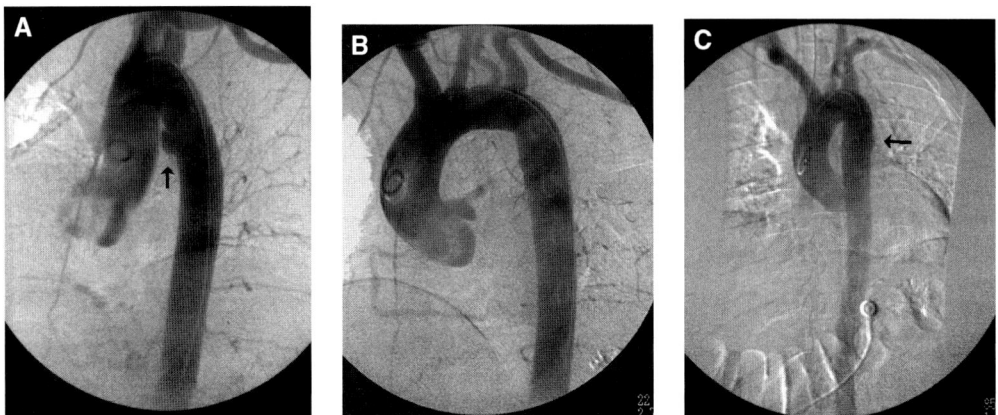

Fig. 2. AP (*A*), right posterior oblique (*B*), and left posterior oblique (*C*) aortograms demonstrate an aortic pseudoaneurysm (*arrows*). The contour defect is seen best in the AP and left posterior oblique views.

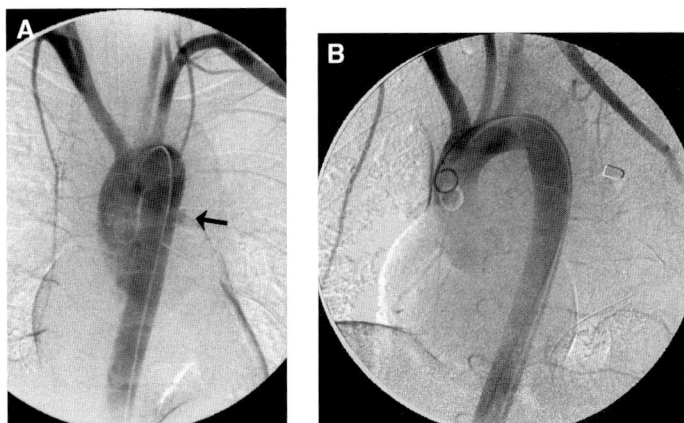

Fig. 3. AP (*A*) and LAO (*B*) aortograms demonstrate a traumatic aortic pseudoaneurysm (*arrow*) in this patient who suffered a gunshot wound to the thorax. The contour defect is seen only in the AP view.

visualization of the small pseudoaneurysms that are common in penetrating trauma.

Thoracic anomalies and normal variants

Imaging of the thoracic aorta in trauma requires a full understanding of nontraumatic developmental and pathologic anatomy. Because trauma is an episodic and essentially random event, over time the trauma radiologist will encounter most forms of anomalies, normal variants, and stable chronic disease, some of which may mimic traumatic injury.

Ductus diverticulum often is referred to as "ductus bump"; it is located at the expected insertion of the ligamentum arteriosum on the anteromedial portion of the thoracic aorta at the point of transition from the transverse arch to the descending thoracic aorta. It is characterized by an eccentric contour abnormality with a smooth, continuous interface with the transverse arch and the descending thoracic aorta. There is rapid flow of contrast without stasis or a double density. The anomaly is seen best on the LAO view, and often is obscured by overlap with the aorta on RAO or AP views (also see elsewhere in this issue) [Fig. 4].

Coarctation of the aorta refers to a developmental anomaly of the proximal descending thoracic aorta located at, or just distal to, the insertion of the ligamentum arteriosum. Coarctation represents a spectrum of anomalies that is characterized by variations in the degree of narrowing of the thoracic aorta. The most severe anomalies are symptomatic and usually are detected in early childhood, whereas the least severe remain asymptomatic and only may be discovered serendipitously [Fig. 5].

A diverticulum of Kommerell is characterized by an ectatic infundibulum at the origin of an anomalous right subclavian artery that originates distal to

the left subclavian artery in a left-sided arch configuration. In this anomaly, the infundibular origin may become aneurysmal, and often exhibits circumferential atherosclerotic changes. The vessel, which most often courses posterior to the esophagus, may create an extrinsic compression on the esophagus and result in the clinical syndrome of "dysphagia lusorum" [Fig. 6]. A diverticular origin of the bronchial artery refers to an anomaly in which there is an infundibulum at the origin of the bronchial or intercostobronchial trunk from the anteromedial portion of the proximal descending thoracic aorta. The anomaly can be distinguished from a true aortic injury by its location caudal to the expected site of the ligamentum arteriosum, small size, smooth contour and interface with the aorta, lack of stasis or double density, and

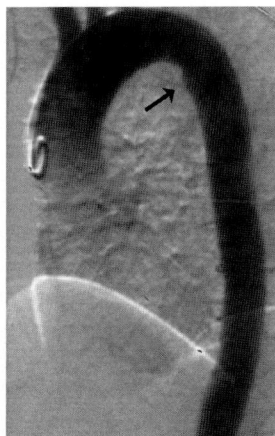

Fig. 4. LAO thoracic arch aortogram demonstrates a prominent ductus bump (*arrow*).

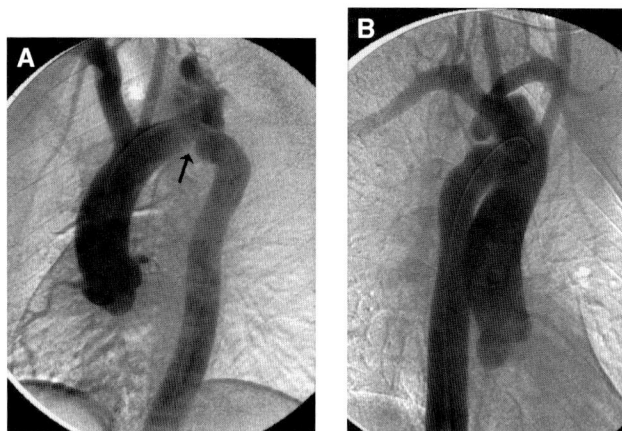

Fig. 5. Right posterior oblique (*A*) and left posterior oblique (*B*) aortograms demonstrate chronic coarctation of the thoracic aorta (*arrow*). Large well collaterals are seen in the region of the left subclavian artery (opposite the arrow).

the identification of a small vessel extending from the apex of the infundibulum [Fig. 7].

Aortic branches

Intercostal, inferior phrenic, subcostal, and internal mammary arteries are the parietal branches of the thoracic aorta. Usually, nine pairs of intercostals arteries arise from the posterior aorta. The first two intercostal arteries are supplied from the highest intercostals arteries, typically branches of the costocervical trunk of the subclavian arteries. The subcostal arteries run below the twelfth ribs. The inferior phrenic arteries arise from the thoracic aorta and supply the posterior part of the upper surface of the diaphragm. The intercostal arteries have anterior and posterior rami. The anterior rami are supplied by the internal mammary or musculo-

phrenic arteries. The internal mammary arteries arise from the subclavian arteries and supply the first six intercostals arteries, whereas the musculophrenic arteries supply the caudal intercostal arteries.

The internal mammary and intercostal arteries lie just inside the rib cage and outside the pleura. They may be injured by blunt or penetrating trauma to the chest wall. With blunt trauma, these vessels usually are injured as the result of fractures of adjacent bones. Alternatively, there may be direct injury by penetrating trauma. When injured, there can be active extravasation, vessel occlusion, arteriovenous fistulization, or dissection.

These injuries can present as an expanding hematoma in the chest wall, but also decompress into the pleural space and cause a hemothorax and associated respiratory embarrassment. The obvious findings of chest wall hematoma on physical exam-

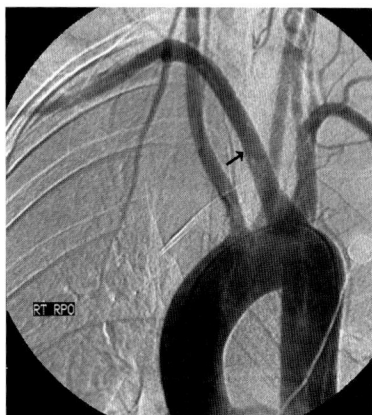

Fig. 6. Aortogram demonstrates an aberrant origin of the right subclavian artery (*arrow*).

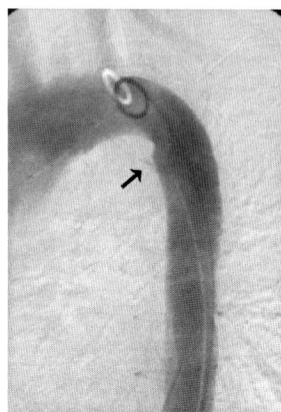

Fig. 7. LAO thoracic aortogram demonstrates a prominent diverticular origin of the bronchial arteries (*arrow*).

ination and hemothorax on chest radiography support the presence of chest wall vascular injury. MDCT units often can diagnose the presence of pseudoaneurysms. Selective angiography should allow for definitive diagnosis and management of these lesions [Fig. 8].

The great vessels arise from the ascending aorta. They comprise the innominate (or brachiocephalic), left common carotid, and left subclavian in the classical branching pattern. These vessels usually originate from the highest point on the arch. They may arise slightly more toward the ascending arch. The number of vessel origins can be variable, and decrease to two or even one as an anatomic variation. The right subclavian arises from the innominate artery and the left arises from the aorta. Hence, the right subclavian has a shorter course. It rises upward and laterally to the medial aspect of the scalene anterior muscle. It ascends slightly above the clavicle. The left subclavian travels through the mediastinum to the medial aspect of the scalene anterior. It also rises above the level of the clavicle. The innominate artery and its continuation as the right common carotid artery and the left common carotid artery arise from the aortic arch and travel through the superior mediastinum.

The great vessels lie in the superior mediastinum where they can be injured by penetrating trauma. Blunt trauma that produces fracture of the sternum or clavicle also can result in injury to the great vessels. When injured, there can be active extravasation, secondary to vessel laceration, arteriovenous fistulization, or vessel truncation. Vessel laceration can result in a pseudoaneurysm or contained hematoma in the superior mediastinum or, in the case of the subclavian, in the base of the neck (zone one). The hematoma can result in compression of the trachea and respiratory embarrassment.

In addition, the vessels can have intimal injury that results in arterial dissection and hemodynamically significant stenosis. Patients who have fracture of the first or second ribs, sternum, or clavicle as detected on physical examination or chest radiograph are at risk for these injuries. Current generation MDCT can diagnose mediastinal hematoma as blood surrounding the great vessel origins in the superior mediastinum. Reformatted evaluation of the great vessels can demonstrate narrowing of these vessels, which raises suspicion for injury. Definitive depiction of injuries can be obtained with aortography and selective angiography of the great vessels.

Thoracic venous injuries

Injuries to the superior vena cava or suprahepatic inferior vena cava are reported infrequently. Injury at either location carries a mortality of more than 60% [13]. The right and left brachiocephalic and subclavian veins make up the large thoracic veins. Although these structures are more superficial than are their accompanying arteries, they are injured less frequently. The venae comitantes to the intercostal, internal mammary, and subcostal veins are among the smaller veins in the thorax. Injuries to these vessels can produce hematoma, hemothorax, or hemomediastinum. The imaging findings on chest radiography and CT mirror those that are seen accompanying the corresponding arterial injury. Often, the definitive diagnosis of thoracic venous injury is obtained by direct visualization at thoracotomy. Because the differential considerations include arterial injury, negative findings on angiography can suggest venous injury as a diagnosis of exclusion.

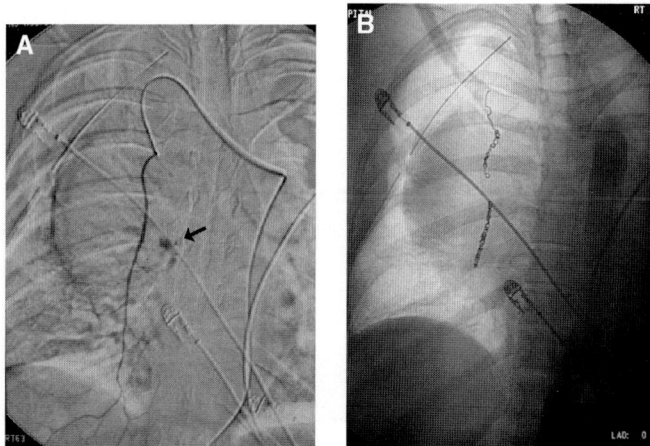

Fig. 8. (A) Initial selective angiogram of the right internal mammary artery demonstrates active extravasation (*arrow*). (B) This lesion was repaired with microcoil embolization.

Interventions

The classic approach to the repair of contained rupture that is due to blunt thoracic trauma is open surgical repair. In young patients without comorbidities or other significant injury, this is the procedure of choice because of its durability and acceptable morbidity and mortality in this population. In older patients, and in the presence of other significant trauma (ie, pelvic, head, spine, extremity trauma) or significant comorbidities, the risk of open surgical repair in the setting of acute trauma is high. Open surgical repair in a stable patient who has a traumatic pseudoaneurysm is associated with a mortality 5% to 18%; most deaths are due to renal failure, blood loss, or congestive heart failure. Open repair in the acute setting and in the presence of comorbidities can increase the mortality significantly [13,14]. Therefore, the recent commercial availability of stent grafts that are designed for the thoracic aorta may be an attractive option for selected patients.

Endovascular treatment for traumatic aortic injury and aortic branch vessel injury is gaining increasing popularity as evidenced by the number of case reports and case series that have appeared in the literature over the past several years [15–25]. The potential advantages of this technique include speed; potential decreased morbidity, such as paraplegia, blood loss, and level of invasiveness; and potential decreased mortality. Dotter [18] reported the first use of endovascular stent grafts in a canine model in 1969. Stent grafting of the thoracic aorta for treatment of aneurysms occurred soon after the initial report on the treatment of an abdominal aortic aneurysm by Parodi and colleagues [19]. Dake and colleagues [20] at Stanford performed the initial work that validated the safety and feasi-

bility of the procedure for aneurysm disease in the thoracic aorta. Their successful use of the "elephant trunk" technique was translated to the use of stent grafts in the treatment of thoracic aortic aneurysms [Fig. 9] [21–23].

The use of endovascular techniques in blunt and penetrating trauma is likely to expand because of the significant advantages that these techniques offer over open repair. Endovascular techniques are associated with decreased anesthetic time and blood loss [24]. Penetrating and blunt trauma, in addition to vascular injury, may result in significant tissue damage and site contamination, which makes a remote entry site for repair attractive [25]. Despite the success of endovascular techniques in the treatment of thoracic aortic aneurysms, significant questions remain about the application of these techniques to the treatment of aortic injury. In particular, this cohort of patients is likely to include significant numbers of young individuals who would bear the anticipated potential longitudinal risk of endoleak and device fatigue or failure. Endovascular treatment has been used as a definitive treatment and as a bridge to open surgical repair. The initial results have been promising; however, long-term data are needed to validate the durability of the technique in traumatic injury, because this subset of patients would be expected to include adults of all ages. Hoffer and colleagues [15] reported a case of endovascular stent grafting that served as a successful bridge to open repair in a young patient. Kasirajan and colleagues [16] reported a series of 27 patients who had TAI; 10 patients underwent open surgical repair and 5 patients had endovascular stent grafting. Overall mortality was lower in the group that had stent grafting (20% versus 50%). There was no paraplegia in any of the survivors. Amabile and colleagues

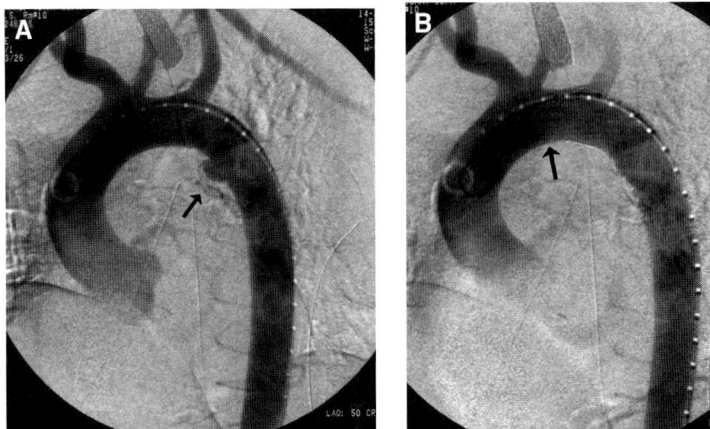

Fig. 9. (*A*) Initial thoracic arch aortogram demonstrates a traumatic pseudoaneurysm (*arrow*). This lesion was repaired with placement of a covered stent. (*B*) Note the noncovered stent apposing the thoracic aorta wall at the level of the left subclavian artery (*arrow*).

[17] reported a series of 20 patients who had acute blunt traumatic aortic rupture over a 5-year period. Eleven patients underwent open surgical repair and 9 had endovascular stent grafting with commercially available devices. In the group that had surgery, one patient died; there were three cases of significant morbidity, including left phrenic nerve palsy, left recurrent laryngeal nerve palsy, and hemopericardium. In the group that had stent grafting, there were no significant periprocedural complications, including paraplegia, and no patient required conversion to open repair. Pseudoaneurysm exclusion was documented in all patients with a mean follow-up of 15.1 months (range 3–41 months).

Intercostal, internal mammary, and subcostal arteries injuries can result in significant chest wall hematoma and hemothorax. These lesions can be suspected based on mechanism of injury and clinical findings. Usually, tube thoracostomy is the initial procedure that is performed in the resuscitation unit. Patients who have hemothorax who lose more than 1500 mL of blood are considered candidates for thoracotomy [26]. In some patients who have significant comorbidities or who are hemodynamically stable with lesser amounts of hemorrhage, selective angiography and embolization is a therapeutic option. Alternatively, patients who continue to have significant bleeding after thoracotomy may benefit from selective angiography and embolization [27].

The internal mammary artery supplies the anterior intercostals arteries and should be evaluated in cases of suspected anterior chest wall injuries [Fig. 10]. In addition, the internal mammary artery can suffer iatrogenic injury in conjunction with placement of subclavian central lines [28]. Injuries of the great vessels can result in significant mediastinal hematoma. These lesions require thoracotomy for surgical management. In patients who have significant comorbidities, selective angiography and covered stent placement is a therapeutic

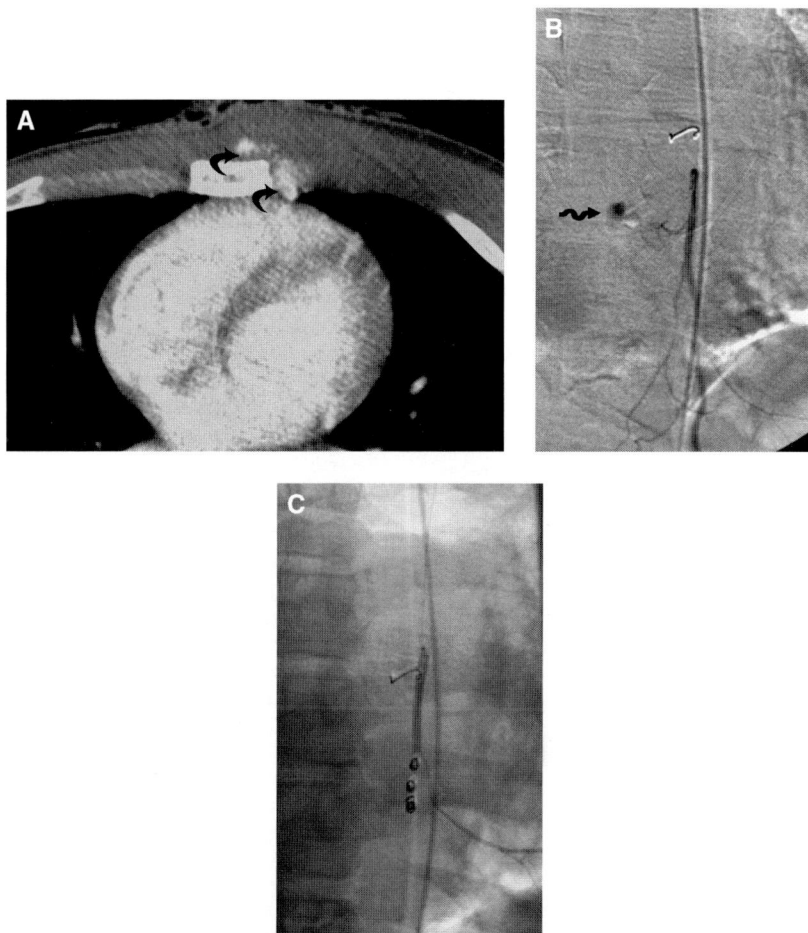

Fig. 10. (*A*) Initial selective angiogram of the subclavian artery demonstrates a traumatic pseudoaneurysm (*curved arrows*). (*B*) This lesion was repaired with placement of a covered stent (Wallgraft). (*C*) Note the bullet and fractured clavicle.

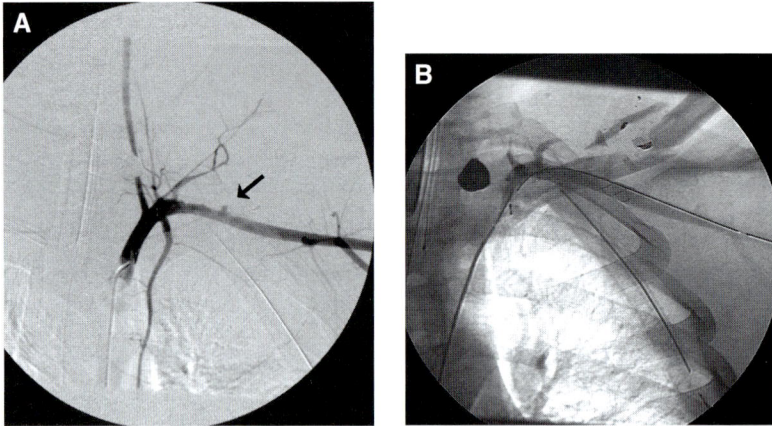

Fig. 11. (*A* and *B*) Vascular stent for intimal injury.

option. Intimal injuries of the great vessels can result in dissections. These injuries can be observed, and if feasible, the patient can be placed on anti-coagulation. Alternatively, vascular stents can be used to repair these vessels [Fig. 11].

Summary

The diagnosis and treatment of traumatic thoracic vascular injury has undergone significant evolution in the past decade, and, in particular, over the past several years. Significant advances in CT provide a rapid, accurate diagnosis in seconds. Continued improvements in stent graft technology have facilitated the use of endovascular techniques for definitive repair of branch vessel and traumatic aortic injury. Angiography, although most often secondary to CT in the diagnostic evaluation, plays a significant role during endovascular repair. In-depth understanding of the technical factors of thoracic angiography is essential to optimize results in the diagnostic and therapeutic settings. Despite the initial optimism over the use of endovascular stent grafts, long-term data on these techniques are lacking. Device size, vascular access, cholesterol embolization, contrast-induced renal failure, radiation injury to patient and operator, endoleak, late rupture, and neointimal hyperplasia are some of the issues that require further investigation and refinements in clinical engineering and management. Despite these obstacles, the use of endovascular techniques in thoracic vascular trauma is likely to continue to expand.

References

[1] Gavant M, Menke P, Fabian T, et al. Blunt traumatic aortic rupture: detection with helical CT of the chest. Radiology 1995;197:125–33.

[2] Mirvis SE, Shanmuganathan K, Miller BH. Traumatic aortic injury: diagnosis with contrast enhanced CT: five-year experience at a major trauma center. Radiology 1996;200:413–22.

[3] Patel NH, Stephens KE, Mirvis SE, et al. Imaging of acute thoracic aortic injury due to blunt trauma: a review. Radiology 1998;209:335–48.

[4] Novelline R, Rhea J, Rao P, et al. Helical CT in emergency radiology. Radiology 1999;213:321–39.

[5] Wicky S, Wintermark M, Denys A, et al. Radiology of blunt chest trauma. Eur Radiol 2000;10: 1524–38.

[6] Dosios TJ, Salemis N, Angouras D, et al. Blunt and penetrating trauma of the thoracic aorta and aortic branches: an autopsy study. J Trauma 2000;49:696–703.

[7] Mattox K, Feliciano D, Burch JM, et al. Five thousand seven hundred sixty cardiovascular injuries in 4459 patients: epidemiologic evolution 1958–1988. Ann Surg 1989;209:698–707.

[8] Chiesa R, Ruettimann M, Lucci C, et al. Blunt trauma of the thoracic aorta: mechanisms involved, diagnosis and management. J Vasc Br 2003;2(3):197–210.

[9] Williams JS, Graff JA, Uku JM, et al. Aortic injury in vehicular trauma. Ann Thorac Surg 1994; 57(3):726–30.

[10] Zehnder M. Delayed posttraumatic rupture of the aorta in a young, healthy individual after closed head injury. Angiology 1956;7:252–67.

[11] Pasic M, Ewert R, Engel M, et al. Aortic rupture and concomitant transaction of the left bronchus after blunt chest trauma. Chest 2000;117: 1508–10.

[12] Esterra A, Mattox KL, Wall MJ. Thoracic aortic injury. Semin Vasc Surg 2000;13(4):345–52.

[13] Mattox KL, Feliciano DV, Burch J, et al. Five thousand seven hundred sixty cardiovascular injuries in 4459 patients: epidemiologic evaluation 1958 to 1987. Ann Surg 1989;209:698–707.

[14] Bacharach JM, Garratt KN, Rooke TW. Chronic traumatic thoracic aneurysm: report of two cases with the question of timing for surgical intervention. J Vasc Surg 1993;17:780–3.

[15] Hoffer E, Karmy-Jones R, Gibson K, et al. Endo-

vascular stent-graft as a bridge to repair of aortic trauma. Emerg Radiol 2001;8(4):233–6.

[16] Kasirajan K, Heffernan D, Langsfeld M. Acute thoracic aortic trauma: a comparison of endoluminal stent grafts with open repair and nonoperative management. Ann Vasc Surg 2003; 17(6):589–95.

[17] Amabile P, Collart F, Gariboldi V, et al. Surgical versus endovascular treatment of traumatic thoracic aortic rupture. J Vasc Surg 2004;40(5):873–9.

[18] Dotter CT. Transluminally placed coilspring endarterial tube grafts. Long-term patency in canine popliteal artery. Invest Radiol 1969;4:329–32.

[19] Parodi JC, Palmaz JC, Barone HD. Transfemoral intraluminal graft implantation for abdominal aortic aneurysm. Ann Vasc Surg 1991;5:491–9.

[20] Dake MD, Miller DC, Semba CP, et al. Transluminal placement of endovascular stent-grafts for the treatment of descending thoracic aortic aneurysms. N Engl J Med 1994;331:1729–34.

[21] Alves C, Fonseca J, Souza J, et al. Endovascular treatment of thoracic disease: patient selection and a proposal of a risk score. Ann Thorac Surg 2002;73:1143–8.

[22] Buffolo E, Palma J, Souza J, et al. Revolutionary treatment of aneurysms and dissection of the descending aorta: the endovascular approach. Ann Thorac Surg 2003;74:S1815–7.

[23] Palma J, Miranda F, Gasques A, et al. Treatment of thoracoabdominal aneurysm with self expandable stent-grafts. Case report. Ann Thorac Surg 2002;74:1685–7.

[24] Marin ML, Veith FJ, Panetta TF. Transluminally placed endovascular stented graft repair for arterial trauma. J Vasc Surg 1994;20:466–73.

[25] Kramer S, Palmer R, Seifarth H, et al. Endovascular grafting of traumatic aortic aneurysms in contaminated fields. J Endovasc Ther 2002;8:262–7.

[26] Karmy-Jones R, Jurkovich GJ, Nathens AB, et al. Timing of urgent thoracotomy for hemorrhage after trauma: a multicenter study. Arch Surg 2001; 136(5):513–8.

[27] Carrillo EH, Heniford BT, Senler SO, et al. Embolization therapy as an alternative to thoracotomy in vascular injuries of the chest wall. Am Surg 1998;64(12):1142–8.

[28] Kulkarni R, Moreyra AE. Left internal mammary artery perforation during Swan-Ganz catheter insertion. Catheter Cardiovasc Diagn 1998;44(3): 317–9.

RADIOLOGIC
CLINICS
OF NORTH AMERICA

Radiol Clin N Am 44 (2006) 251–258

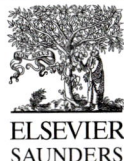

Nonvascular Mediastinal Trauma

Juntima Euathrongchit, MD, Nisa Thoongsuwan, MD,
Eric J. Stern, MD*

- Tracheobronchial injury
  Clinical findings
  Radiologic findings of tracheobronchial injury
- Esophageal injury
  Clinical findings
  Radiologic findings of esophageal trauma
- Tracheoesophageal fistula
  Clinical and radiologic findings of tracheoesophageal fistula
- Thoracic duct injury
  Clinical and radiologic findings of thoracic duct injury
- Miscellaneous
- Summary
- References

This article discusses the radiologic and clinical features of nonvascular mediastinal trauma, and focuses on the tracheobronchial tree, the esophagus, and the thoracic duct. Blunt chest and penetrating trauma account for most of the causes of such nonvascular injuries, but iatrogenic and inhalation injuries are other well-known causes. The injury distribution and clinical manifestations are different for each structure. In our combined experience at a level 1 trauma center, the overall prevalence of injury in each organ is low compared with vascular injuries. As such, and given the frequent nonspecific nature of clinical signs and symptoms of nonvascular mediastinal injuries, the diagnosis often is delayed and results in poor treatment outcome [1].

Tracheobronchial injury

The trachea can be divided arbitrarily at the thoracic inlet into two parts: the cervical trachea and the intrathoracic trachea. The intrathoracic trachea courses in the midline with a slight deviation to the right, which is caused by the aortic arch. It bifurcates into the left and right main bronchi at the tracheal carina at approximately the T4 vertebral body level [Fig. 1]. Both main bronchi are considered mediastinal structures before exiting by way of each hilum to divide into the major lobar bronchi. Tracheobronchial injury (TBI) is reported to occur in only 1% to 3% of patients who have blunt chest trauma, and in 2% to 9% of those who suffer penetrating chest injuries [2,3]. The tracheobronchial tree is protected from injury to some extent by surrounding structures, including the sternum, both lungs, and the great vessels anterolaterally, and the thoracic vertebrae and esophagus, posteriorly. As such, injuries to these surrounding structures are seen in association with TBI. Similarly, given potentially violent injury mechanisms, TBI is associated with closed head injury, spinal cord injury, facial fractures, lung injury, aortic traumatic injury, chest

Harborview Medical Center, Department of Radiology, University of Washington School of Medicine, Seattle, WA, USA
* Corresponding author. Harborview Medical Center, Department of Radiology, University of Washington School of Medicine, Box 359728, Seattle, WA 98104-2499.
E-mail address: estern@u.washington.edu (E.J. Stern).

doi:10.1016/j.rcl.2005.10.001

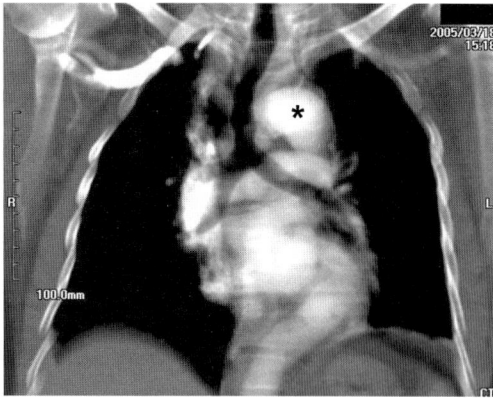

Fig. 1. Coronal reconstruction of the chest CT scan shows normal course of the trachea deviation to the right from the aortic arch (*) and division into the left and right main bronchus at the T4 vertebral level.

wall injury, and abdominal injuries in from 40% to 100% of cases. Combined esophageal and tracheal rupture is seen in approximately 20% of cases of TBI [4].

The two primary causes of trauma to the tracheobronchial tree are penetrating injuries (in ~70% of cases) and blunt trauma (in the remainder) [5]. The other causes of injury, such as foreign body aspiration, inhalation, and iatrogenic injuries from intubation or tracheostomy, are uncommon.

Penetrating trauma is seen more commonly in the cervical, rather than the intrathoracic, trachea [2,6,7], and usually involves the anterior portion of tracheal cartilage and intercartilaginous ligament. For the intrathoracic airway, the distal trachea, just above the carina, and the right lower bronchus are the regions that are involved most commonly [7].

In contrast to penetrating injuries, 80% of cases of blunt TBI occur within 2.5 cm of the carina [7,8]. The right main stem bronchus tends to be injured more commonly than the left because there is less protection from surrounding structures [7,8].

Mechanisms of blunt tracheal injury include the following [7,9,10]:

- Rapid increased intraluminal tracheal pressure from sudden chest compression against a closed glottis, typically during high-speed crashes. In these cases, rupture usually occurs in the membranous portion.
- Separation and stretching of the tracheobronchial tree due to anteroposterior chest compression and hyperextension of the neck or direct crushing of the trachea between the sternum and thoracic vertebrae, causing tracheobronchial disruption.
- Rapid deceleration with shearing forces passed to the relative fixed cricoid cartilage and ca-

rina, resulting in rupture of the trachea and bronchi, especially near the lower tracheal–carinal junction.

A single, transverse rupture of the tracheobronchial tree is seen much more commonly than a longitudinal or complex tear. Iatrogenic tracheal rupture from intubation commonly occurs at the posterior membranous wall. Inhalation injury, such as inspired hot gases, steam, or toxic fumes (eg, chlorine gas), can result in severe damage to the tracheal mucosa, starting with edema and followed by necrosis, ulceration, scar formation, and finally, tracheal stenosis [7].

Clinical findings

Diagnosis of TBI is delayed in up to two thirds of patients because the airway column is maintained by intact peritracheobronchial tissue [7,8]. Common symptoms of TBI are nonspecific and include dyspnea, cough, hoarseness, and hemoptysis. Clinical signs also are nonspecific and include subcutaneous emphysema, hemoptysis, respiratory distress, and hypoxia. Persistent pneumomediastinum; pneumothorax; subcutaneous emphysema, despite treatment; fractures of the first three ribs; or posterior dislocation of sternoclavicular joint are suggestive of, or associated with, TBI [10]. Endo/bronchoscopy can confirm the diagnosis when the clinical and radiologic features are suspected. Late effects of undiagnosed TBI may be tracheobronchial stenosis from granulation tissue and fibrosis that leads to chronic airway obstruction.

Radiologic findings of tracheobronchial injury

The most direct radiologic sign of tracheal rupture is demonstration of a tracheal wall defect or tracheal deformity. These findings are seen far more readily using CT than conventional radiography. Indirect signs of injury include an airway leak into the surrounding mediastinal tissue, an abnormal configuration of the endotracheal tube balloon cuff, and distal lung parenchymal abnormalities (eg, persistent atelectasis). The most common radiologic features of TBI are pneumomediastinum (60%) and pneumothorax (≤70%) that result from air escaping through a tracheal tear into the mediastinum and pleural space [11]. Persistent subcutaneous emphysema, pneumothorax, or atelectasis, despite appropriate therapy, should be considered suspicious for TBI in the proper clinical setting.

Deviation of an endotracheal tube from its expected course, and focal overdistension of the endotracheal tube balloon cuff or protrusion of the balloon through a tracheal laceration are highly suggestive radiologic findings for tracheal injury [Figs. 2 and 3] [9]. The lung distal to the injury

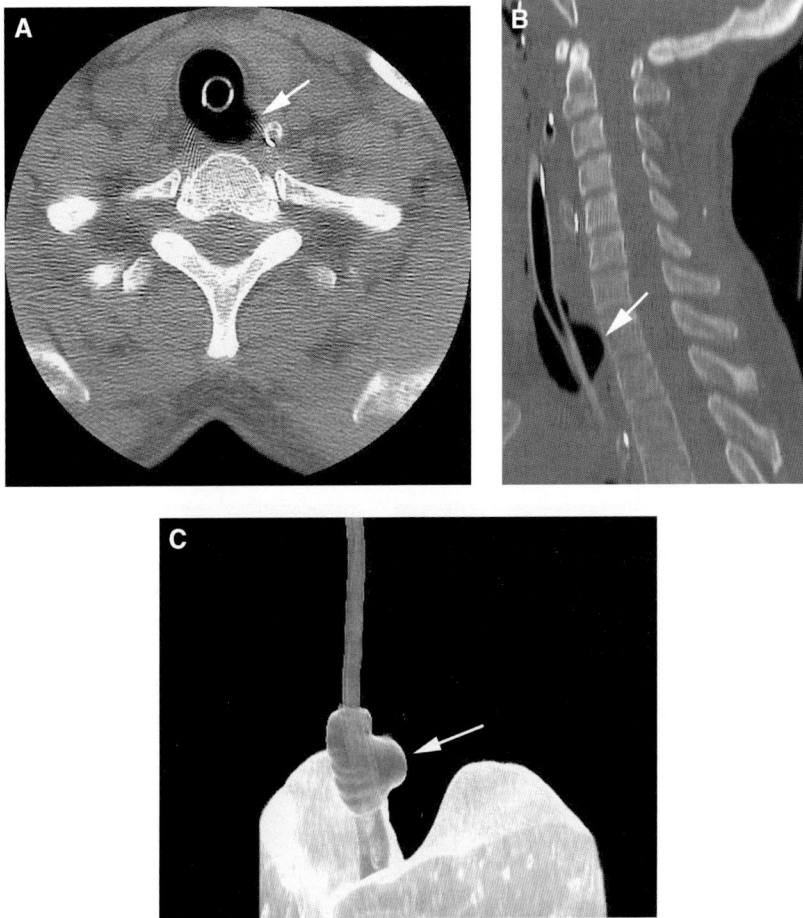

Fig. 2. Tracheal rupture from a high-speed vehicle accident. (*A*) The axial CT scan of the cervical spine shows the focal left posterolateral protrusion of the endotrachial tube balloon cuff (*arrow*). (*B*) The sagittal CT scan of the cervical spine again shows the focal protrusion of the balloon cuff (*arrow*). (*C*). With the three-dimensional reconstruction, the abnormal figure of the balloon cuff is demonstrated well (*arrow*).

can be atelectatic, especially with complete disruption of the airway. The distal collapsed lung will "fall" to the most dependent portion of the pleural space, which produces the so-called "fallen lung sign." Although essentially pathognomonic for the diagnosis of TBI, it is a rare finding [10,11].

Whereas conventional chest radiograph is the initial imaging study for the evaluation of blunt chest trauma, and typically establishes the diagnoses of pneumothorax and pneumomediastinum, the direct diagnosis of TBI is made more much confidently and commonly with CT [9]. Multidetector CT (MDCT) has improved markedly our ability to make this diagnosis, particularly when supplemented by the use of thin-slice collimation, multiplanar reformation, mini–maximum intensity projection rendering, and virtual CT bronchoscopy. The increasing use of screening chest CT in patients who have blunt chest trauma should increase the

number of patients who have TBI who are diagnosed in the acute trauma setting.

Esophageal injury

The esophagus can be divided into three portions: cervical, thoracic, and intra-abdominal. The intrathoracic esophagus is located along the right lateral descending aorta in the middle mediastinum, behind the trachea and in front of the thoracic spine. Protected by the thoracic cage, the incidence of esophageal injury from external chest trauma is rare, typically less than 1% [4,12,13]. The most common cause of esophageal perforation is medical procedures [14,15], such as endoscopy and dilation procedures. Typically, these procedures are performed for esophageal pathology that results in a weaker wall that is more prone to perforation. The remaining causes of esophageal injury include

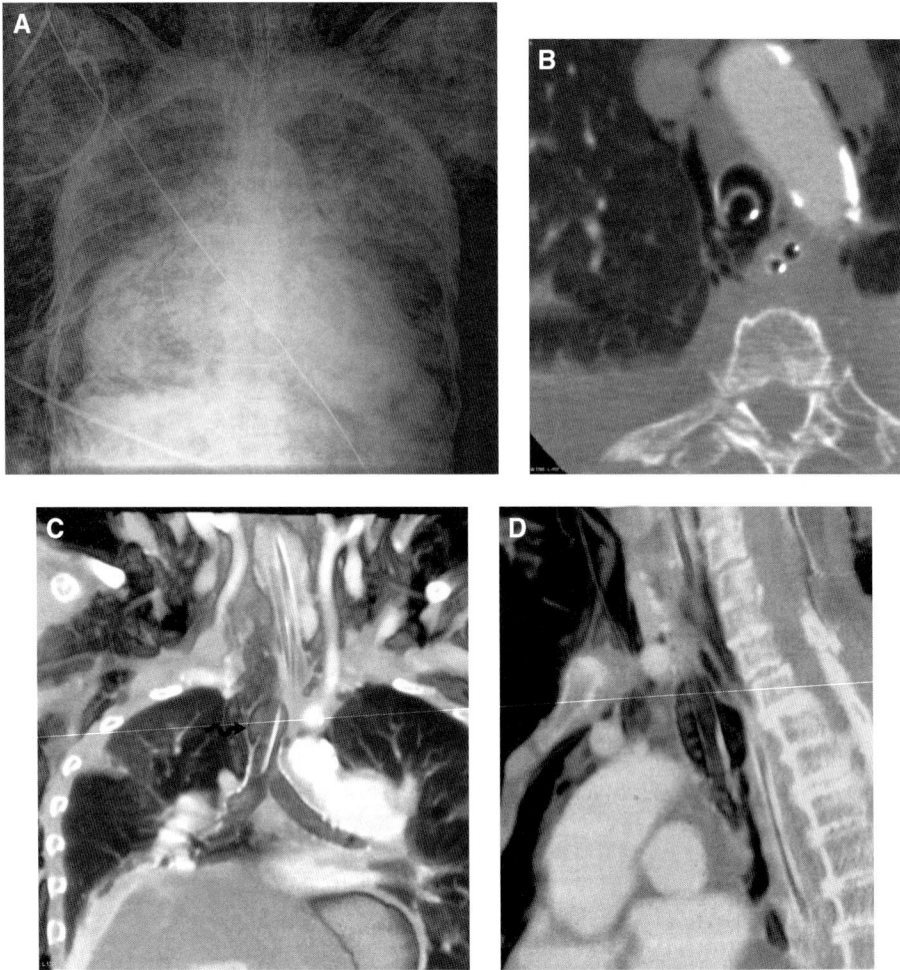

Fig. 3. Tracheal rupture after blunt trauma. (*A*) Admission chest radiograph of elderly woman shows diffuse soft tissue air and huge hiatal hernia. (*B*) CT shows air surrounding thoracic trachea with apparent bulging of endotracheal balloon posteriorly. (*C* and *D*). Coronal and sagittal volume rendered images confirm endotracheal balloon bulging through membranous tracheal tear (*arrow* in *C*).

certain toxic ingestions, emetic injury (Boerhaave's syndrome), and external penetrating trauma.

Penetrating esophageal injuries result mainly from gun shot, shotgun, and stab wounds [16]. Penetrating and blunt esophageal ruptures often are associated with injury to the surrounding organs, such as heart, great vessels, trachea, and spine [17].

Clinical findings

Esophageal injuries have a high morbidity and mortality, and early diagnosis and treatment improve outcome. Symptoms and signs of esophageal injury are dependent on the depth of esophageal wall involvement. The most common symptom of esophageal injury is retrosternal chest pain. Other nonspecific symptoms include dysphagia, odynophagia, pleuritic chest pain, and dyspnea. Signs of full-thickness tear without tracheal trauma include

subcutaneous emphysema, pneumomediastinum, pneumothorax, and demonstration of gastric contents in pleural fluid. Most cases of blunt or penetrating esophageal injury are delayed in diagnosis, which leads to a poor outcome [4,16].

Radiologic findings of esophageal trauma

Patients who have a penetrating injury track through the mediastinum should be evaluated by esophagography, starting with water-soluble contrast media, and if negative, followed by barium swallow; the higher density contrast allows detection of smaller lesions or contrast leaks. Flexible fiber optic or rigid esophagoscopy also can be performed with a diagnostic sensitivity that ranges from 50% to 90% [4].

The depth of esophageal penetration directly affects radiologic findings. In superficial penetrating injury, esophagography will not demonstrate a tear easily; however, if the injury extends to the lumen, a full-thickness perforation potentially produces pneumomediastinum, pneumothorax, pleural effusion, and leakage of contrast medium during a swallowing study. Malposition of a surgical appliance (eg, stent) or demonstration of a foreign body in or near the course of the esophagus on radiography indicates a potential esophageal perforation. Progressive leakage of esophageal fluid content with superimposed inflammation and infection gradually alters the mediastinal contour and produces widening and indistinct borders. The anatomic position of the esophagus in the thorax results in preferential injury patterns; injury to the superior two thirds usually results in

right pleural effusion, whereas injury of the lower one third results in a left pleural effusion [18].

The chest radiograph, as the usual initial imaging examination to evaluate suspected esophageal perforation, is used to demonstrate air collections in the mediastinum and subcutaneous soft tissues [Fig. 4]. For confirmation and localization of the site of rupture, contrast study of the esophagus can be performed under fluoroscopy with complimentary conventional radiographs. CT can readily show a small leak of contrast material from the esophagus that may be difficult to visualize on conventional radiography, and can detect a small metallic foreign body from accidental ingestion [17]. Other CT abnormalities include extraluminal air, periesophageal fluid, and esophageal thicken-

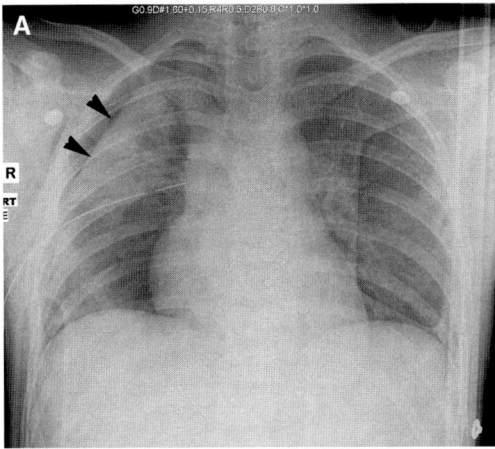

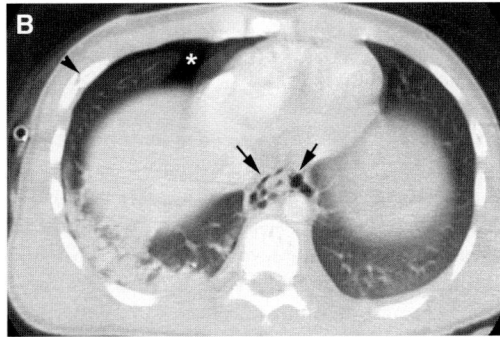

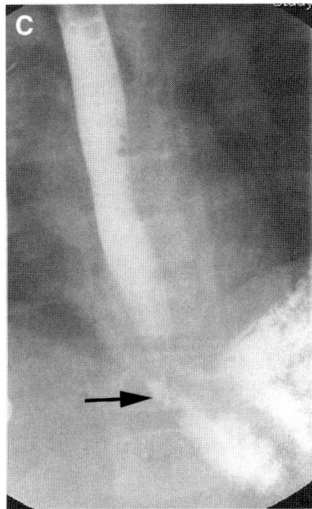

Fig. 4. Esophageal rupture from an all-terrain vehicle accident. (*A*) Chest radiograph shows the right pneumothorax (arrowheads) with the chest tube. The lung contusion at the right lung apex also is noted. (*B*) CT scan of the chest shows air leakage around the esophagus (*arrows*). The right pneumothorax (*) and the right rib fracture (arrowhead) also are demonstrated. (*C*) The esophagography confirms the leakage at the esophagogastric junction (*arrow*).

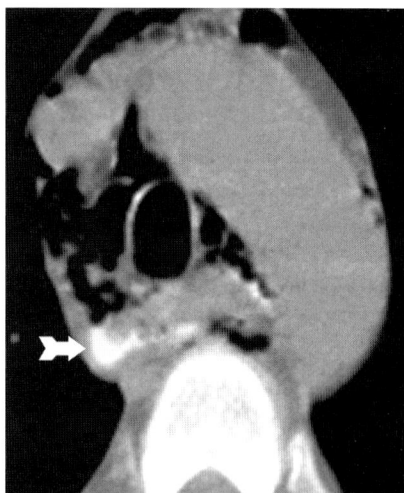

Fig. 5. Esophageal contrast leak. CT was performed after esophagram for penetrating mediastinal injury and shows leak of contrast from the esophagus (*arrow*). Pneumomediastinum is observed and the trachea had a full-thickness injury at surgery. (*From* Mirvis SE. Diagnostic imaging of thoracic trauma. In: Mirvis SE, Shanmuganathan K, editors. Imaging in trauma and critical care. 2nd edition. Philadelphia: WB Saunders; 2003. p. 297–367).

ing that can be clues to esophageal perforation [see Figs. 4 and 5]. Recently, CT has played an increasing role in evaluating esophageal injury because it has come into general use as a common method to evaluate patients who have acute chest pain. CT techniques include imaging with and without intravenous contrast medium injection and, when possible, distending the esophagus with water and ingestion of effervescent granules [19,20].

Tracheoesophageal fistula

Acquired tracheoesophageal fistula after chest trauma is rare, and occurs in just 0.2% of patients who have blunt chest injury [7,21]. Most cases involve young adult patients. In cases of penetrating trauma, injury usually involves the trachea and esophagus [22].

Typically, the mechanism of the blunt traumatic tracheoesophageal fistula is a compression of the trachea and esophagus between the sternum and the vertebrae, which results in injury to the membranous portion of the trachea and the anterior esophageal wall. Because most young patients have a highly elastic chest wall, concurrent fracture of the thoracic cage is infrequent. The most common traumatic cause of tracheoesophageal fistula is long-term use of an endotracheal tube and nasogastric tube, with esophageal and tracheal wall is-

chemia producing focal necrosis of the esophageal and tracheal walls and subsequent formation of a fistula [21,23].

Clinical and radiologic findings of tracheoesophageal fistula

The most common site of a tracheoesophageal fistula is at or just above the carina. Classic symptoms and signs are evidence of pneumonia or coughing after swallowing that occur in the 3 to 10 days after chest trauma [23,24]. Esophagography and CT can diagnose and demonstrate the fistula location directly. Otherwise, radiologic findings are indirect, and include pneumonia, gaseous dilatation of the esophagus, pneumomediastinum, and subcutaneous emphysema.

Thoracic duct injury

The thoracic duct is a lymphatic drainage system that arises from the cisterna chyli, passes into the thoracic cavity by way of the aortic hiatus, and courses to the right side of the spine between the azygos vein and the aorta. At the carinal level, the course of the thoracic duct changes to the left—just lateral to the left side of the trachea—and is directed between the esophagus and the left subclavian artery, where it drains into the venous system at the junction of the left brachiocephalic and internal jugular veins. Understanding this course helps to locate the points of potential injury, because the lower third of the duct lies mainly to the right of midline and leads to right-sided chylothorax, as opposed to injury to the upper thoracic portion, which causes a left-sided chylothorax [25,26]. Bilateral chylothoraces may be seen when injury occurs near the carina. Isolated external penetrating and nonpenetrating thoracic duct injuries are rare and usually occur in association with the vascular or tracheoesophageal injury [27].

Proposed mechanisms of blunt thoracic duct rupture include shearing of lymphatic channels from hyperflexion and extension of the vertebral column, and disruption of the chyle-containing lymphatic system from stretching and tearing motion during acute compression [28].

Clinical and radiologic findings of thoracic duct injury

Thoracic duct injury results in a chylothorax or chylopericardium. Prolonged leakage of lymph may lead to nutritional deficiencies, respiratory dysfunction, and immunosuppression with a mortality of up to 50% [29]. Chylous effusions contain a high triglyceride content—greater than 110 mg/dL—that produces a milky appearance [25]. Demonstration of a chylothorax or chylous fluid from a surgical wound is most likely due to thoracic duct perforation [26]. If chylothorax is noted after blunt chest trauma, esophageal injury should be sought carefully [4].

Lymphangiography is the imaging procedure of choice to diagnose and localize a laceration point. Abnormal lymphangiography shows leakage of contrast from the thoracic duct, a lymphocele, or lymphatic obstruction. An indirect sign of leakage that is seen on CT is a low-attenuation (negative Hounsfiled units) intrathoracic fluid collection [1].

Miscellaneous

The remaining traumatic nonvascular mediastinal structural injuries are seen rarely, except as case reports. Phrenic nerve injury may be seen after chest surgery, especially cardiac surgery, thoracotomy, or laparotomy [30,31].

Summary

Although nonvascular mediastinal injuries are rare, they are associated with a high morbidity and mortality and always should be considered in the appropriate clinical setting. Although chest radiographic screening may permit detection of indirect signs of injury to the nonvascular mediastinal structures, CT, particularly MDCT, may allow definitive diagnosis which leads to earlier treatment, and should be obtained with a low threshold in major blunt trauma or penetrating injury that may or definitely involves the mediastinum.

References

[1] Sachs PB, Zelch MG, Rice TW, et al. Diagnosis and localization of laceration of the thoracic duct: usefulness of lymphangiography and CT. AJR Am J Roentgenol 1991;157:703–5.

[2] Lee RB. Traumatic injury of the cervicothoracic trachea and major bronchi. Chest Surg Clin N Am 1997;7:285–304.

[3] Symbas PN, Justicz AG, Ricketts RR. Rupture of the airways from blunt trauma: treatment of complex injuries. Ann Thorac Surg 1992;54:177–83.

[4] Karmy-Jones R, Jurkovich GJ. Blunt chest trauma. Curr Probl Surg 2004;41:211–380.

[5] Huh J, Milliken JC, Chen JC. Management of tracheobronchial injuries following blunt and penetrating trauma. Am Surg 1997;63:896–9.

[6] Baillot R, Dontigny L, Verdant A, et al. Penetrating chest trauma: a 20-year experience. J Trauma 1987;27:994–7.

[7] Stark P. Imaging of tracheobronchial injuries. J Thorac Imaging 1995;10:206–19.

[8] Kiser AC, O'Brien SM, Detterbeck FC. Blunt tracheobronchial injuries: treatment and outcomes. Ann Thorac Surg 2001;71:2059–65.

[9] Chen JD, Shanmuganathan K, Mirvis SE, et al. Using CT to diagnose tracheal rupture. AJR Am J Roentgenol 2001;176:1273–80.

[10] Stern EJ. Airway rupture/laceration. In: Stern EJ, Hunter JC, Mann FA, et al, editors. Trauma radiology companion, methods, guidelines, and imaging fundamentals. Philadelphia: Lippincott-Raven; 1997. p. 130–1.

[11] Karmy-Jones R, Avansino J, Stern EJ. CT of blunt tracheal rupture. AJR Am J Roentgenol 2003; 180:1670.

[12] Asensio JA, Berne J, Demetriades D, et al. Penetrating esophageal injuries: time interval of safety for preoperative evaluation–how long is safe? J Trauma 1997;43:319–24.

[13] Wicky S, Wintermark M, Schnyder P, et al. Imaging of blunt chest trauma. Eur Radiol 2000; 10:1524–38.

[14] Eroglu A, Can Kurkcuogu I, Karaoganogu N, et al. Esophageal perforation: the importance of early diagnosis and primary repair. Dis Esophagus 2004;17:91–4.

[15] Ghahremani GG. Esophageal trauma. Semin Roentgenol 1994;29:387–400.

[16] Asensio JA, Chahwan S, Forno W, et al. Penetrating esophageal injuries: multicenter study of the American Association for the Surgery of Trauma. J Trauma 2001;50:289–96.

[17] Bastos RB, Graeber GM. Esophageal injuries. Chest Surg Clin N Am 1997;7:357–71.

[18] Kshettry VR, Bolman III RM. Chest trauma. Assessment, diagnosis, and management. Clin Chest Med 1994;15:137–46.

[19] Fadoo F, Ruiz DE, Dawn SK, et al. Helical CT esophagography for the evaluation of suspected esophageal perforation or rupture. AJR Am J Roentgenol 2004;182:1177–9.

[20] Lee S, Mergo PJ, Ros PR. The leaking esophagus: CT patterns of esophageal rupture, perforation, and fistulization. Crit Rev Diagn Imaging 1996; 37:461–90.

[21] Sebastian MW, Wolfe WG. Traumatic thoracic fistulas. Chest Surg Clin N Am 1997;7:385–400.

[22] Feliciano DV, Bitondo CG, Mattox KL, et al. Combined tracheoesophageal injuries. Am J Surg 1985;150:710–5.

[23] Layton TR, DiMarco RF, Pellegrini RV. Tracheoesophageal fistula from nonpenetrating trauma. J Trauma 1980;20:802–5.

[24] Stephens TW. Traumatic tracheo-oesophageal fistula following steering-wheel type of injury. Br J Surg 1965;52:370–2.

[25] Hillerdal G. Chylothorax and pseudochylothorax. Eur Respir J 1997;10:1157–62.

[26] Whiteford MH, Abdullah F, Vernick JJ, et al. Thoracic duct injury in penetrating neck trauma. Am Surg 1995;61:1072–5.

[27] Worthington MG, de Groot M, Gunning AJ, et al. Isolated thoracic duct injury after penetrating chest trauma. Ann Thorac Surg 1995;60:272–4.

[28] Skala J, Witte C, Bruna J, et al. Chyle leakage after blunt trauma. Lymphology 1992;25: 62–8.

[29] Kumar S, Kumar A, Pawar DK. Thoracoscopic management of thoracic duct injury: is there a place for conservatism? J Postgrad Med 2004;50: 57–9.

[30] DeVita MA, Robinson LR, Rehder J, et al. Incidence and natural history of phrenic neuropathy occurring during open heart surgery. Chest 1993;103:850–6.

[31] Cullen ML. Pulmonary and respiratory complications of pediatric trauma. Respir Care Clin N Am 2001;7:59–77.

RADIOLOGIC
CLINICS
OF NORTH AMERICA

Radiol Clin N Am 44 (2006) 259–271

ELSEVIER
SAUNDERS

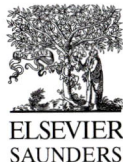

Acute Pulmonary Embolism: Imaging in the Emergency Department

Paul G. Kluetz, MD[a], Charles S. White, MD[b],*

- Chest radiography
- Serum markers
- Nuclear ventilation-perfusion scintigraphy
- Conventional pulmonary angiography
- CT pulmonary angiography
- Magnetic resonance pulmonary
  angiography
- Ultrasound
- Echocardiography in the unstable patient
- Special considerations
  Pregnancy
  Increased use
- Summary
- References

Venous thromboembolic disease (VTE) represents a continuum of disease from deep venous thrombosis (DVT) to pulmonary embolism (PE). PE is a common and deadly illness with a reported annual U.S. incidence of between 0.7 and 1 case/1000 population [1,2]. PE continues to affect hospitalized patients, with an estimated 170,000 cases of DVT or PE per year [3]. Autopsy studies have shown that up to 10% of in-hospital deaths are caused by PE [4,5]. All-cause mortality of patients with the diagnosis of PE was reported to be as high as 17.4% at 3 months [6], and likely accounts for 100,000 to 200,000 annual deaths. Treatment with unfractionated or low molecular weight heparin reduced mortality from PE to as low as 0.6% to 1.0% [7]; this makes accurate diagnosis a matter of life or death.

Despite its high prevalence, acute PE is difficult to diagnose. It was reported that 62% to 83% of autopsy-proven PEs were not diagnosed clinically [4,8]. History and physical examination findings for PE or DVT are neither sensitive nor specific [9,10]. For instance, one study revealed that as few as 19% of those who had autopsy-proven PE

had symptomatic DVT [5]. Currently, the diagnostic work-up of PE uses a combination of clinical scoring algorithms, serum tests, ECG, chest radiography (CXR), and further diagnostic imaging studies. Current imaging modalities include nuclear ventilation-perfusion (V/Q) scanning, lower extremity ultrasound, CT pulmonary angiography (CTPA), and, less frequently, echocardiography, magnetic resonance and conventional pulmonary angiography (PA).

Chest radiography

A common misconception is that the CXR frequently is normal in PE. On the contrary, in the Prospective Investigation of Pulmonary Embolism Diagnosis [PIOPED] study, only 12% of the radiographs from nearly 400 patients were interpreted as normal [11]. A prospective observational study by Elliott and colleagues [12] further characterized the radiographic abnormalities that are seen in PE. Cardiomegaly was the most common finding (occurred in 29% of patients), and was followed by pleural effusion, elevated hemidiaphragm, pul-

[a] Department of Internal Medicine, University of Maryland, Baltimore, MD, USA
[b] Department of Diagnostic Radiology, University of Maryland School of Medicine, Baltimore, MD, USA
* Corresponding author. Department of Diagnostic Radiology, University of Maryland School of Medicine, 655 West Baltimore Street, Baltimore, MD 21201.
E-mail address: cwhite@umm.edu (C.S. White).

doi:10.1016/j.rcl.2005.10.004

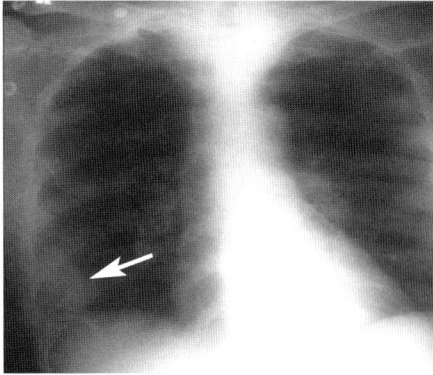

Fig. 1. Posteroanterior upright CXR revealing focal peripheral consolidation in the right lower lobe (*arrow*). This is the classic "Hampton's hump" sign that is seen in a minority of patients who have PE, and is suggestive of pulmonary infarction in the lung parenchyma supplied by the artery occluded by embolus.

monary arterial enlargement, and parenchymal pulmonary infiltrates. Each of these findings is nonspecific. The classic CXR findings of PE include focal subpleural density (Hampton's hump) [Fig. 1] and regional oligemia (Westermark's sign); however, these signs also suffer from poor specificity and even worse sensitivity. Despite being a poor screening test for PE, CXR continues to be used as a preliminary diagnostic test. The examination is safe and inexpensive and may identify unrelated and possibly deadly causes of chest pain, such as pneumothorax. Additionally, CXR should be used for proper interpretation of nuclear V/Q scans if that examination is indicated.

Serum markers

A key component of the diagnostic work-up for PE involves the use of blood tests. Traditionally, arterial blood gas measurements were obtained to assess for an increase in the alveolar–arterial oxygen gradient. A review of several studies that analyzed this test showed it to be insensitive and nonspecific [13,14]. More recently, the D-dimer test has become a viable screening tool for VTE disease. D-dimer is a by-product of fibrinolysis that is sensitive for VTE with a high negative predictive value [15,16]. Additionally, one study suggested that a quantitative D-dimer level, as well as other clinical signs, can predict the extent of perfusion defects on VQ, and thus, the size of PE [17]. The D-dimer assay has been used in combination with pretest clinical scoring models (eg, Well's criteria), which assess a patient's risk of PE using history and physical examination findings (eg, history of malignancy or recent surgery, heart rate, and evidence of DVT). The use of an accurate and reproducible D-dimer assay with a pretest clinical scoring model, like the Well's criteria, had a negative predictive value as high as 99.5% and can safely rule out VTE without subsequent imaging studies [18,19].

Nuclear ventilation-perfusion scintigraphy

Historically, the V/Q scan has been an important tool in the diagnosis of PE. Typically, V/Q scan results are classified as normal, low, intermediate, and high probability for PE. Patients with high-probability VQ scans warrant anticoagulation [Fig. 2]. Although only a minority of scans are interpreted as normal, this category has excellent negative predictive value; only 0.3% of patients had recurrent PE according to a recent meta-analysis [20]. Furthermore, withholding anticoagulation in those with normal VQ scans was safe [21]. In contrast, the clinical significance of low-probability scans is less certain. Whereas several investigators reported morbidity and mortality from undiag-

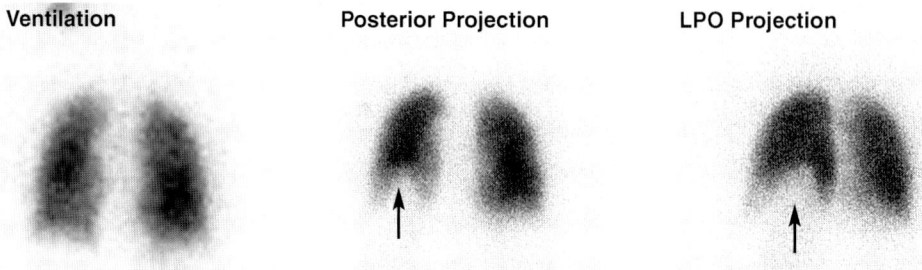

Fig. 2. High-probability V/Q scan obtained with dual head single-photon emission CT using xenon-133 gas and intravenous injection of 4 mCi of technetium–99-m macroaggregated albumin particles. Ventilation is homogeneous; however, left posterior oblique (LPO) and posterior projections of the perfusion scan reveal large defects in the lateral basal and posterior basal segments of the left lower lobe (*arrows*). (Courtesy of Faazia Mahmoud, MD, Baltimore, MD.)

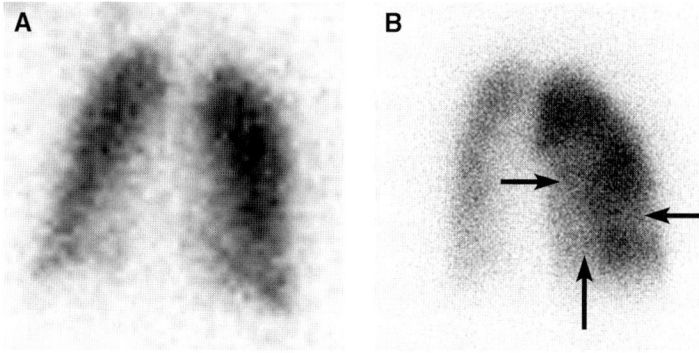

Fig. 3. Intermediate-probability V/Q scan obtained with dual head SPECT using xenon-133 gas and intravenous injection of 4 mCi of technetium–99-m macroaggregated albumin particles. (*A*) Anterior projection of single breath ventilation scan reveals mild decreased ventilation at the bases. (*B*) Right posterior oblique projection of perfusion scan shows multiple defects in the right lung (*arrows*). CXR revealed a right lower lobe infiltrate. This combination was read as intermediate probability. (Courtesy of Faazia Mahmoud, MD, Baltimore, MD.)

nosed PEs in this group [22,23], a more recent series reported no deaths attributed to PE in 536 patients with low-probability scans [24]. Until a greater consensus is reached, it seems evident that a low-probability scan, in the presence of cardio-pulmonary disease or high clinical suspicion for PE, should be evaluated further. The intermediate (indeterminate) probability category is the most problematic [Fig. 3]. In the PIOPED study, nearly 40% of results were classified as indeterminate. PE was present in 33% of this group [10], which mandates further study for those with intermediate VQ results. Some investigators support the use of CTPA after indeterminate or inconclusive VQ scans [25]. The high percentage of intermediate studies is a major limitation of V/Q scanning.

Like any imaging modality, sensitivity and specificity of nuclear VQ scanning depends on the technology that is being used. More recent studies that used advanced nuclear imaging, demonstrated improved sensitivity and specificity for VQ scanning [26]. A recent study by Reinartz and colleagues [27] revealed that VQ scans using single-photon emission CT (SPECT) with ultrafine aerosol was comparable to four-slice tomographic imaging, and exceeded CT in sensitivity, but not in specificity. The investigators noted that the more commonly available conventional planar lung scintigraphy does not compare favorably with CT.

Interobserver agreement has been fair for VQ scans; however, interpretation of nuclear medicine studies can be made more reproducible by using predefined criteria. A 2003 study by Hagen and colleagues [28] found that interobserver agreement was in the 0.65 to 0.79 range; the highest agreement used a predefined interpretation criterion that was developed by Hull.

Despite improvements in technology and interpretation, the VQ scan is limited by indeterminate results, long scan times, and the need to assemble a team to perform the study. The combination of a high number of indeterminate VQ scans and the ability of CTPA to pick up alternative diagnoses has led some investigators to conclude that CTPA confidently establishes a diagnosis more often [26,29,30]. Nonetheless, VQ scanning has a role in the diagnosis of PE. The British Thoracic Society recently recommended that VQ scanning is a reasonable alternative to CTPA if CXR is normal, there is no cardiopulmonary disease, the readers use predefined criteria, and a nondiagnostic result is followed up by further studies [31].

Conventional pulmonary angiography

Conventional PA identifies PE by observation of a filling defect or vessel cutoff [Fig. 4]. Conventional

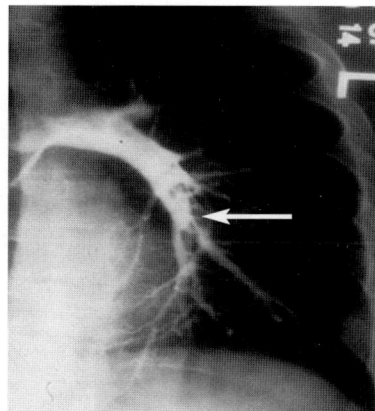

Fig. 4. Conventional invasive PA. Anteroposterior projection of pulmonary angiographic image is coned down to the left lung revealing intraluminal defect and vessel cutoff at the central and segmental portion of the left pulmonary arterial circulation (*arrow*).

angiography is less attractive than other modalities because it is invasive, expensive, regarded by some as dangerous, and requires a team to assemble. Advances in the use of nonionic contrast media and technique have improved the safety of the procedure [32,33]; however, it remains a time consuming examination with a small risk of significant morbidity. Despite long being considered the gold standard for detection of PE, the accuracy of PA continues to be scrutinized. PA lacks sensitivity for detecting subsegmental PE, with reported interreader agreement as low as 66% using data from the PIOPED study [34]. Furthermore, a recent study on porcine models revealed that the sensitivity of PA for subsegmental clot was only 87%, which is similar to that for CT [35]. Although many investigators question the usefulness of conventional PA in the evaluation of acute PE, the technique may play a role in critically ill patients in whom CT has been reported to be less accurate [36]. Additionally, PA offers the advantage of intervention by way of direct thrombus fragmentation in the setting of massive PE [37], but this requires special training and is not available in all settings. As noninvasive modalities improve, the indications for diagnostic conventional angiography are likely to narrow.

CT pulmonary angiography

CTPA is rapidly becoming the first-line imaging modality for PE. Reports of increased use of CTPA for PE in emergency room and in-patient settings confirm the recognition of this modality as an important diagnostic tool for PE [38]. CTPA offers many advantages over competing modalities, including availability, cost-effectiveness, volumetric data acquisition, identification of alternate diagnoses, and the ability to image pelvic and lower extremity veins in the same study. Additionally, CT

can be used in the setting of an abnormal CXR or underlying cardiopulmonary disease, which can make interpretation of nuclear studies challenging. The accuracy and interobserver agreement of CT are well described and compares favorably with other modalities.

CTPA directly visualizes emboli by observation of a filling defect within the enhanced pulmonary arteries [Fig. 5]. Precise techniques reported for CTPA in the literature vary. Our CT protocol uses 100 mL to 150 mL of contrast material with an injection rate of 3 mL/sec. The authors use multislice scanners (16-slice) for evaluation of PE with a protocol that consists of 1- to 2-mm collimation and 50% overlap. We routinely obtain thinslab reformations in axial and coronal planes. The multidetector CT (MDCT) scanners are capable of bolus timing, using a region of interest on the pulmonary arteries. Scanning is initiated automatically when a preselected threshold attenuation value (usually 150 HU) is reached in the pulmonary arteries after contrast injection. Further modifications are necessary for the new generation of 40- and 64-slice scanners.

The advantage of volumetric data acquisition can be realized by using several reformations, including sagittal and coronal planar, curved planar, volume, maximal intensity projection, and paddle wheel views. In particular, the paddle wheel reformation may lead to increased sensitivity for PE [Fig. 6]. In paddle wheel views, planar slab reformations are obtained in multiple planes around a selected horizontal axis pivot point [39]. In a small retrospective study of five patients with known PE, Chiang and colleagues [40] reported that the paddle wheel reformations had a significantly higher percentage of overall detection of PE than did coronal reformations that were obtained with equivalent slab thickness. Further research is needed to de-

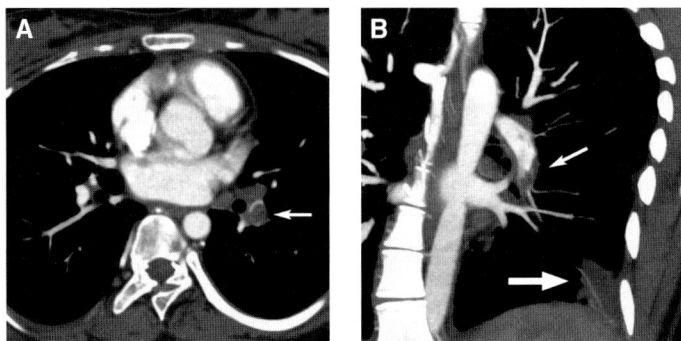

Fig. 5. Contrast-enhanced 16-detector CTPA with maximal intensity projection in axial (*A*) and coronal (*B*) projections. Clot is visualized directly in the left lower lobe pulmonary artery (*small arrows*). A wedge-shaped area of consolidation in the corresponding left lower lobe (*large arrow, B*) is consistent with pulmonary infarct—the CT version of "Hampton's hump."

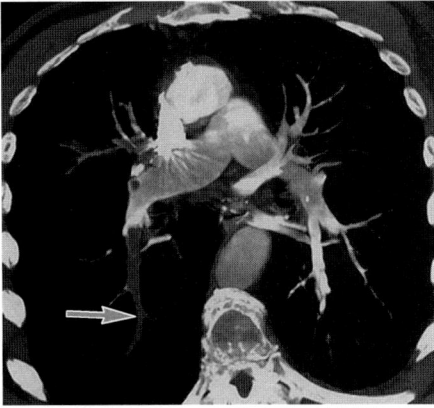

Fig. 6. Contrast-enhanced CTPA using paddle wheel reformation reveals PE in the right segmental pulmonary arterial tree (arrow). The paddle wheel view can depict branching structures like the pulmonary arteries in a more continuous manner from hilum to pleura. (Courtesy of Philippe Boiselle, MD, Boston, MA.)

termine the optimal reformation that will provide the highest sensitivity for PE in the most efficient manner.

Interobserver reliability of CTPA is good with an agreement rate of 74% to 77% [41]. In a 1999 review by Holbert and colleagues [42], this compared favorably with agreement rates of 39% and 46% for V/Q and conventional PA, respectively. In terms of accuracy, CTPA exhibited excellent sensitivity and specificity for central and segmental PE [43,44]; however, like PA and magnetic resonance PA (MRPA), CT is least sensitive in the assessment of small emboli that are isolated to the subsegmental vessels [45]. Baile and colleagues [35] compared PA with spiral CT with 1-mm collimation using a porcine model as the gold standard. In this study, the overall sensitivities of CT and PA were equal, and it was concluded that CTPA is comparable to PA for the detection of emboli. There was no difference between the two techniques in the detection of subsegmental emboli. Further validity of the accuracy of CTPA in the detection of PE is forthcoming with the PIOPED II trial. Rather than using conventional PA as a gold standard, this trial is using a combination of multiple imaging modalities to determine whether patients have PE [46].

The fact that PA and CT lack sensitivity for isolated subsegmental emboli has raised the question of the clinical relevance of these findings. To elucidate this, recent studies have focused on outcome-based measures. Multiple studies using 3- and 6-month follow-up after negative CT showed that the incidence of VTE or PE in those patients is low. Negative predictive values from these studies have been in the 96% to 99% range [47–51]. In a study by Goodman and colleagues [21], the follow-up

results for CT were not significantly different from low-probability and normal VQ scans. In addition, unlike VQ scans, underlying pulmonary disease does not seem to affect the negative predictive value of CTPA [52]. Musset and colleagues [53] added pretest clinical probability to their algorithm for withholding anticoagulation. For patients with low or intermediate clinical probability, negative CT, and negative ultrasound of lower extremities, only 1.8% had VTE at 3-month follow-up. A multicenter prospective trial by van Strijen and colleagues [54] assessed 3-month clinical follow-up after negative CT and serial compression ultrasound. The incidence of VTE in this group was only 0.4%. These data compare favorably with PA outcome data from 1-year follow-up which revealed a 1.6% rate of PE in those not who were anticoagulated after normal angiography [55]. Many investigators believe that there seems to be adequate support to withhold anticoagulation after a negative CT scan in the absence of signs or symptoms of DVT.

A further advantage of spiral CT over traditional techniques for evaluation of PE is its ability to suggest an alternative diagnosis [Fig. 7]. Kim and colleagues [56] found CT useful in suggesting a different etiology in 57 of 85 (67%) patients who did not have PE. Other investigators cited alternative diagnosis rates of between 25% and 53% [29,47,54]. A recent multicenter study by Richman and colleagues [57] looked at the clinical significance of alternative diagnoses. Seven percent of patients that were seen in the emergency department with CT scans that were negative for PE had an alternate diagnosis that required "specific and immediate action." Diagnoses included infiltrate or

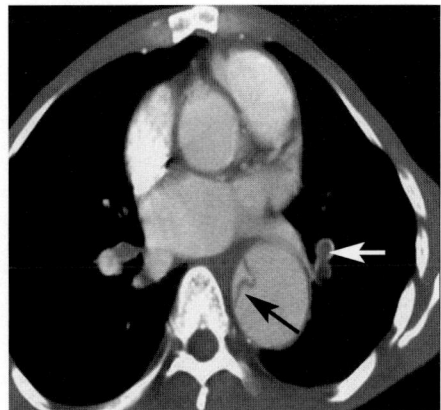

Fig. 7. Axial projection of contrast-enhanced 16-detector CTPA reveals PE in the left segmental pulmonary circulation (white arrow). An important benefit of CTPA is the identification of alternate or additional diagnoses; in this case, aortic dissection was identified (black arrow).

consolidation that suggested pneumonia (81%), aortic aneurysm or dissection (7%), and mass that suggested undiagnosed malignancy (7%). If these data are generalized, CTPA may have the ability to discover aortic aneurysm or dissection in 1 out of every 200 negative PE studies that are performed in the emergency setting. The incidental finding of clinically relevant disease is a powerful benefit to this modality.

Cost is a concern when attempting to find the ideal test for a disease entity. Recent studies suggested that CT is the most cost-effective modality to diagnose PE. For instance, after a careful cost analysis of several diagnostic algorithms, Doyle and colleagues [58] reported that CT scanning is the least expensive imaging technique for the diagnosis of PE per life saved.

An additional use of spiral CT is its ability to image the deep venous system to detect thrombus—a procedure that is termed CT venography (CTV).

Like ultrasound evaluation of the lower extremities, the presence of thrombus indicates a high risk that PE has or will occur [Fig. 8]. This evaluation is performed with the same bolus as the pulmonary artery study after a delay of approximately 2 minutes. CTV has the added benefit, over ultrasound, of imaging the pelvic veins [Fig. 9]. Multiple studies showed good sensitivity of CTV when compared with ultrasound of the lower extremities [59–61]. Additional studies are warranted to determine whether combined CTPA/CTV can improve the diagnostic yield of CTPA alone.

Despite its many benefits, CTPA has several limitations. Many interpretation pitfalls [Figs. 10 and 11] require considerable expertise in CTPA interpretation [62]. The impact of expertise is not trivial; one study reporting that the interobserver agreement between general radiologists and experienced chest radiologists was 0.76 and 0.93, respectively [63]. Technical hurdles that are caused by

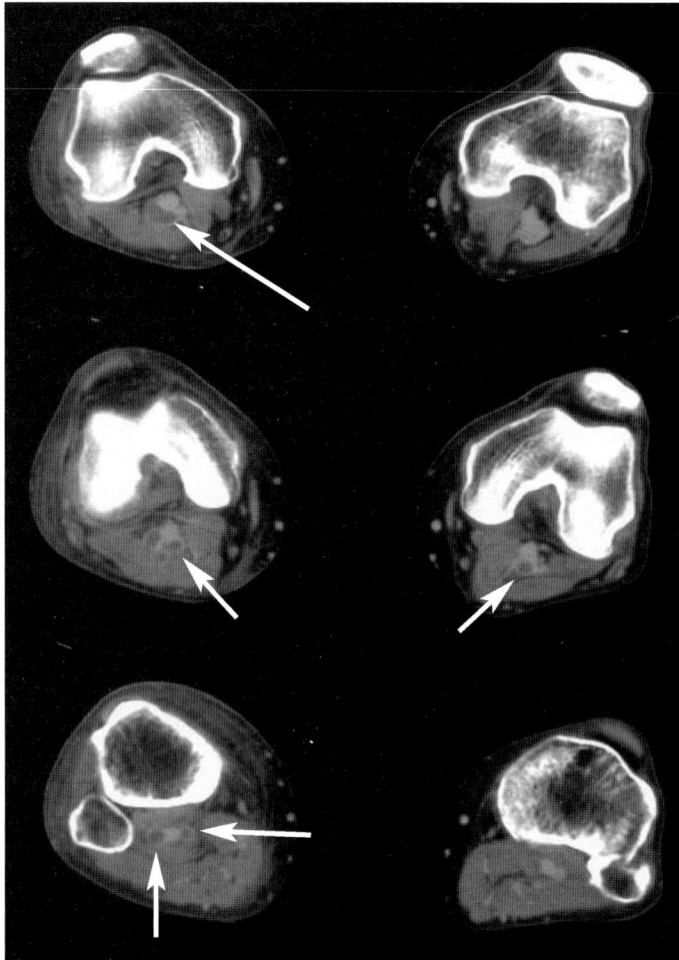

Fig. 8. Axial projections of contrast-enhanced 16-detector CTV reveal bilateral deep venous thrombosis in the area of the popliteal fossa. CTV identifies clot by direct visualization (*arrows*) in the same manner as CTPA.

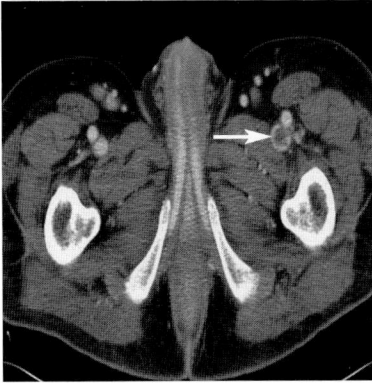

Fig. 9. Axial image of contrast-enhanced 16-detector CTV reveals pelvic venous thrombosis in the left iliac venous circulation (*arrow*). The evaluation of pelvic veins is a significant advantage of CTV over ultrasonography.

respiratory motion artifact; intrathoracic hardware, including mechanical valves and pacemakers; bolus timing; and scanning artifacts also must be considered. Additionally, CTPA requires a large-bore peripheral IV that can be problematic in obese patients or those who use intravenous drugs. Finally, patients who have renal insufficiency or contrast allergies may not be good candidates for CTPA.

Magnetic resonance pulmonary angiography

MRPA and magnetic resonance perfusion [Fig. 12] are other noninvasive imaging modalities that show promise in the evaluation of acute PE. MRPA shares with CT the ability to acquire volumetric data of the lung vasculature with subsequent reconstruction and visualization in multiple planes. Unlike CT, MRPA provides no ionizing radiation to the patient. In addition, the use of gadolinium provides a less nephrotoxic alternative to iodinated contrast material, and seems to produce fewer allergic reactions. The examination also can include lower extremity and pelvic vasculature for the assessment of DVT, and can identify alternative diagnoses. Drawbacks to MRPA, as compared with CT, include limited availability, longer acquisition time, poor signal-to-noise ratio, respiratory and cardiac motion artifacts, and limited spatial resolution. In addition, the examination is contraindicated for some patients with older metallic hardware because of the powerful field strength of MR magnets. Finally, patients who are claustrophobic may need to be sedated to complete the study.

Initial studies of MRPA were disappointing, and revealed reasonable sensitivity but poor specificity for proximal and segmental clots [64,65]. Advances in MR hardware and gadolinium intravenous contrast enhancement have provided better results. Meaney and colleagues [66] reported that three

independent reviewers had sensitivities of 75% to 100% and specificities of 95% to 100% in a 30-patient prospective study that compared MRPA with conventional PA. However, there were no patients in the series with small, more difficult-to-detect subsegmental PE. Multiple studies have documented the difficulty of using MRPA to assess distal segmental and subsegmental emboli. A 1994 study by Loubeyre and colleagues [67] reported that all six patients who had emboli in distal arteries were missed by MRPA when compared with conventional PA. A study by Gupta and col-

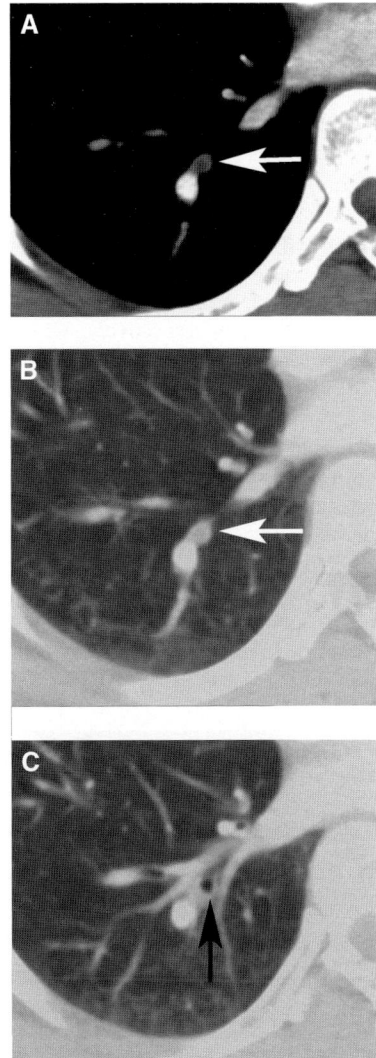

Fig. 10. Axial views of contrast-enhanced 16-detector CTPA coned down over the right lung reveals what appears to be a filling defect (*arrow, A*) in or near a right-sided segmental vessel using tissue windows. On lung windows, the abnormality is seen again (*arrow, B*); however, on the adjacent axial slice, continuity of the abnormality with an airway (*arrow, C*) reveals that the finding is a mucous plug.

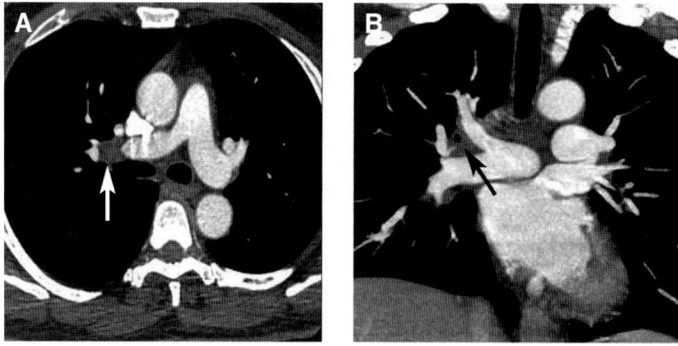

Fig. 11. Axial view (*A*) of a contrast-enhanced 16-detector CTPA reveals what appears to be a filling defect (*white arrow*) in the right main pulmonary artery. Careful examination of this study in axial and coronal (*B*) projections reveals that the abnormality is hilar lymphadenopathy (*black arrow*), another common CTPA pitfall.

leagues [68] revealed that four of five subsegmental clots were missed when compared with conventional PA. More recently, a prospective study of 141 patients by Oudkerk and colleagues [69] reported accuracy approaching that of CT for gadolinium-enhanced MRPA in the identification of proximal and segmental PE. In this study, sensitivity for subsegmental, segmental, and central PE was 40%, 84%, and 100% respectively, which again highlights the difficulty of this modality in detecting subsegmental clot. The accuracy of MRPA, like that of CT, is dependent on the radiologist's training. In one study, the sensitivity and specificity of MRPA improved from 46% to 71% and 90% to 97%, respectively, when interpreted by a vascular MR-trained radiologist as compared with a general radiologist [70].

In addition to the evaluation of pulmonary arteries, MR imaging of the veins of the pelvis and lower extremities has been described [65]. Sensitivity and specificity of MRA for proximal DVT and extension into the pelvis was reported to be between 94% and 100% and 90% and 100%, respectively [71–73]. Research into newer contrast agents that have longer intravascular half-lives also is promising. The use of these agents may allow for better concentration of contrast in the pulmonary vasculature, which provides better resolution. The newer contrast also may permit the simultaneous imaging of lungs and the pelvic/lower extremity system, much like the combined CTA/CTV. Other advances in MRPA, including functional MR (fMR) imaging V/Q scanning [74], blood-pooling contrast agents (eg, gadomer [75]), and real-time true fast imaging with steady-state precession (TrueFisp) [76], are promising areas of research for MRPA in the evaluation of PE.

Although prospective data on the accuracy of MRPA for PE are limited, existing studies have shown that sensitivity and specificity of this modality approach that of CTPA when compared with conventional PA. Like earlier studies of CT, MRPA suffers most in the detection of subsegmental emboli. With the increasing availability and sophistication of MR scanners, this modality may become more useful for the detection of PE, particularly in pregnant patients and those who have renal insufficiency or iodinated contrast allergies.

Ultrasound

The use of lower extremity ultrasound in the evaluation of PE is limited. Although the examination is insensitive for asymptomatic DVT [77], a positive result can be used to institute anticoagulation. In addition to its poor sensitivity for lower extremity thrombus in asymptomatic patients, only approximately half of patients with known PE have DVT [17,78], which may be secondary to the majority of the thrombus migrating proximally to the lungs. By itself, lower extremity ultrasound is not sensi-

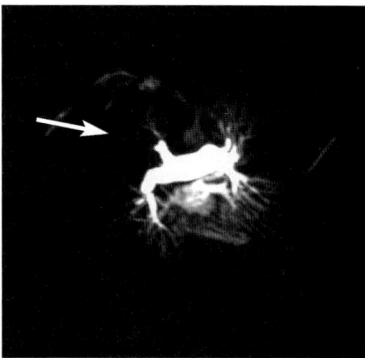

Fig. 12. Coronal view of contrast-enhanced MR perfusion study obtained using a three-dimensional fast low-angle shot sequence with ultrashort repetition time and echo time on a 1.5-Tesla magnet reveals vessel cutoff and loss of vascularity in the right upper lung zone (*arrow*). This finding is consistent with PE. (Courtesy of Robert C. Gilkeson, MD, Cleveland, OH.)

tive enough for the evaluation of PE; however, it is a reasonable preliminary study in pregnant patients or when other modalities are not available. Additionally, several investigators have included serial ultrasound of the lower extremities to diagnostic algorithms that are aimed at screening patients who remain at elevated risk after a PE work-up [53,79]. It must be emphasized that evaluation cannot stop after an isolated negative ultrasound of the extremities.

Echocardiography in the unstable patient

Whereas echocardiography is of limited use in the standard work-up of PE, there are some unique benefits to this study. Because of its speed and portability, bedside echocardiography can be useful in patients who are suspected of having PE and are who are too unstable for CT scan or further evaluation [80]. Transesophageal and transthoracic echo were reported to visualize the clot directly [81]; however, it is far more likely that indirect evidence of PE will be seen in the form of right ventricular (RV) dilation and septal bowing. Echocardiographic evidence of PE in the acutely unstable patient is a compelling reason to consider thrombolytic therapy.

Evidence of RV strain also may offer prognostic information for the hemodynamically stable patient who has PE. Although controversial, right heart strain that was visualized on echocardiography was reported to increase the risk of PE-related mortality as much as twofold [82]. Some studies reported that thrombolytic therapy in hemodynamically stable patients with known PE who show echocardiographic evidence of RV strain can improve RV function rapidly, and may lead to a lower rate of recurrent PE [83,84]. Aggressive management with thrombolytics in stable patients who have PE is controversial, and several investigators reported a lack of sufficient evidence to support this approach [85,86].

Because of the possible role of RV strain on patient management, investigators have looked at CTPA's ability to assess RV function in patients who have documented PE. In a retrospective study by Contractor and colleagues [87] in 2002, CT had a positive predictive value of 100% for RV dysfunction as defined by RV:left ventricular ratio of greater than 0.6 or septal bowing. More recently, Schoepf and colleagues [88] demonstrated that enlargement of the RV on CT helps to predict early death in patients who have PE. In a CTPA study that is positive for PE, it may add important clinical information to include a description of RV size and septal anatomy.

Special considerations

Pregnancy

Pregnancy is a known risk factor for thromboembolic disease. Diagnosis of PE in the pregnant patient is a challenge because there is concern about iodinizing radiation to the developing fetus. It is generally agreed that the risk of misdiagnosis of PE outweighs the risk of radiation. In a 2002 study of 120 pregnant women who were imaged with VQ scans, there were no adverse effects on 110 live births that were followed to a median of 20.5 months of age [89]. Although the concern for fetal radiation has led some investigators to dismiss CT as a diagnostic tool in pregnancy, a 2002 study found that the average fetal radiation dose for CTPA was less than VQ scans during all trimesters [90]. Despite limited data on CT scan radiation in pregnant women, a survey of thoracic radiologists reported that more than 75% of practices use CTPA in pregnant patients for the diagnosis of PE. Of those, 53% perform CTPA without a nuclear study first [91]. The use of MR imaging has been considered for the pregnant patient because of its lack of radiation; however, until MR imaging improves in availability and accuracy, it seems that helical CTPA with adequate shielding and dose-reduction protocols is likely to be used. Further study is warranted in the diagnosis of PE in the pregnant patient.

Increased use

With the increasing availability of CT scanners and the acceptance of CTPA by emergency departments and referring physicians, there is a risk that CTPA will add a significant strain to radiology departments that already are struggling to keep up with demand. The use of CT for diagnosis of PE was examined recently by Prologo and colleagues [38]. They reported that CTPA volume has increased from 1997–1998 to 2002–2003, whereas the rates of CT-detected PE and ancillary findings have decreased. Although much of this likely is secondary to the greater availability of CT scanning as well as movement away from V/Q scanning, the judicious use of CT would be optimal. Use of CT scanning is most appropriate when indicated after clinical pretest probability and D-dimer evaluation. Using clinical tools, such as the Wells criteria and sensitive D-dimer assays, it was shown that imaging can be reduced substantially while maintaining patient safety [18,92]. Regardless of what clinical algorithm is instituted, all patients with concern for PE must have pretest probability assessed. It even was suggested that clinical probability be included on every CTPA request in order for the CT to be completed [93]. Despite the continued acceptance of CTPA for diagnosis of PE, nuclear VQ scanning still makes up a large percentage of studies for PE [94], and when indicated, can help to decompress the strain on CT resources.

Summary

There continue to be great advances in imaging technologies for the diagnosis of PE. Improvements in noninvasive imaging techniques, including CT and MR and nuclear V/Q scanning, have decreased the indication for conventional PA. In particular, the increasing availability, speed, and accuracy of multi-detector CT has led to growing acceptance of this modality as the primary diagnostic study of choice. The increasing sensitivity of CT and other modalities for isolated subsegmental emboli require continued investigation into the clinical significance of these findings. Preliminary data question the clinical relevance of these small subsegmental emboli. Patients who present with pregnancy, renal insufficiency, or claustrophobia require that the radiologist be familiar with the strengths and weaknesses of the current imaging arsenal so that the safest and most accurate study can be performed. Further prospective studies, such as the PIOPED II trial, are warranted, and will continue to allow us to optimize our approach to the diagnosis of PE.

References

[1] Silverstein MD, Heit JA, Mohr DN, et al. Trends in the incidence of deep vein thrombosis and pulmonary embolism: a 25-year population-based study. Arch Intern Med 1998;158(6):585–93.

[2] Gray HW. The natural history of venous thromboembolism: impact on ventilation/perfusion scan reporting. Semin Nucl Med 2002;32(3):159–72.

[3] Anderson Jr FA, Wheeler HB, Goldberg RJ, et al. A population-based perspective of the hospital incidence and case-fatality rates of deep vein thrombosis and pulmonary embolism. The Worcester DVT Study. Arch Intern Med 1991; 151(5):933–8.

[4] Karwinski B, Svendsen E. Comparison of clinical and postmortem diagnosis of pulmonary embolism. J Clin Pathol 1989;42(2):135–9.

[5] Sandler DA, Martin JF. Autopsy proven pulmonary embolism in hospital patients: are we detecting enough deep vein thrombosis? J R Soc Med 1989;82(4):203–5.

[6] Goldhaber SZ. Epidemiology of pulmonary embolism. Semin Vasc Med 2001;1(2):139–46.

[7] Simonneau G, Sors H, Charbonnier B, et al. A comparison of low-molecular-weight heparin with unfractionated heparin for acute pulmonary embolism. The THESEE Study Group. Tinzaparine ou Heparine Standard: Evaluations dans l'Embolie Pulmonaire. N Engl J Med 1997;337(10): 663–9.

[8] Modan B, Sharon E, Jelin N. Factors contributing to the incorrect diagnosis of pulmonary embolic disease. Chest 1972;62(4):388–93.

[9] Carson JL, Kelley MA, Duff A, et al. The clinical course of pulmonary embolism. N Engl J Med 1992;326(19):1240–5.

[10] The PIOPED Investigators. Value of the ventilation/perfusion scan in acute pulmonary embolism. Results of the Prospective Investigation of Pulmonary Embolism Diagnosis (PIOPED). JAMA 1990;263(20):2753–9.

[11] Worsley DF, Alavi A, Aronchick JM, et al. Chest radiographic findings in patients with acute pulmonary embolism: observations from the PIOPED Study. Radiology 1993;189(1): 133–6.

[12] Elliott CG, Goldhaber SZ, Visani L, et al. Chest radiographs in acute pulmonary embolism. Results from the International Cooperative Pulmonary Embolism Registry. Chest 2000;118(1): 33–8.

[13] Kline JA, Johns KL, Colucciello SA, et al. New diagnostic tests for pulmonary embolism. Ann Emerg Med 2000;35(2):168–80.

[14] Rodger MA, Carrier M, Jones GN, et al. Diagnostic value of arterial blood gas measurement in suspected pulmonary embolism. Am J Respir Crit Care Med 2000;162(6):2105–8.

[15] Dunn KL, Wolf JP, Dorfman DM, et al. Normal D-dimer levels in emergency department patients suspected of acute pulmonary embolism. J Am Coll Cardiol 2002;40(8):1475–8.

[16] Abcarian PW, Sweet JD, Watabe JT, et al. Role of a quantitative D-dimer assay in determining the need for CT angiography of acute pulmonary embolism. AJR Am J Roentgenol 2004;182(6): 1377–81.

[17] Galle C, Papazyan JP, Miron MJ, et al. Prediction of pulmonary embolism extent by clinical findings, D-dimer level and deep vein thrombosis shown by ultrasound. Thromb Haemost 2001;86(5):1156–60.

[18] Wells PS, Anderson DR, Rodger M, et al. Excluding pulmonary embolism at the bedside without diagnostic imaging: management of patients with suspected pulmonary embolism presenting to the emergency department by using a simple clinical model and d-dimer. Ann Intern Med 2001;135(2):98–107.

[19] Kruip MJ, Slob MJ, Schijen JH, et al. Use of a clinical decision rule in combination with D-dimer concentration in diagnostic work-up of patients with suspected pulmonary embolism: a prospective management study. Arch Intern Med 2002;162(14):1631–5.

[20] van Beek EJ, Brouwers EM, Song B, et al. Lung scintigraphy and helical computed tomography for the diagnosis of pulmonary embolism:

a meta-analysis. Clin Appl Thromb Hemost 2001; 7(2):87–92.

[21] Goodman LR, Lipchik RJ, Kuzo RS, et al. Subsequent pulmonary embolism: risk after a negative helical CT pulmonary angiogram—prospective comparison with scintigraphy. Radiology 2000;215(2):535–42.

[22] Hull RD, Raskob GE, Pineo GF, et al. The low-probability lung scan. A need for change in nomenclature. Arch Intern Med 1995;155(17): 1845–51.

[23] Bone RC. The low-probability lung scan. A potentially lethal reading. Arch Intern Med 1993; 153(23):2621–2.

[24] Rajendran JG, Jacobson AF. Review of 6-month mortality following low-probability lung scans. Arch Intern Med 1999;159(4):349–52.

[25] Radan L, Mor M, Gips S, et al. The added value of spiral computed tomographic angiography after lung scintigraphy for the diagnosis of pulmonary embolism. Clin Nucl Med 2004;29(4): 255–61.

[26] Coche E, Verschuren F, Keyeux A, et al. Diagnosis of acute pulmonary embolism in outpatients: comparison of thin-collimation multi-detector row spiral CT and planar ventilation-perfusion scintigraphy. Radiology 2003;229(3):757–65.

[27] Reinartz P, Wildberger JE, Schaefer W, et al. Tomographic imaging in the diagnosis of pulmonary embolism: a comparison between V/Q lung scintigraphy in SPECT technique and multislice spiral CT. J Nucl Med 2004;45(9):1501–8.

[28] Hagen PJ, Hartmann IJ, Hoekstra OS, et al. Comparison of observer variability and accuracy of different criteria for lung scan interpretation. J Nucl Med 2003;44(5):739–44.

[29] Cross JJ, Kemp PM, Walsh CG, et al. A randomized trial of spiral CT and ventilation perfusion scintigraphy for the diagnosis of pulmonary embolism. Clin Radiol 1998;53(3):177–82.

[30] Garg K, Welsh CH, Feyerabend AJ, et al. Pulmonary embolism: diagnosis with spiral CT and ventilation-perfusion scanning—correlation with pulmonary angiographic results or clinical outcome. Radiology 1998;208(1):201–8.

[31] British Thoracic Society guidelines for the management of suspected acute pulmonary embolism. Thorax 2003;58(6):470–83.

[32] Nilsson T, Carlsson A, Mare K. Pulmonary angiography: a safe procedure with modern contrast media and technique. Eur Radiol 1998;8(1): 86–9.

[33] Zuckerman DA, Sterling KM, Oser RF. Safety of pulmonary angiography in the 1990s. J Vasc Interv Radiol 1996;7(2):199–205.

[34] Stein PD, Henry JW, Gottschalk A. Reassessment of pulmonary angiography for the diagnosis of pulmonary embolism: relation of interpreter agreement to the order of the involved pulmonary arterial branch. Radiology 1999;210(3): 689–91.

[35] Baile EM, King GG, Muller NL, et al. Spiral computed tomography is comparable to angiography for the diagnosis of pulmonary embolism. Am J Respir Crit Care Med 2000;161(3 Pt 1): 1010–5.

[36] Velmahos GC, Toutouzas KG, Vassiliu P, et al. Can we rely on computed tomographic scanning to diagnose pulmonary embolism in critically ill surgical patients? J Trauma 2004; 56(3):518–25.

[37] Murphy JM, Mulvihill N, Mulcahy D, et al. Percutaneous catheter and guidewire fragmentation with local administration of recombinant tissue plasminogen activator as a treatment for massive pulmonary embolism. Eur Radiol 1999; 9(5):959–64.

[38] Prologo JD, Gilkeson RC, Diaz M, et al. CT pulmonary angiography: a comparative analysis of the utilization patterns in emergency department and hospitalized patients between 1998 and 2003. AJR Am J Roentgenol 2004;183(4): 1093–6.

[39] Simon M, Boiselle PM, Choi JR, et al. Paddlewheel CT display of pulmonary arteries and other lung structures: a new imaging approach. AJR Am J Roentgenol 2001;177(1):195–8.

[40] Chiang EE, Boiselle PM, Raptopoulos V, et al. Detection of pulmonary embolism: comparison of paddlewheel and coronal CT reformations—initial experience. Radiology 2003;228(2):577–82.

[41] van Rossum AB, Pattynama PM, Ton ER, et al. Pulmonary embolism: validation of spiral CT angiography in 149 patients. Radiology 1996; 201(2):467–70.

[42] Holbert JM, Costello P, Federle MP. Role of spiral computed tomography in the diagnosis of pulmonary embolism in the emergency department. Ann Emerg Med 1999;33(5):520–8.

[43] Mullins MD, Becker DM, Hagspiel KD, et al. The role of spiral volumetric computed tomography in the diagnosis of pulmonary embolism. Arch Intern Med 2000;160(3):293–8.

[44] Remy-Jardin M, Remy J, Deschildre F, et al. Diagnosis of pulmonary embolism with spiral CT: comparison with pulmonary angiography and scintigraphy. Radiology 1996;200(3):699–706.

[45] Goodman LR, Curtin JJ, Mewissen MW, et al. Detection of pulmonary embolism in patients with unresolved clinical and scintigraphic diagnosis: helical CT versus angiography. AJR Am J Roentgenol 1995;164(6):1369–74.

[46] Gottschalk A, Stein PD, Goodman LR, et al. Overview of Prospective Investigation of Pulmonary Embolism Diagnosis II. Semin Nucl Med 2002;32(3):173–82.

[47] Garg K, Sieler H, Welsh CH, et al. Clinical validity of helical CT being interpreted as negative for pulmonary embolism: implications for patient treatment. AJR Am J Roentgenol 1999; 172(6):1627–31.

[48] Lomis NN, Yoon HC, Moran AG, et al. Clinical outcomes of patients after a negative spiral CT pulmonary arteriogram in the evaluation of

acute pulmonary embolism. J Vasc Interv Radiol 1999;10(6):707–12.

[49] Gottsater A, Berg A, Centergard J, et al. Clinically suspected pulmonary embolism: is it safe to withhold anticoagulation after a negative spiral CT? Eur Radiol 2001;11(1):65–72.

[50] Ost D, Rozenshtein A, Saffran L, et al. The negative predictive value of spiral computed tomography for the diagnosis of pulmonary embolism in patients with nondiagnostic ventilation-perfusion scans. Am J Med 2001;110(1):16–21.

[51] Friera A, Olivera MJ, Suarez C, et al. Clinical validity of negative helical computed tomography for clinical suspicion of pulmonary embolism. Respiration (Herrlisheim) 2004;71(1):30–6.

[52] Tillie-Leblond I, Mastora I, Radenne F, et al. Risk of pulmonary embolism after a negative spiral CT angiogram in patients with pulmonary disease: 1-year clinical follow-up study. Radiology 2002;223(2):461–7.

[53] Musset D, Parent F, Meyer G, et al. Diagnostic strategy for patients with suspected pulmonary embolism: a prospective multicentre outcome study. Lancet 2002;360(9349):1914–20.

[54] van Strijen MJ, de Monye W, Schiereck J, et al. Single-detector helical computed tomography as the primary diagnostic test in suspected pulmonary embolism: a multicenter clinical management study of 510 patients. Ann Intern Med 2003;138(4):307–14.

[55] Henry JW, Relyea B, Stein PD. Continuing risk of thromboemboli among patients with normal pulmonary angiograms. Chest 1995;107(5):1375–8.

[56] Kim KI, Muller NL, Mayo JR. Clinically suspected pulmonary embolism: utility of spiral CT. Radiology 1999;210(3):693–7.

[57] Richman PB, Courtney DM, Friese J, et al. Prevalence and significance of nonthromboembolic findings on chest computed tomography angiography performed to rule out pulmonary embolism: a multicenter study of 1,025 emergency department patients. Acad Emerg Med 2004;11(6):642–7.

[58] Doyle NM, Ramirez MM, Mastrobattista JM, et al. Diagnosis of pulmonary embolism: a cost-effectiveness analysis. Am J Obstet Gynecol 2004;191(3):1019–23.

[59] Garg K, Kemp JL, Wojcik D, et al. Thromboembolic disease: comparison of combined CT pulmonary angiography and venography with bilateral leg sonography in 70 patients. AJR Am J Roentgenol 2000;175(4):997–1001.

[60] Loud PA, Katz DS, Klippenstein DL, et al. Combined CT venography and pulmonary angiography in suspected thromboembolic disease: diagnostic accuracy for deep venous evaluation. AJR Am J Roentgenol 2000;174(1):61–5.

[61] Cham MD, Yankelevitz DF, Shaham D, et al. Deep venous thrombosis: detection by using indirect CT venography. The Pulmonary Angiography-Indirect CT Venography Cooperative Group. Radiology 2000;216(3):744–51.

[62] Aviram G, Levy G, Fishman JE, et al. Pitfalls in the diagnosis of acute pulmonary embolism on spiral computer tomography. Curr Probl Diagn Radiol 2004;33(2):74–84.

[63] Chartrand-Lefebvre C, Howarth N, Lucidarme O, et al. Contrast-enhanced helical CT for pulmonary embolism detection: inter- and intraobserver agreement among radiologists with variable experience. AJR Am J Roentgenol 1999;172(1):107–12.

[64] Erdman WA, Peshock RM, Redman HC, et al. Pulmonary embolism: comparison of MR images with radionuclide and angiographic studies. Radiology 1994;190(2):499–508.

[65] Grist TM, Sostman HD, MacFall JR, et al. Pulmonary angiography with MR imaging: preliminary clinical experience. Radiology 1993;189(2):523–30.

[66] Meaney JF, Weg JG, Chenevert TL, et al. Diagnosis of pulmonary embolism with magnetic resonance angiography. N Engl J Med 1997;336(20):1422–7.

[67] Loubeyre P, Revel D, Douek P, et al. Dynamic contrast-enhanced MR angiography of pulmonary embolism: comparison with pulmonary angiography. AJR Am J Roentgenol 1994;162(5):1035–9.

[68] Gupta A, Frazer CK, Ferguson JM, et al. Acute pulmonary embolism: diagnosis with MR angiography. Radiology 1999;210(2):353–9.

[69] Oudkerk M, van Beek EJ, Wielopolski P, et al. Comparison of contrast-enhanced magnetic resonance angiography and conventional pulmonary angiography for the diagnosis of pulmonary embolism: a prospective study. Lancet 2002;359(9318):1643–7.

[70] Sostman HD, Layish DT, Tapson VF, et al. Prospective comparison of helical CT and MR imaging in clinically suspected acute pulmonary embolism. J Magn Reson Imaging 1996;6(2):275–81.

[71] Fraser DG, Moody AR, Morgan PS, et al. Diagnosis of lower-limb deep venous thrombosis: a prospective blinded study of magnetic resonance direct thrombus imaging. Ann Intern Med 2002;136(2):89–98.

[72] Evans AJ, Sostman HD, Witty LA, et al. Detection of deep venous thrombosis: prospective comparison of MR imaging and sonography. J Magn Reson Imaging 1996;6(1):44–51.

[73] Laissy JP, Cinqualbre A, Loshkajian A, et al. Assessment of deep venous thrombosis in the lower limbs and pelvis: MR venography versus duplex Doppler sonography. AJR Am J Roentgenol 1996;167(4):971–5.

[74] Yang J, Wan MX, Guo YM. Pulmonary functional MRI: an animal model study of oxygen-enhanced ventilation combined with Gd-DTPA-enhanced perfusion. Chin Med J (Engl) 2004;117(10):1489–96.

[75] Fink C, Ley S, Puderbach M, et al. 3D pulmonary perfusion MRI and MR angiography of pulmonary embolism in pigs after a single injection of a blood pool MR contrast agent. Eur Radiol 2004; 14(7):1291–6.

[76] Kluge A, Muller C, Hansel J, et al. Real-time MR with TrueFISP for the detection of acute pulmonary embolism: initial clinical experience. Eur Radiol 2004;14(4):709–18.

[77] Wells PS, Lensing AW, Davidson BL, et al. Accuracy of ultrasound for the diagnosis of deep venous thrombosis in asymptomatic patients after orthopedic surgery. A meta-analysis. Ann Intern Med 1995;122(1):47–53.

[78] Turkstra F, Kuijer PM, van Beek EJ, et al. Diagnostic utility of ultrasonography of leg veins in patients suspected of having pulmonary embolism. Ann Intern Med 1997;126(10):775–81.

[79] Wells PS, Ginsberg JS, Anderson DR, et al. Use of a clinical model for safe management of patients with suspected pulmonary embolism. Ann Intern Med 1998;129(12):997–1005.

[80] Madan A, Schwartz C. Echocardiographic visualization of acute pulmonary embolus and thrombolysis in the ED. Am J Emerg Med 2004; 22(4):294–300.

[81] Casazza F, Bongarzoni A, Centonze F, et al. Prevalence and prognostic significance of right-sided cardiac mobile thrombi in acute massive pulmonary embolism. Am J Cardiol 1997; 79(10):1433–5.

[82] ten Wolde M, Sohne M, Quak E, et al. Prognostic value of echocardiographically assessed right ventricular dysfunction in patients with pulmonary embolism. Arch Intern Med 2004;164(15): 1685–9.

[83] Goldhaber SZ, Haire WD, Feldstein ML, et al. Alteplase versus heparin in acute pulmonary embolism: randomised trial assessing right-ventricular function and pulmonary perfusion. Lancet 1993;341(8844):507–11.

[84] Kreit JW. The impact of right ventricular dysfunction on the prognosis and therapy of normoten-sive patients with pulmonary embolism. Chest 2004;125(4):1539–45.

[85] Hamel E, Pacouret G, Vincentelli D, et al. Thrombolysis or heparin therapy in massive pulmonary embolism with right ventricular dilation: results from a 128-patient monocenter registry. Chest 2001;120(1):120–5.

[86] Davidson BL, Lensing AW. Should echocardiography of the right ventricle help determine who receives thrombolysis for pulmonary embolism? Chest 2001;120(1):6–8.

[87] Contractor S, Maldjian PD, Sharma VK, et al. Role of helical CT in detecting right ventricular dysfunction secondary to acute pulmonary embolism. J Comput Assist Tomogr 2002;26(4): 587–91.

[88] Schoepf UJ, Kucher N, Kipfmueller F, et al. Right ventricular enlargement on chest computed tomography: a predictor of early death in acute pulmonary embolism. Circulation 2004;110(20): 3276–80.

[89] Chan WS, Ray JG, Murray S, et al. Suspected pulmonary embolism in pregnancy: clinical presentation, results of lung scanning, and subsequent maternal and pediatric outcomes. Arch Intern Med 2002;162(10):1170–5.

[90] Winer-Muram HT, Boone JM, Brown HL, et al. Pulmonary embolism in pregnant patients: fetal radiation dose with helical CT. Radiology 2002; 224(2):487–92.

[91] Schuster ME, Fishman JE, Copeland JF, et al. Pulmonary embolism in pregnant patients: a survey of practices and policies for CT pulmonary angiography. AJR Am J Roentgenol 2003;181(6): 1495–8.

[92] Wells PS, Rodger M. Diagnosis of pulmonary embolism: when is imaging needed? Clin Chest Med 2003;24(1):13–28.

[93] Miller AC, Boldy DA. Pulmonary embolism guidelines: will they work? Thorax 2003;58(6):463.

[94] Stein PD, Kayali F, Olson RE. Trends in the use of diagnostic imaging in patients hospitalized with acute pulmonary embolism. Am J Cardiol 2004; 93(10):1316–7.

RADIOLOGIC
CLINICS
OF NORTH AMERICA

Radiol Clin N Am 44 (2006) 273–293

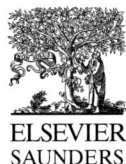

Nontraumatic Thoracic Emergencies

Jean Jeudy, MD, Stephen Waite, MD[1], Charles S. White, MD*

Acute chest pain is one of the most common complaints of patients who present to an emergency department (ED), and accounts for up to 5% of all visits [1]. It also is one of the most complex issues in an emergency setting because, although clinical signs and symptoms often are nonspecific, rapid diagnosis and therapy are of great importance. Accuracy in the diagnosis and treatment of chest pain remains a challenging task for the emergency physician.

The chest radiograph (CXR) remains an important component of the evaluation of chest pain, and usually is the first examination to be obtained. Nevertheless, cross-sectional imaging has added greatly to the ability to characterize the wide constellation of clinical findings into a distinct etiology. The potential for an "all-in-one" test for the work-up of these patients has led to the increasingly predominant role of CT imaging in defining nontraumatic thoracic emergencies. This article reviews how the various entities that can present as nontraumatic chest pain can manifest radiographically.

Cardiac assessment

The clinical scenarios of unstable angina, non ST-segment elevated myocardial ischemia, and ST-segment elevated myocardial ischemia make up the acute coronary syndrome (ACS) [2]. These entities encompass the most significant and potentially lethal causes of chest pain in the ED. In 2005, the estimated direct and indirect costs of coronary heart disease are $142 billion.

More than 335,000 people die of heart disease in an ED or before reaching a hospital every year. Of patients who die suddenly because of coronary heart disease, 50% of men and 64% of women have no previous symptoms. Patients who have classic symptoms of ischemia are stratified quickly and receive reperfusion therapy, including thrombolysis and coronary angioplasty. Patients who have unstable angina and atypical chest pain present a greater diagnostic dilemma because they may be at risk for a lethal event, despite symptoms that seem to be less critical.

The CXR usually is the first imaging technique that is used in assessing the patient who has cardiac disease in the ED. Although it remains sensitive for various noncardiac causes of chest pain (eg, pneumonia or pneumothorax), direct evidence of myocardial ischemia often is absent. Indirect signs include atherosclerotic calcifications in the coronary vessels and in the aorta, calcification of the

Department of Diagnostic Radiology, University of Maryland School of Medicine, Baltimore, MD, USA
* Corresponding author. Department of Diagnostic Radiology, University of Maryland School of Medicine, 655 West Baltimore Street, Baltimore, MD 21201.
E-mail address: cwhite@umm.edu (C.S. White).
[1] *Present address:* Department of Radiology, State University of New York Downstate, Brooklyn, NY.

0033-8389/06/$ – see front matter © 2006 Elsevier Inc. All rights reserved.
doi:10.1016/j.rcl.2005.10.008
radiologic.theclinics.com

heart borders that may represent previous infarction, or mediastinal widening [Fig. 1]. Cephalization and an enlarged cardiac silhouette suggest congestive heart failure. The rapid availability of the CXR and quick exclusion of many noncardiac causes of chest pain make it unlikely that the CXR will be supplanted for the initial imaging assessment.

New frontiers in cardiac imaging may open because of recent advances in multidetector CT (MDCT) technology. Thin section imaging with spatial resolution of approximately 1 mm and temporal resolution of less than 100 milliseconds have enabled imaging with cessation of heart motion. This has allowed sufficient anatomic detail to discern coronary stenoses secondary to calcified and noncalcified plaque [Fig. 2]. Current clinical guidelines dictate that patients who have classic signs of cardiac ischemia and additional EKG changes should undergo immediate catheterization with intervention as needed. Many clinicians look to the promise of a noninvasive technique with an

equivalent clinical impact as an attractive alternative. The added power to elicit secondary or alternative diagnoses creates the potential for a comprehensive evaluation of chest pain.

The ACS refers to sudden rupture of vulnerable plaque with occlusion of a coronary vessel. The consequence is myocardial ischemia or infarction that may be transmural or subendocardial [Fig. 3]. Approximately 10% to 30% of such patients have normal coronary angiograms [3].

Effective imaging of the coronary arteries requires, at minimum, a multidetector scanner with cardiac gating capability. A retrospective technique is used with segmented reconstruction of the diastolic phase of the cardiac cycles [4]. Overlapping axial sections also are reconstructed with a minimum slice thickness of as little as 0.75 mm and a maximum in-plane spatial resolution of approximately 0.4 mm × 0.4 mm [5].

Temporal resolution is optimized by scanning at heart rates of 50 to 65 beats per minute, with the

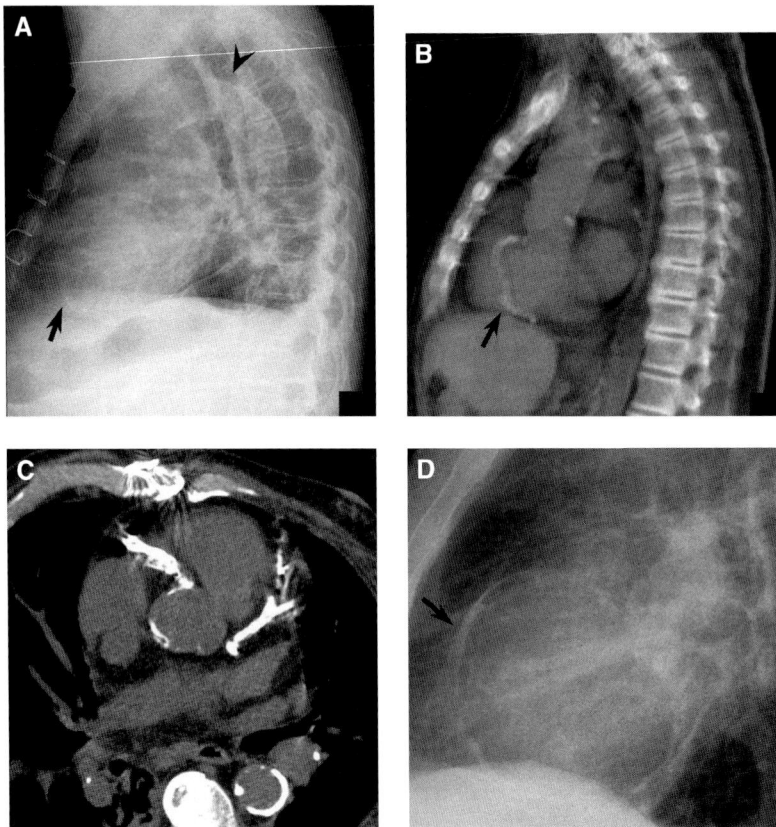

Fig. 1. Patient who had chronic chest pain and renal disease. (*A*) Lateral radiograph demonstrates extensive aortic calcification (*arrowhead*) and calcification in the distribution of the right coronary artery (*arrow*). (*B*) Sagittal ray-sum image better displays the attenuation difference between tissues, and highlights the calcification that is seen on the CXR (*arrow*). (*C*) Caudal oblique view of the aortic root displaying dense calcifications in all three coronary distributions. (*D*) Another patient who had pericardial calcification seen on the lateral radiograph (*arrow*), which suggests the diagnosis of constrictive pericarditis, and which was confirmed on later cardiac catheterization.

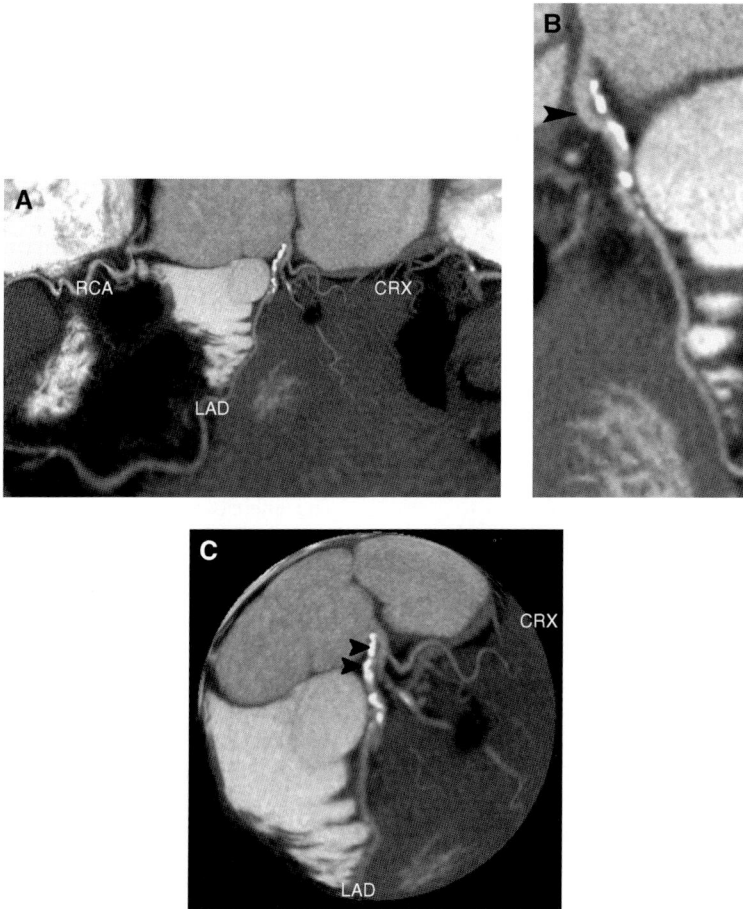

Fig. 2. Patient who had recurrent episodes of chest pain and family history of coronary artery disease. (A) Postprocessed two-dimensional view of the coronary arteries demonstrates extensive calcified plaque and subtle noncalcified plaque in the left main and anterior descending (LAD) coronary arteries. CRX, lateral circumflex artery; RCA, right coronary artery. Curved multiplanar reformat (B) and globe view (C) of the LAD confirm the presence of plaque and approximately 50% stenosis of the LAD (arrowheads). The stenosis was confirmed on cardiac catheterization and the patient received a coronary artery bypass.

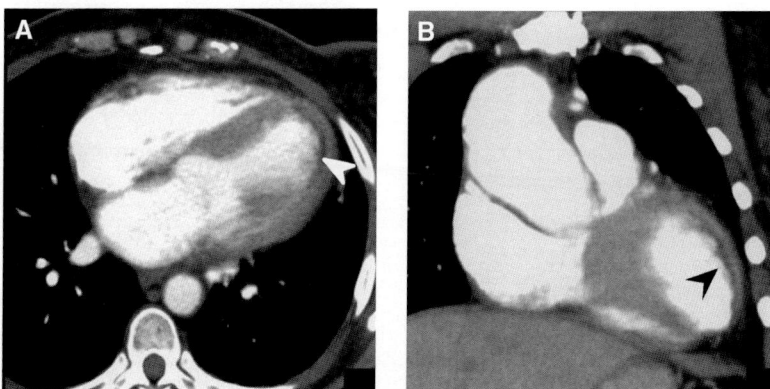

Fig. 3. Patient who had a history of substernal chest pain and increasing anginal symptoms. Contrast-enhanced axial (A) and (B) reformatted coronal CT images demonstrate a focal zone of myocardial thinning and decreased attenuation (arrowheads) within the anteroapical portion of the heart, compatible with ischemia, that was confirmed with nuclear stress testing.

additional administration of oral or intravenous β-blockers as necessary to control rate. The breath-hold requirement on 16-channel MDCT is 16 to 20 seconds, on average, and less than 10 seconds on a 64-channel MDCT.

Intravenous injection of contrast medium can be optimized by using a test bolus or an automatic bolus-triggering technique. Approximately 150 mL of iodinated contrast is injected at 4 to 5 mL/s through an antecubital vein. With optimal enhancement, noncalcified and calcified plaque in the coronary artery wall can be identified.

Studies comparing 4-channel MDCT and conventional coronary angiography found that 30% to 32% of vessels depicted by MDCT were unable to be analyzed; the proximal coronary segments were visualized adequately most often. The sensitivity for analyzable segments were 83% to 85% and specificities ranged from 76% to 93% [6,7]. More recent studies that examined the capability of 16-channel MDCT to evaluate the coronary vessels demonstrated improved spatial and temporal resolution that resulted in more analyzable segments compared with 4-channel detector scans, and better correlation with conventional angiography [8,9]. Ropers and colleagues [8] correctly detected 73% of significant stenoses in their study group, and determined an absence of stenosis with a sensitivity of 92%, specificity of 93%, and accuracy of 93%. Their positive and negative predictive values were 79% and 97%, respectively. Nieman and colleagues [9] found similar results, with sensitivity, specificity, and positive and negative predictive values of 95%, 86%, 80%, and 97%, respectively.

Electron beam CT (EBT) has been used to assess cardiac risk by demonstrating coronary calcium. Quantification can be achieved by using the method of Agatston and colleagues [10], which accounts for the amount and density of the calcium. In the ED setting, several studies have evaluated EBT as a means to stratify risk among patients who present with chest pain and have an indeterminate initial work-up [11,12]. A sensitivity of 98% to 100% has been found using coronary calcium as a marker. EBT also has a high negative predictive value. Laudon and colleagues [12] found no patient with a negative EBT who had a cardiac event in the 4 months after presentation to the ED. Georgiou [13] studied 192 patients who underwent EBT as part of their ED evaluation, and noted a strong correlation between coronary calcium score and a subsequent cardiac event. On average, patients were followed for 50 ± 10 months.

The increasing capabilities of MDCT and its already established indications for many other causes of chest pain have created interest in providing a comprehensive evaluation of cardiac and noncardiac chest pain. The term "triple rule-out" has been used to encompass contrast-enhanced MDCT evaluation of coronary artery disease, pulmonary embolism, and aortic dissection; however, the examination also may assess occult pneumonia or pneumothorax, rib fractures, and mediastinal disease (eg. esophageal perforation) [Fig. 4] [14].

Using 16-channel MDCT, a complete evaluation for chest pain requires a protocol compromise. Typically, ECG gating is not used to assess for pulmonary embolism, but is necessary for delineation of the coronary arteries. A wide field-of-view (FOV) is used for pulmonary embolism and aortic dissection evaluation, whereas a narrow FOV that is centered on the heart provides the best spatial resolution for the coronary arteries.

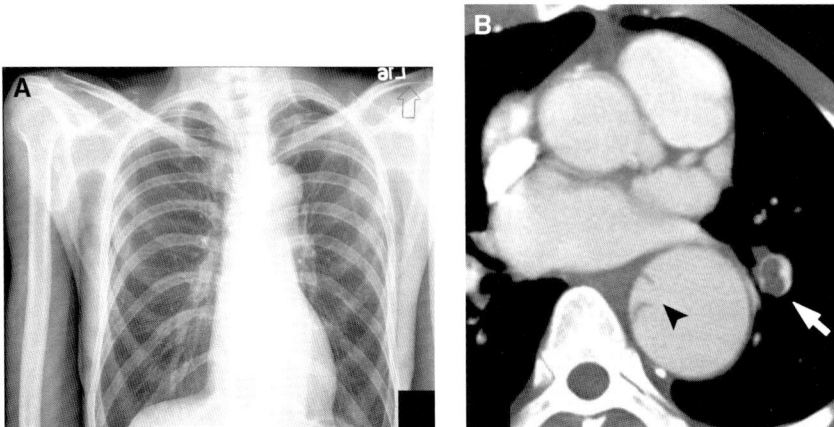

Fig. 4. Patient who had acute tearing chest pain and previously had intermittent shortness of breath. (*A*) Initial CXR is unrevealing for specific abnormalities. (*B*) Contrast-enhanced axial CT reveals aneurysmal dilatation of the descending aorta and intimomedial rupture of a dissection flap (*arrowhead*). An intraluminal filling defect is observed in the left lower lobe pulmonary artery that is compatible with pulmonary emboli (*arrow*).

In the authors' practice at University of Maryland, they have studied patients who presented to the ED with chest pain and an intermediate level of suspicion for cardiac ischemia after initial evaluation [13]. The authors' 16-channel MDCT protocol consisted of 16 × 0.75 mm retrospectively ECG triggered acquisition with reconstruction at 1 mm, pitch of 0.25, and a contrast bolus of 120 to 150 mL injected intravenously at 4 mL/s using bolus tracking. Initially, images were reconstructed at 75% of the R-R interval using a large FOV to assess noncardiac causes of chest pain. Subsequently, 10 equal phases were reconstructed at 10% intervals using a narrow FOV to assess the coronary arteries and heart. Phases between 40% and 90% and curved planar reconstructions of the three major coronary arteries were produced. Two radiologists evaluated each reconstructed image for significant coronary stenosis. Ground truth was defined by relevant imaging studies, such as cardiac catheterization when available or final clinical impression. Of 69 patients who met the criteria for enrollment, 13 (18%) had significant CT findings that were confirmed by a standard reference technique, of which 10 were cardiac and three were noncardiac. There were two false positive and two false negative results. Overall, sensitivity and specificity were 83% and 96%, respectively.

Although the study showed the feasibility of a comprehensive MDCT evaluation for chest pain in the ED, which may be especially useful to exclude significant disease, substantial limitations must be overcome. Each examination in the authors' protocol required 30 to 35 seconds to complete, so that most patients could not maintain a breathhold. Reconstruction of the 10 cardiac phases, consisting of 2500 to 3000 images, required 20 to 30 minutes and postprocessing often required more than 30 minutes. Many of these difficulties can be solved with the use of 64-channel MDCT in conjunction with faster reconstruction and postprocessing capabilities. Nevertheless, the precise role of CT for a comprehensive evaluation of chest pain in the ED remains to be defined.

Coronary CT angiography also has other clinical applications. Its role in verifying coronary artery bypass graft patency has been well demonstrated [Fig. 5] [15–19]; however, imaging of internal mammary grafts is more challenging because of their small size. Visualization of in-graft stenoses within stents also is difficult because of metallic artifact. Cardiac functional analysis and plaque characterization are other potential applications, although their use may be limited in the acute setting.

Radiation exposure is one of the most controversial issues that is related to MDCT. Retrospective cardiac ECG gating—the imaging reconstruction technique of choice to acquire coronary artery data—results in higher radiation doses to the patient as compared with an uncomplicated coronary angiogram. Current scanners permit modulation of the radiation dose given during systole to reduce exposure to the patient; however, this limits the evaluation of systolic cardiac phases that may contain useful diagnostic information. Dosimetry will continue to be an important factor because the future generation of scanners with thinner collimation may require higher radiation doses to maintain an appropriate contrast to noise ratio.

Multiple studies have validated the usefulness of radionuclide myocardial perfusion imaging for providing diagnostic and prognostic information [19–22]. Sestamibi (Bristol-Myers Squibb, North Billerica, Massachusetts) and Tc^{99m} have been the most common agents used in these studies. Among

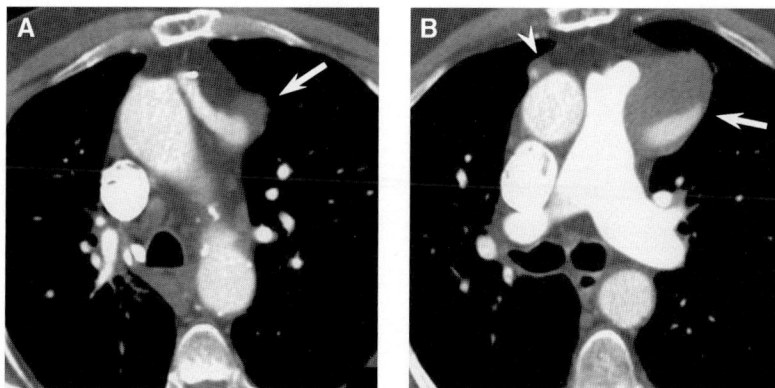

Fig. 5. Patient who had increasing chest discomfort and a history of coronary artery bypass. (*A*) Contrast CT demonstrates aneurysmal dilatation of a saphenous vein graft (*arrow*) originating from the aortic arch and inserting on a diagonal branch of the left anterior descending coronary artery. Note limited patency (*B*) of a second saphaneous vein graft to the posterior descending artery branching from the right coronary artery (*arrowhead*).

patients who have ACS with ST elevation myocardial ischemia, non-ST elevation myocardial ischemia, or unstable angina, the typical role for radionuclide imaging is to identify the location and extent of myocardial injury early in the disease, and to quantify final infarct size and extent of myocardial salvage later. In patients who have suspected ACS but no definite ECG changes, the primary role for radionuclide imaging is risk stratification. Observational studies have demonstrated a negative predictive value of close to 100% for excluding myocardial ischemia in these patients [19]. The American College of Cardiology/American Heart Assocation/American Society of Nuclear Cardiology Radionuclide Guidelines classify myocardial perfusion imaging in this setting as a class I, level A indication—a designation of strong clinical evidence and general agreement for its usefulness and benefit [14]. Investigators have attempted to apply these findings in a clinical setting. Two prospective studies showed that when radionuclide imaging is added to the diagnostic algorithm, patients incurred lower hospital costs and shorter lengths of hospital stay without adverse clinical outcome, as compared with usual ED evaluation strategies [21,22].

Aorta/vascular

Acute aortic syndrome describes the subset of aortic emergencies that is characterized by the symptoms of chest pain and hypertension [23]. These entities include aortic dissection (AD), intramural hematoma (IMH), and penetrating atherosclerotic ulcer. Aortic aneurysm leak and rupture have been included in this categorization [24]. Although the pathogenesis of each entity varies, the unifying theme is a disruption of the medial layer of the aorta that can extend circumferentially or longitudinally along the vessel. This leads to a predisposition to further disrupt the remaining layers of the aortic wall.

Aortic dissection

Acute AD is a cardiovascular emergency that requires prompt diagnosis and treatment [25]. AD usually occurs in the presence of hypertension. The event arises as an intimal tear of the aorta, and blood later dissects into the aortic media to form a false and true lumen. Tears that develop in the descending aorta (Stanford type B) are managed pharmacologically with antihypertensive therapy [Fig. 6]. The primary aim is to reduce blood pressure, and thereby, decrease the force of left ventricular contraction and vessel wall tension [26].

Intimal tears that involve the ascending aorta, whether or not there is extension into the descending aorta (Stanford type A), are associated with a higher mortality that necessitates emergent surgical repair [Fig. 7]. One of the most life-threatening complications that leads to this increased mortality is dissection into the pericardial space that may lead to rapid hemorrhagic extravasation, cardiac tamponade, and death. Up to 50% of patients who have dissection that involves the ascending aorta, have complicating aortic regurgitation. Coronary artery dissection or obstruction is another ominous complication that can lead to myocardial ischemia [26].

The survival for patients who have uncomplicated distal AD is approximately 75%, whether they are treated medically or surgically. The additional risk of surgery and paraplegia from interruption of the spinal arteries makes surgical repair of

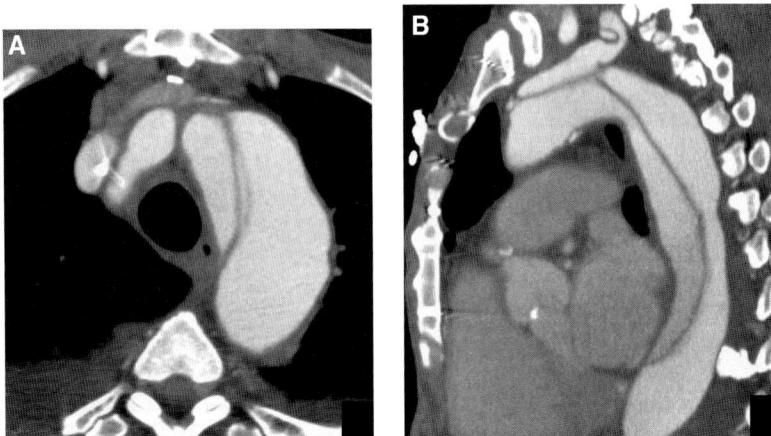

Fig. 6. Patient who had tearing chest pain. Axial CT (*A*) and sagittal multiplanar reconstruction (MPR) (*B*) demonstrate a dissection flap starting from the origin of the left subclavian artery and extending into the descending aorta, which is compatible with type B dissection.

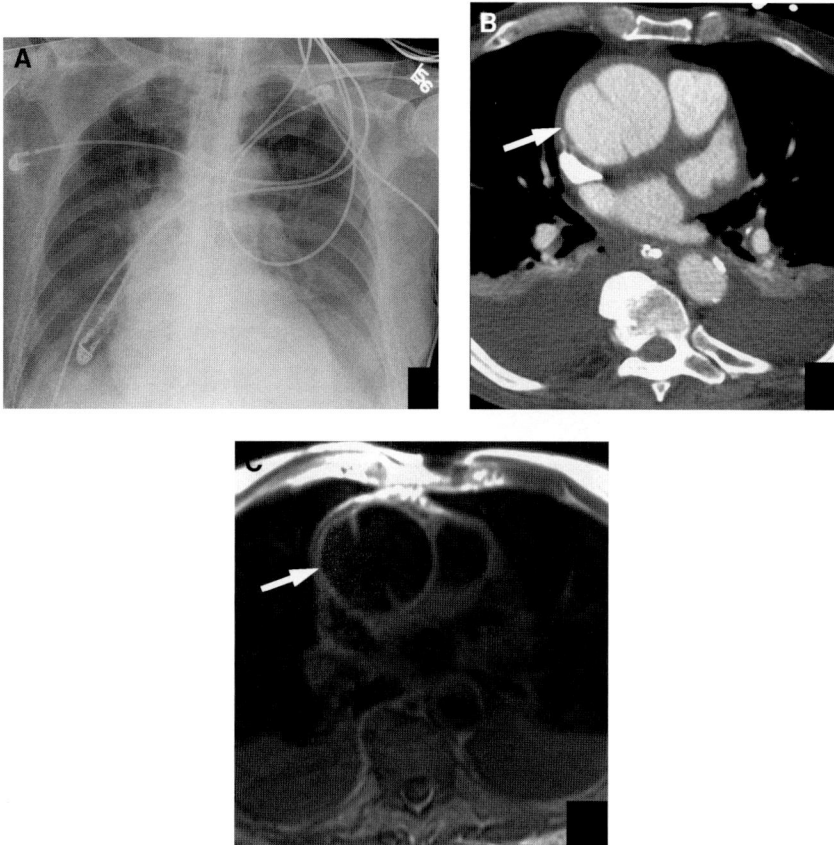

Fig. 7. Patient who had an acute onset of chest pain. (A) Plain radiograph demonstrates mild pulmonary edema and bilateral pleural effusions. Mild prominence is suggested along the contour of the ascending aorta. Contrast-enhanced CT (B) and T1-weighted axial MR imaging (C) demonstrate aneurysmal dilatation of the aorta (arrow) as well as an intimomedial flap that are compatible with a type A dissection.

the descending aorta a less attractive approach [27]. Surgical management for type B dissections is reserved for complications, such as rapidly expanding aortic diameter, acute or impending aortic rupture, intractable pain, ischemia of limbs and organ systems, and uncontrolled hypertension [28].

Plain CXRs, although not specific, usually are abnormal in cases of dissection. An abnormal aortic or mediastinal contour is seen most commonly. Up to 59% of patients demonstrate mediastinal widening [29]. Pleural effusion is another frequent finding; however as many of 12% of patients have normal CXRs [28,29]. Other imaging options that are available for the diagnosis of AD include conventional angiography, CT, MR imaging, and transesophageal echocardiography (TEE) [30–32].

CT is the most widely used modality, particularly if sited in or near the ED, and it has a sensitivity and specificity of nearly 100% [33,34]. The primary finding on a contrast-enhanced CT is the identification of the intimomedial flap that separates the true and false lumens. Dissection usually originates at points of maximal hydraulic stress, commonly in

the descending aorta just proximal to the ligamentum arteriosum or at the right lateral wall of the ascending aorta [24]. In 8% of patients, direct visualization of the intimomedial entrance tear is identified in which the free edges are seen pointing toward the false lumen [Fig. 8] [35]. Additional findings include displacement of intimal calcifications that is caused by the false lumen dissecting through the media, and compression of the true lumen by the larger false lumen.

Although CT typically provides sufficient diagnostic information, lack of availability of CT or equivocal imaging findings may dictate another diagnostic approach. In such cases, TEE and MR imaging may prove valuable. In some institutions, TEE is used as a primary technique for the evaluation of AD. Because of the high sensitivity of this triad of noninvasive techniques, conventional aortography is used infrequently. Another factor that limits invasive angiography's use is its insensitivity for the presence of IMH.

MR imaging of the aorta plays a lesser role in the evaluation of acute AD because it is available less

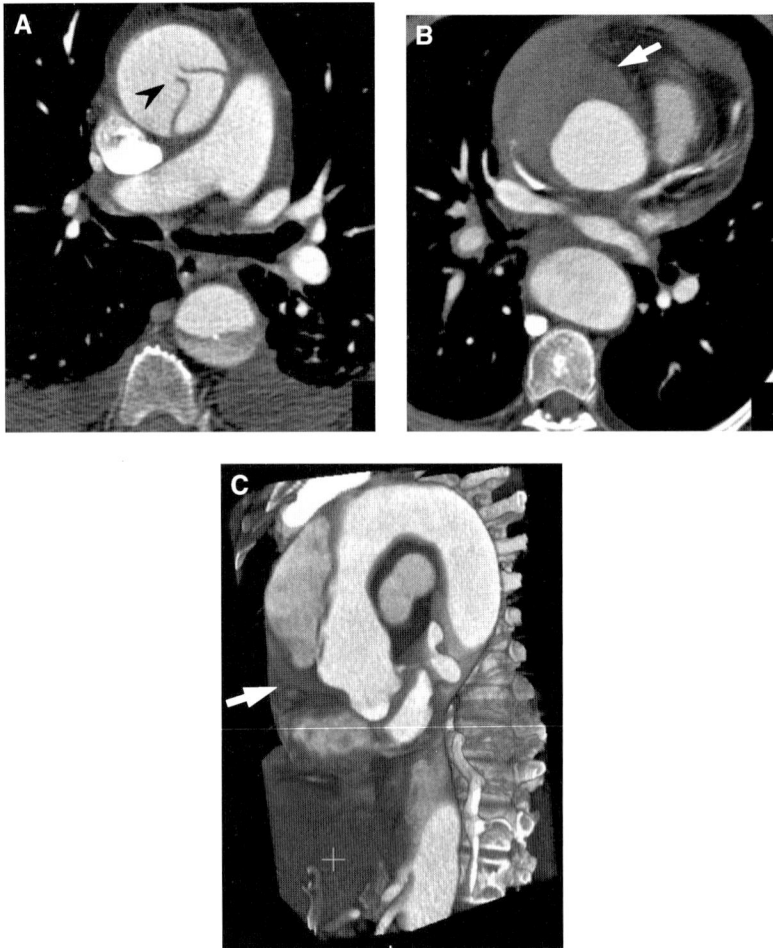

Fig. 8. Patient who had acute chest pain due to type A dissection. (*A*) The communication between true and false lumen is illustrated by the site of intimomedial rupture (*arrowhead*). Contrast-enhanced CT (*B*) and obliqued-sagittal volume-rendered (*C*) images demonstrate IMH that extends to the aortic root (*arrows*) and pericardium, an often life-threatening complication of type A dissection.

widely and is more cumbersome in critically ill patients [36]. In select patients, such as those who have renal insufficiency or contrast allergy, MR imaging can identify the dissection flap and the extent of dissection, and provide functional information regarding valvular insufficiency. With developments in fast-imaging MR techniques, MR imaging may play an increased diagnostic role in the future [Fig. 9] [37–39]. TEE is used as a secondary imaging study in as many as one third of patients. The presence of an undulating intimomedial flap that separates the true and false lumens is the primary finding that is sought. The different flow patterns of the true and false lumen also can be illustrated with color Doppler techniques. The functional information that is gained from TEE also is valuable. This includes assessment of aortic valvular disturbance, aortic root dilatation, coronary involvement, and pericardial effusion [28]. Strong dependence on perfor-

mance and interpretation by an experienced operator remain major disadvantages of the technique.

Intramural hematoma

IMH represents a clinically indistinguishable variant of AD in which no discrete intimal flap is identified, and no flowing blood is observed within the false channel. Spontaneous hemorrhage of the vasa vasorum weakens the media without an intimal tear [40]. The resultant hemorrhage can extend longitudinally along the aorta and may progress to frank dissection [41]. IMH is classified in a manner similar to conventional AD; involvement of the ascending aorta is considered a Stanford type A lesion. Increasingly, surgery is being recommended for type A IMH [41].

The primary finding of IMH on noncontrast CT is a crescentic region of increased attenuation, which

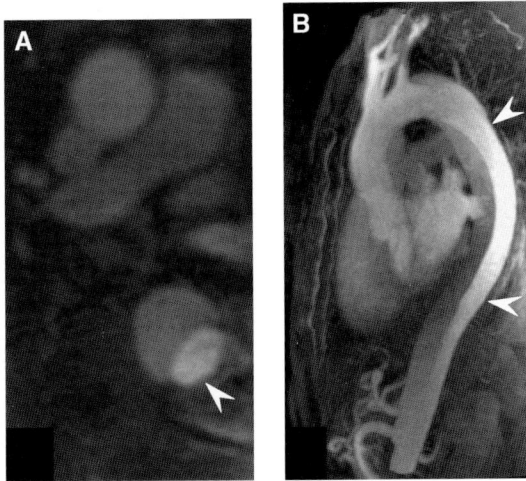

Fig. 9. Patient who had chest pain. Axial (*A*) and sagittal (*B*) T1-weighted fat-saturated images with gadolinium enhancement show type B dissection. Note the differential of flow seen in true and false lumens (*arrowheads*).

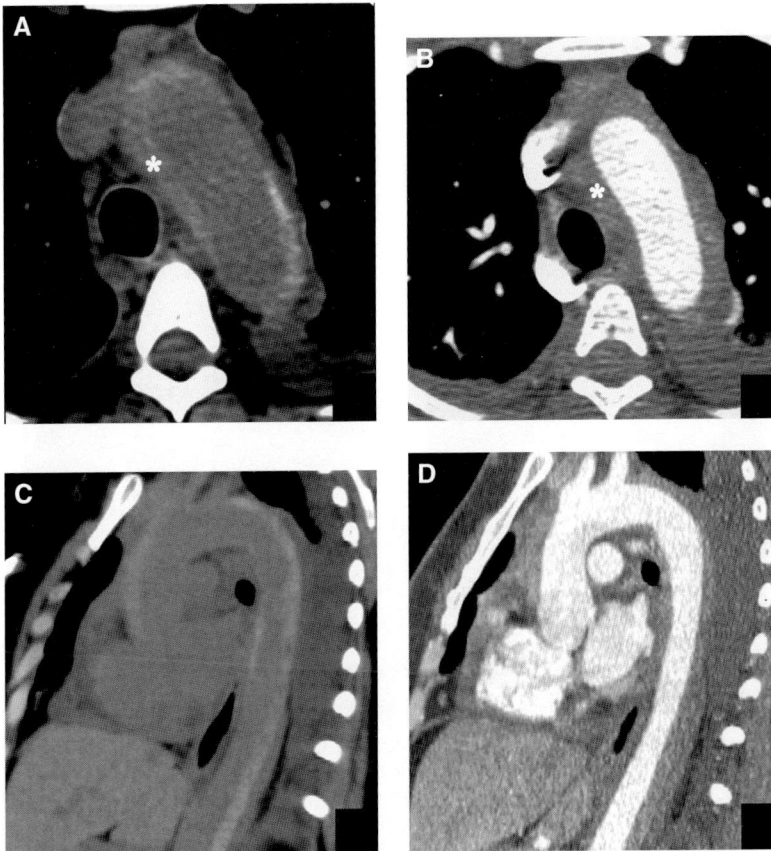

Fig. 10. Patient who had a history of tearing chest pain. Noncontrast (*A*) and contrast-enhanced (*B*) images, at the level of the aortic arch, demonstrate intramural soft tissue density starting just beyond the origin of the left subclavian artery. The noncontrast image illustrates the increased attenuation of the IMH compared with intraluminal blood (*asterisks*) and represents a key element when making the diagnosis. (*C* and *D*) Obliqued-sagittal MPR image shows the extent of IMH and relative conspicuity of the extent of IMH on contrast enhanced images.

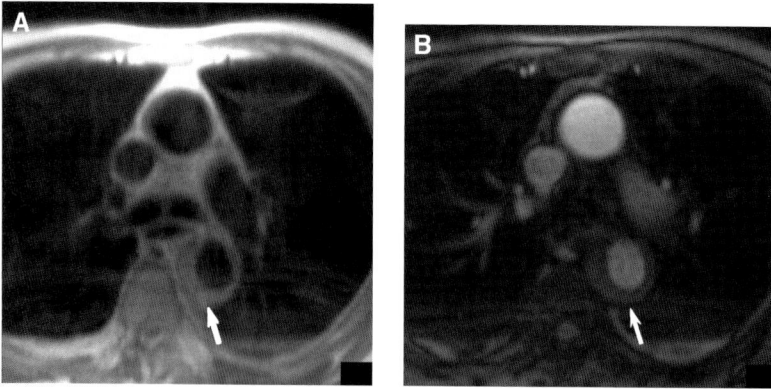

Fig. 11. Patient who had tearing chest pain and renal insufficiency. T1- (A) and T2-weighted (B) MR images demonstrate the characteristic crescentic appearance of IMH (arrows) within the descending aorta.

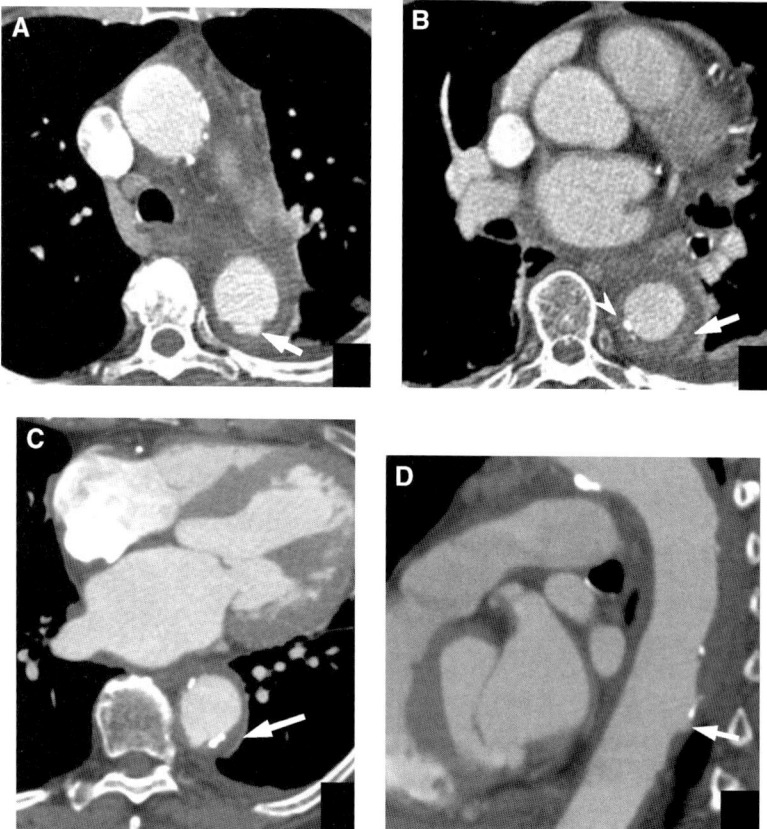

Fig. 12. Patient who had acute onset of sharp back pain. (A) Contrast-enhanced axial CT image demonstrates atherosclerosis and a small area of contrast that extends outside the true lumen of the descending aorta, which is compatible with a small penetrating ulcer (arrow). (B) Eccentric high-attenuation density is seen surrounding the lumen, which represents the resultant IMH (arrow). Note the focal intimal calcification (arrowhead) that identifies the density as an intramural process as opposed to mural thrombus. (C and D) Patient who had new onset chest pain. (C) Contrast CT image shows an eccentric rim of soft tissue density that involves the descending aorta. Intimal atherosclerotic calcifications are observed anterior to soft tissue density, which suggest an intramural component instead of mural thrombus. The arrow points to a small outpouching that passes beyond the expected intima, which is compatible with a small penetrating atherosclerotic ulcer. (D) Sagittal MPR shows the small penetrating ulcer and adjacent IMH (arrow).

represents a hematoma in an intramural location [Fig. 10]. The potential for this finding to be occult and overlooked on contrast enhanced CT imaging necessitates the addition of a noncontrast study when an acute aortic syndrome is suggested [42]. Additional findings include displacement of intimal calcifications that aids in distinguishing IMH from mural thrombus, lack of intramural enhancement excluding free flow from classic acute dissection, and compression of the true aortic lumen by the hematoma. IMH can be identified on MR imaging as crescentic thickening of the aortic wall with increased signal on T1-weighted images, often in the subacute phase [Fig. 11]. Slow flow of an acute dissection and absence of flow in an IMH also can be shown using gradient echo or phase-contrast techniques [43]. IMH associated with ulceration tends to predominate in the descending aorta. One series showed the distribution of all IMHs to be 48% in the ascending aortic, 8% in the aortic arch, and 44% in the descending aorta [32,44].

Many investigators have examined the usefulness of CT to predict progression from IMH to AD. Type A IMH is more likely to progress to dissection if the initial CT demonstrates an aortic diameter of more than 5 cm [45,46]. The thickness of the hematoma also may be indicative of the amount of intramural bleeding, which leads to increased intimal weakness and risk for rupture [41]. Measurements of aortic root movement and aortic wall stiffness also may play a prognostic role for stratifying risk for dissection in the future [47].

Penetrating ulcer

Stanson and colleagues [48] first described penetrating atherosclerotic aortic ulcer (PAU) as a distinct entity in 1986, and over the last 2 decades investigators have continued to provide a more complete characterization of the condition. PAU is regarded as an entity of aging that may precipitate AD, particularly IMH. Penetrating ulcer usually occurs in the elderly with concomitant severe atherosclerosis.

A calcified atheromatous plaque, easily identified on unenhanced CT images, ulcerates and disrupts the internal elastic lamina and then penetrates the underlying intimal and medial layers [Fig. 12]. A contrast-filled outpouching often extends beyond the plaque and wall of the aortic lumen. The resul-

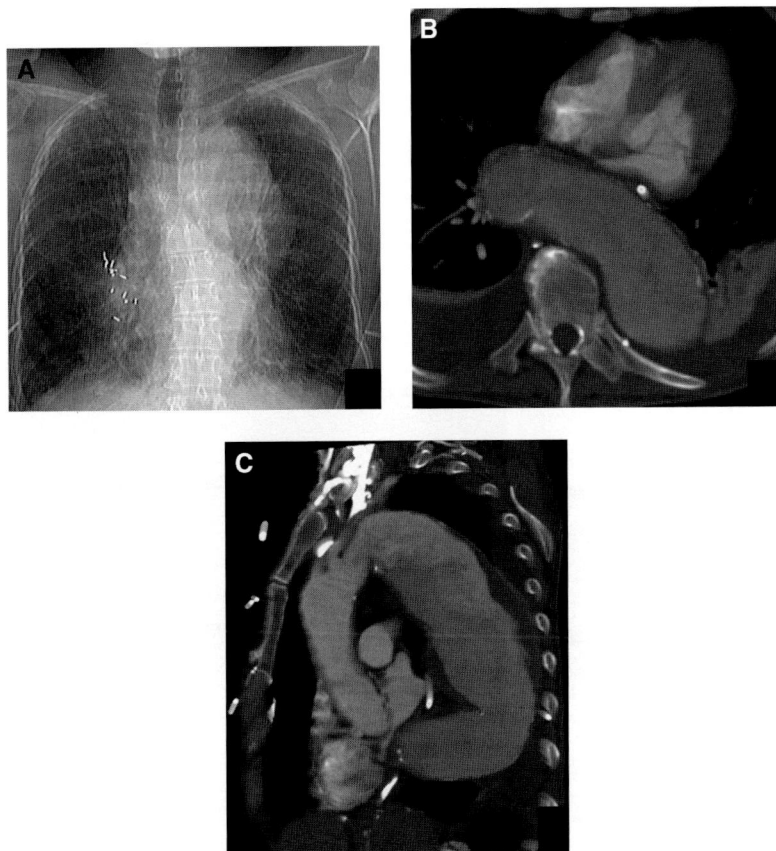

Fig. 13. Patient who had intermittent chest pain. (*A*) Chest radiograph demonstrates a marked abnormality of the aortic contour. (*B*) A tortuous aorta is seen with aneurysmal dilatation occurring beyond the origin of the left subclavian artery. (*C*) Obliqued-sagittal thick slab MPR shows the extent of aneurysmal dilatation.

tant hemorrhage in the media leads to IMH [49]. Thickening and enhancement of the involved aortic wall also can be seen [44]. Additional complications include focal dissection, disruption of the adventitia that leads to pseudoaneurysm, or aortic rupture.

Two controversies surrounding this entity include the timing of intervention, and the ability to identify those who are at risk for complications of a PAU. Investigators have described an increased risk for aortic rupture in patients who have PAU as compared with patients who have a Stanford type A or B AD [49,50]. Endovascular stent placement has become a widely accepted method of treatment in these patients; however, these patients tend to have comorbid medical problems that place them at high surgical risk [51]. Because these patients also have atherosclerosis of the aorta, management often is conservative with close follow-up, and surgery is reserved for complications (eg, aortic rupture) or if medical therapy has failed.

Some investigators consider the development of the IMH to be the first complication of PAU; however, few studies have demonstrated findings that are prognostic factors for fatal complications. Some studies showed that aortic diameter or ulcer size was a predictor of clinical behavior, but other studies have not found such an association [45,51–53].

Aortic aneurysm

A true aortic aneurysm involves all three layers of the aortic wall and most commonly is due to atherosclerosis. False aortic aneurysms (pseudoaneurysms) often are the result of trauma to the intimal wall and containment of the resultant hemorrhage by the outer layers of media or adventitia. Infection can lead to a mycotic aneurysm that also may form a pseudoaneurysm (see later discussion).

Thoracic aortic aneurysm (TAA) occurs most frequently in men who are between 50 and 70 years of age. Of these, approximately 50% originate in the ascending aorta, 10% originate at the aortic arch, and 40% originate in the descending aorta [54,55]. TAA has been estimated to expand at a rate of 0.5 cm per year, with a significant increased risk for rupture when greater than 5 cm in diameter [56,57]. Although many aortic aneurysms are asymptomatic, approximately one third of patients who are diagnosed with an intact TAA experience an aortic rupture within a month of diagnosis [58]. Other patients who are at risk present with pain that is related to mass effect or enlarging size [Fig. 13].

Imaging of thoracic aneurysms has been extremely helpful to distinguish patients who are at risk for rupture from those who can be followed more conservatively. Initial radiographic findings may demonstrate enlargement of the thoracic aorta. CT imaging, with sensitivity and specificity that is comparable to conventional aortography, offers the best evaluation because it is noninvasive, readily available in most EDs, and allows for detailed assessment of the aorta with three-dimensional reconstruction techniques [Fig. 14]. Most aneurysms are followed sequentially with

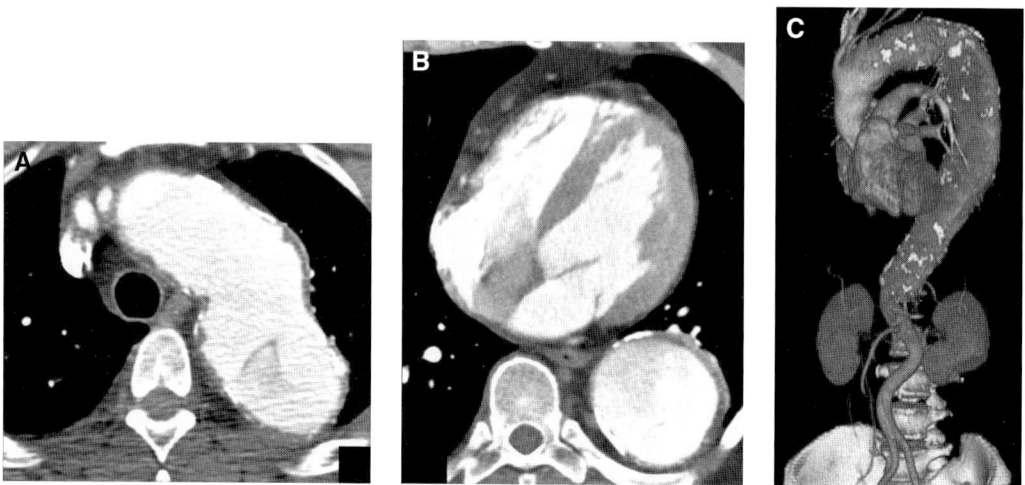

Fig. 14. Patient who had intermittent chest pain. (*A* and *B*) Contrast-enhanced CT at the level of the aortic arch and at the level of left ventricle demonstrate a markedly dilated and tortuous aorta, that involves the ascending and descending portions. (*C*) Three-dimensional volume-rendered image demonstrates the extent of aortic aneurysmal dilatation and comparison with adjacent anatomic structures.

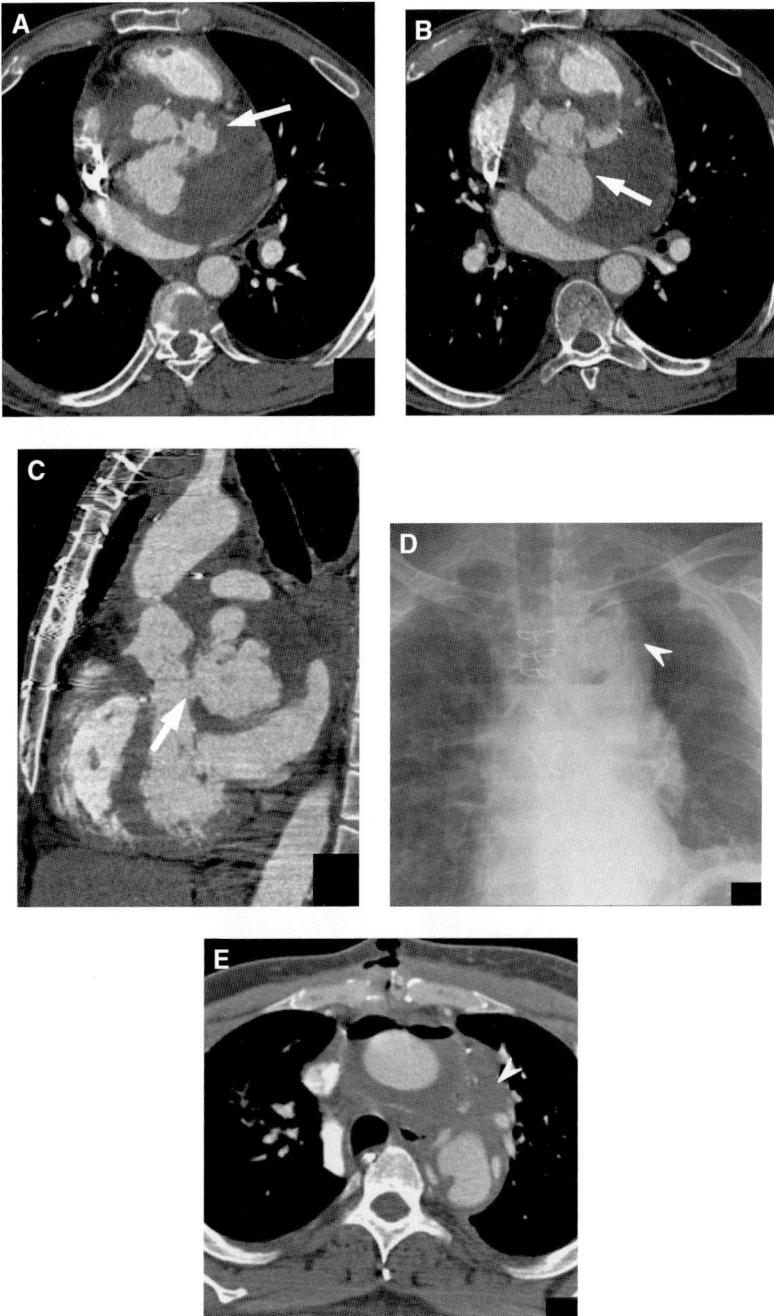

Fig. 15. Patient who had a history of aortic valve replacement and recurrent intravenous drug use. (*A* and *B*) Axial contrast-enhanced CT images demonstrate extravasation of contrast and hemorrhagic collection below the root of the aorta (*arrows*). Periaortic soft tissue density represents inflammation and infection that is due to endocarditis. Note the mass effect on the left atrium. (*C*) Sagittal multiplanar reformatted image demonstrates the point of extravasation (*arrow*) and anatomic relationship of the subsequent collection with the aorta. (*D* and *E*) A different patient who had a history of coronary artery bypass grafts. (*D*) Chest radiograph shows mediastinal widening and lucency surrounding the aortic arch (*arrowhead*). (*E*) Contrast CT shows extension of sternal infection into the mediastinum (*arrowhead*) which led to the development of a mycotic aneurysm of the aorta.

cross-sectional imaging to document rapid changes in diameter. Endovascular stent-graft placement usually is timed to occur when the risk of rupture outweighs the potential risk of intervention [51].

Infectious vascular process (mycotic aneurysm)

Mycotic aneurysm, originally a term for fungal vascular infection, is now used generally to describe aneurysms that result from bacteremia and embolization of any infectious material, with superinfection of an atheromatous plaque [59]. Bacteria also may seed the intact vascular wall through hematogenous spread to the vasa vasorum, where the resultant focal suppurative process weakens the arterial wall and allows formation of an aneurysm. Alternatively, direct extension from an extravascular infectious focus, such as vertebral osteomyelitis, may penetrate into an adjacent vascular structure

and lead to necrosis, bleeding, and pseudoaneurysm formation [Fig. 15] [60].

Staphylococcus and *Salmonella* species are the organisms that are implicated most commonly in the development of a mycotic aneurysm [60,61]. Several other organisms, including *Streptococcus* species, *Mycobacterium tuberculosis*, fungi, and various gram-negative and positive-bacteria, occasionally may cause a mycotic aneurysm in immune-competent and immune-suppressed patients [61–63].

Patients present with nonspecific symptoms, and thus, a diagnosis of infected aortic aneurysm may not be suspected during the initial clinical evaluation. Usually, CT is the initial imaging technique because of its availability, rapid imaging capabilities, and ability to uncover alternative diagnoses in the setting of a nonspecific clinical scenario. Characteristic findings include a periaortic soft tissue mass, stranding, and fluid [64]. TEE im-

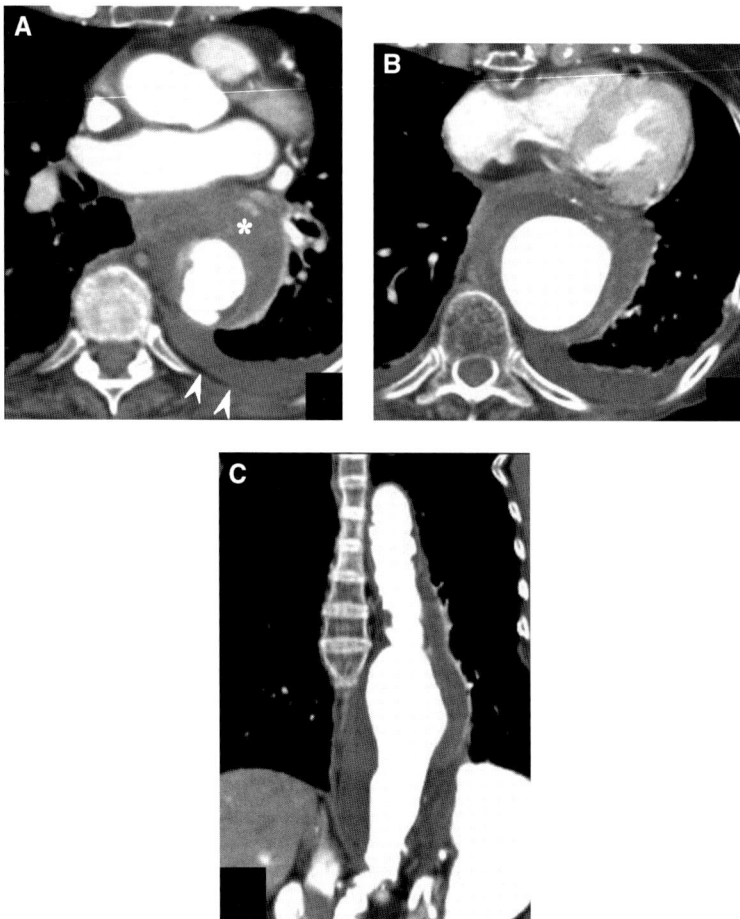

Fig. 16. Patient who had intermittent chest pain that became acutely severe. (*A* and *B*) Contrast-enhanced axial CT images demonstrate aneurysmal dilatation of the aorta with extensive surrounding infiltrative changes (*asterisk*). High-attenuation periaortic fluid and pleural fluid is confirming aortic rupture (*arrowheads*). (*C*) Coronal MPR further illustrates the level of acute dilatation and level of the periaortic collection.

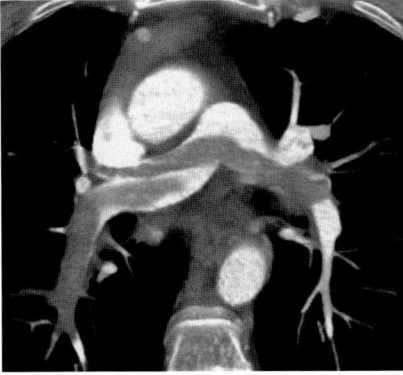

Fig. 17. Patient who had severe chest pain and tachycardia. On the obliqued-axial volume intensity projection, multiple "cords" of thrombus are seen extending into all vessels branching off from the main pulmonary trunk.

ages heart valves, and thus, is helpful in ruling out bacterial endocarditis as a precipitating etiology. Disadvantages that are inherent to the technical limitations and aspects of this modality, such as patient body habitus, overlying bowel gas, and operator-dependent examination quality, limit the usefulness of this modality in the diagnosis of mycotic aneurysm [64].

Spontaneous aortic rupture

Rupture of the aorta often is the fatal natural history of any aortic syndrome. Periaortic hematoma is one of the hallmark findings. Another sign of impending rupture is hyperdense mediastinal, pericardial, or pleural fluid that is compatible with hemorrhage on unenhanced CT of the chest. The presence of IMH, focal defect in a calcified aortic wall, and extravasation of contrast material also are ominous signs on a contrast-enhanced study [Fig. 16] [65].

Pulmonary embolism

Pulmonary embolism (PE) is the third leading cause of death in the United States, with approximately 50,000 to 100,000 deaths per year—an incidence that exceeds 1 per 1000 and a mortality of greater than 15% in the first 3 months after diagnosis [66,67]. CT pulmonary angiography has become the primary method by which PE is evaluated in most institutions. The primary imaging feature of PE is identification of an intraluminal full or partial pulmonary arterial filling defect [Fig. 17]. Other findings include pleural-based, wedge-shaped consolidation; oligemia; and pleural

effusion [Fig. 18]. PE is discussed in detail elsewhere in this issue.

Pleuroparenchymal lung disease

Pleural and parenchymal lung disease commonly manifest with symptoms of chest pain. Usually, a typical history and corroborating clinical findings discriminate pulmonary entities from cardiac or vascular pathology. The CXR often permits refinement of the differential diagnosis, but CT scanning often is obtained early in the evaluation. Two common pulmonary entities that can present as nontraumatic emergencies include spontaneous pneumothorax or pneumomediastinum and esophageal rupture. Spontaneous pneumothorax occurs in the absence of trauma, and is classified as primary or secondary, depending on the precipitating cause. Primary spontaneous pneumothorax usually presents in young adults and is caused most commonly by apical blebs [68]. Smoking seems to play a considerable role in the development of these blebs [69]. Secondary causes include chronic obstructive pulmonary disease, metastases (primary sarcomas, particularly osteogenic sarcoma) [70], infectious etiologies (tuberculosis, *Pneumocystis jiroveci* infection), cystic lung disease (pulmonary Langerhans cell histiocytosis and lymphangiomyomatosis), and endometriosis.

The classic radiographic sign is identification of the pleural line separated from the chest wall, which leaves an area of lucency absent of parenchymal vessels. Recumbent patients also can develop a deep sulcus sign as air layers anteriorly and projects as an area of increased lucency that outlines the costophrenic sulcus [Fig. 19]. CT scan provides a more thorough assessment of the dis-

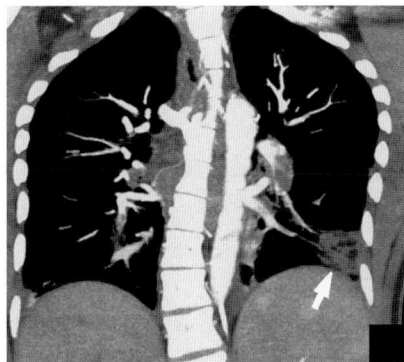

Fig. 18. Patient who had chest pain and shortness of breath. Wedge- shaped parenchymal density in left lower lobe (*arrow*), which is compatible with Hampton's hump, is seen commonly on plain radiographs.

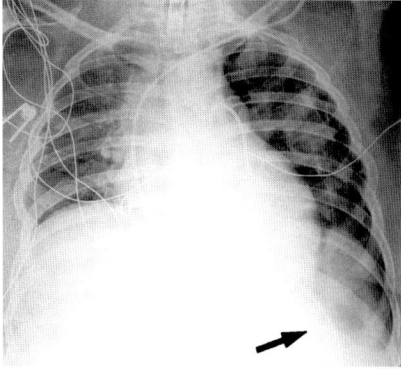

Fig. 19. Patient who had chest pain and desaturation on pulse oximetry. Portable CXR demonstrates increased lucency at the base of the left chest, which is compatible with a deep sulcus sign of pneumothorax (*arrow*). Typically, this is seen in a patient in the recumbent position.

tribution of pleural air. CT may show apical blebs or subpleural metastases as the etiology of the pneumothorax [Fig. 20]. Life-threatening tension pneumothorax occurs if intrapleural pressure increased to a point where gas exchange and cardiac function become affected adversely. Imaging findings include contralateral mediastinal shift and diaphragmatic depression.

Pneumomediastinum or migration of air into the mediastinum generally results from extrathoracic (ie, iatrogenic, penetrating trauma) or intrathoracic causes (ie, alveolar rupture, Valsalva maneuver, tracheal rupture, esophageal rupture, or blunt trauma). Spontaneous pneumomediastinum has been described with rupture of pleural blebs, marijuana or cocaine inhalation, labor, respiratory infection, emesis, and athletic competition [71–73]. The most common symptoms are chest pain and dyspnea, and subcutaneous emphysema is the most common clinical finding. The radiographic signs are a depiction of air outlining the nor-

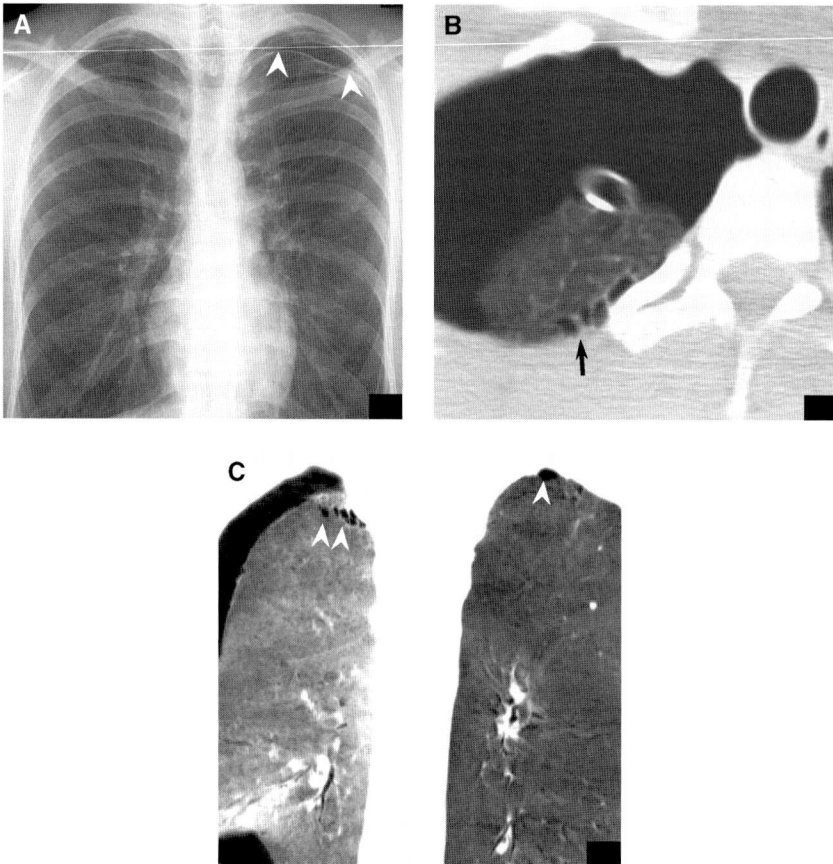

Fig. 20. Young male patient who had a history of recurrent pneumothoraces. (*A*) Chest radiograph demonstrates left apical pneumothorax (*arrowheads*). (*B*) One month later, the patient developed a right-sided pneumothorax. Small blebs are observed at the right lung apex (*arrow*), which suggest the underlying the causative factor. (*C*) Minimal intensity projection images demonstrate increased sensitivity when identifying small blebs (*arrowheads*).

mal mediastinal anatomy. Such signs include the continuous diaphragm sign, air surrounding the pulmonary artery, double bronchial wall sign, and air around the pulmonary ligament [Fig. 21] [73]. Rarely, pneumomediastinum may progress to tension pneumomediastinum, which may be life threatening. This occurs most often in mechanically ventilated patients with positive pressure in whom pneumopericardium also is visible on the CXR.

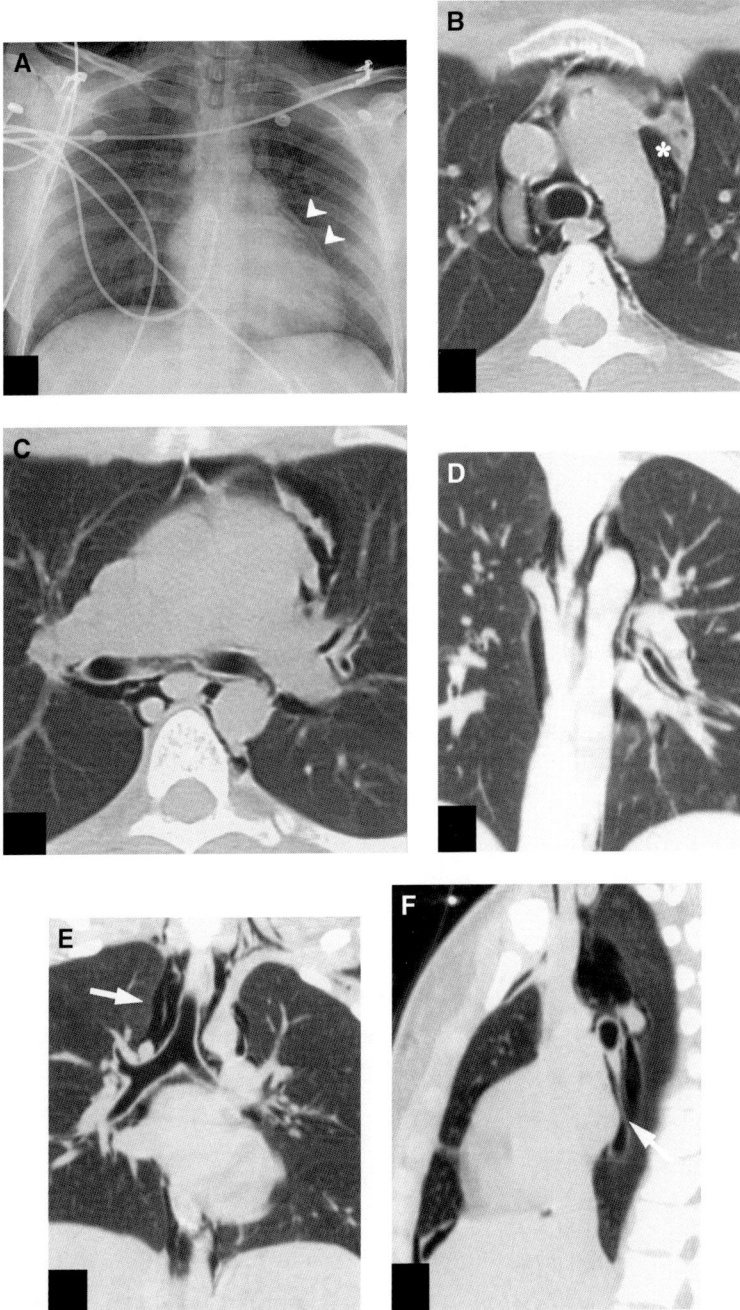

Fig. 21. Patient who had acute chest pain. (*A*) Chest radiograph demonstrates a thin area of lucency adjacent to the left heart border (*arrowheads*). (*B* and *C*) Axial CT images with lung windowing reveal gas surrounding all of the mediastinal structures (*asterisk*) and both main bronchi, which is compatible with pneumomediastinum. (*D* and *E*) Coronal MPR further illustrates how the mediastinal anatomy is outlined by gas (*arrow*) and explains the appearance on plain radiographs. (*F*) Sagittal MPR demonstrates gas outlining the right pulmonary ligament (*arrow*).

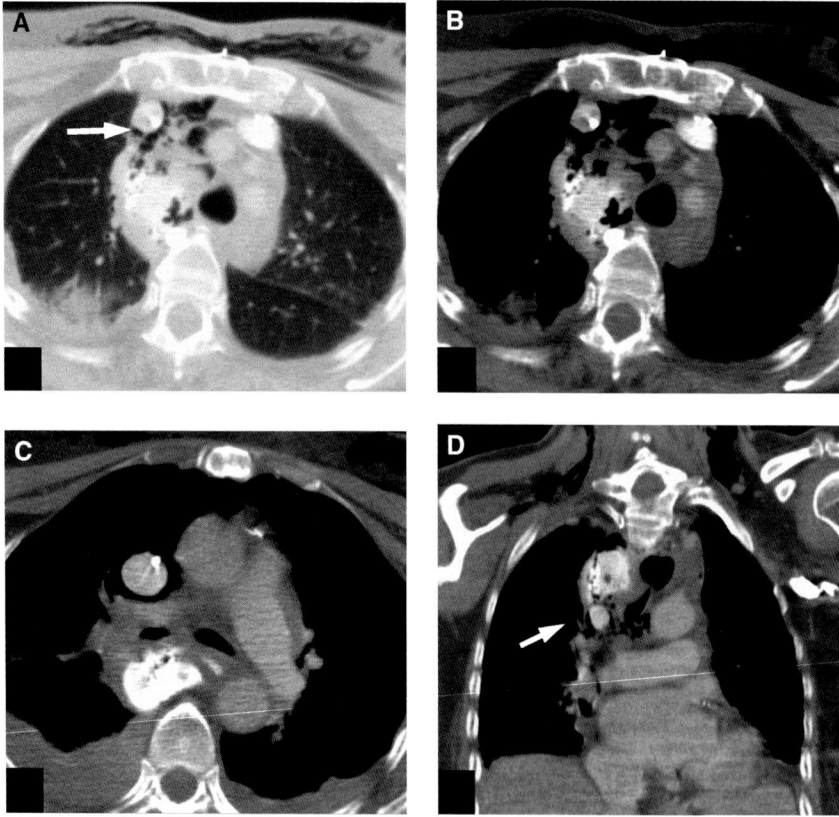

Fig. 22. Patient who had several bouts of retching and recent TEE. (A) Axial CT image with lung windows demonstrates significant subcutaneous emphysema in the anterior mediastinum (*arrow*) and anterior chest wall. (B and C) Similar images with mediastinal windows reveal a large collection of extraluminal contrast in the posterior mediastinum—which extended from the root of the neck to the diaphragm—that was compatible with an esophageal perforation. (D) Coronal MPR further illustrates the extent of the extraluminal extravasation (*arrow*).

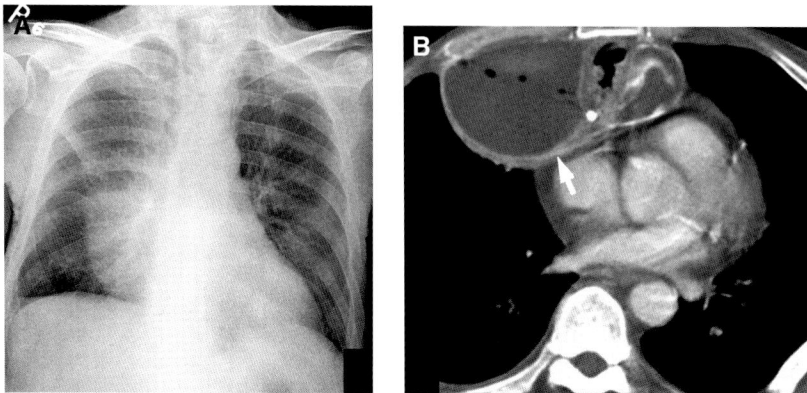

Fig. 23. Patient who had a history of gastric bypass procedure presented with increasing chest pain. (A) Chest radiograph demonstrates an abnormal right heart border and mediastinal contour. (B) Contrast-enhanced axial CT demonstrates a wall-enhancing complex fluid collection in the right anterior mediastinal space. These features, plus the presence of small foci of gas in the collection, are compatible with a mediastinal abscess that was drained percutaneously.

Esophageal rupture

Perforation can occur from violent retching (Boerhaave's syndrome) or from trauma (including iatrogenic causes, such as endoscopy). Prompt recognition and proper clinical management are necessary to reduce morbidity and mortality. Esophageal perforation should be suspected on the basis of the history in association with vomiting, chest pain, fever, and subcutaneous emphysema. Patients do not always appear ill on presentation. Subcutaneous emphysema is uncommon within the first 12 hours, and fever may occur in only 50% of presenting patients [74]. Radiographic studies may reveal mediastinal emphysema, mediastinal widening, left-sided pleural effusion, pneumomediastinum, or pneumothorax [Fig. 22] [61]. Fluoroscopic evaluation of the esophagus is the examination of choice; water-soluble contrast is used initially, with the subsequent administration of barium for a more definitive assessment [75].

MDCT has played a greater role in evaluating esophageal rupture because of the ability to elicit an alternative diagnosis while looking for primary and secondary signs of rupture. Findings that raise suspicion for esophageal injury include mediastinal gas or fluid, esophageal thickening, or pleural effusion, particularly left-sided effusion [75,76]. Mediastinitis and mediastinal abscess formation were reported in 1% of patients who had esophageal perforation. CT findings of acute mediastinitis secondary to esophageal perforation may include esophageal thickening, extraluminal gas, pleural effusion, single or multiple abscesses, and extraluminal contrast medium [Fig. 23] [76].

Summary

Acute chest pain in the absence of trauma remains a diagnostic challenge because it encompasses a wide spectrum of cardiac and noncardiac disease. Although accurate clinical history and physical examination are essential, diagnostic imaging continues to be indispensable in helping physicians to navigate nonspecific signs and symptoms and reach a more refined assessment. With newer technologic advancements on the horizon, the role of imaging is likely to play an even greater role in the clinician's diagnostic armamentarium.

References

[1] Jagminas L, Partridge R. A comparison of emergency department versus inhospital chest pain observation units. Am J Emerg Med 2005;23: 111–3.

[2] Pollack Jr CV, Gibler WB. 2000 ACC/AHA guidelines for the management of patients with unstable angina and non-ST-segment elevation myocardial infarction: a practical summary for emergency physicians. Ann Emerg Med 2001;38:229–40.

[3] Kern MJ. Syndrome X: understanding and evaluating the patient with chest pain and normal coronary arteriograms. Heart Dis Stroke 1992;1: 299–302.

[4] Halliburton SS, Stillman AE, Flohr T, et al. Do segmented reconstruction algorithms for cardiac multi-slice computed tomography improve image quality? Herz 2003;28:20–31.

[5] Schoenhagen P, Halliburton SS, Stillman AE, et al. Noninvasive imaging of coronary arteries: current and future role of multi-detector row CT. Radiology 2004;232:7–17.

[6] Achenbach S, Giesler T, Ropers D, et al. Detection of coronary artery stenoses by contrast-enhanced, retrospectively electrocardiographically-gated, multislice spiral computed tomography. Circulation 2001;103:2535–8.

[7] Nieman K, Rensing BJ, van Geuns RJ, et al. Usefulness of multislice computed tomography for detecting obstructive coronary artery disease. Am J Cardiol 2002;89:913–8.

[8] Ropers D, Baum U, Pohle K, et al. Detection of coronary artery stenoses with thin-slice multidetector row spiral computed tomography and multiplanar reconstruction. Circulation 2003;107: 664–6.

[9] Nieman K, Cademartiri F, Lemos PA, et al. Reliable noninvasive coronary angiography with fast submillimeter multislice spiral computed tomography. Circulation 2002;106:2051–4.

[10] Flohr T, Bruder H, Stierstorfer K, et al. New technical developments in multislice CT, part 2: sub-millimeter 16-slice scanning and increased gantry rotation speed for cardiac imaging. RoFo 2002;174:1022–7.

[11] Agatston AS, Janowitz WR, Hildner FJ, et al. Quantification of coronary artery calcium using ultrafast computed tomography. J Am Coll Cardiol 1990;15:827–32.

[12] Laudon DA, Vukov LF, Breen JF, et al. Use of electron-beam computed tomography in the evaluation of chest pain patients in the emergency department. Ann Emerg Med 1999;33:15–21.

[13] Georgiou D, Budoff MJ, Kaufer E, et al. Screening patients with chest pain in the emergency department using electron beam tomography: a follow-up study. J Am Coll Cardiol 2001;38:105–10.

[14] White CS, Kuo D, Kelemen M, et al. Chest pain evaluation in the emergency department: can MDCT provide a comprehensive evaluation? AJR Am J Roentgenol 2005;185:533–40.

[15] Chiurlia E, Menozzi M, Ratti C, et al. Follow-up of coronary artery bypass graft patency by multislice computed tomography. Am J Cardiol 2005; 95:1094–7.

[16] Schlosser T, Konorza T, Hunold P, et al. Noninvasive visualization of coronary artery bypass grafts using 16-detector row computed tomography. J Am Coll Cardiol 2004;44:1224–9.

[17] Ropers D, Ulzheimer S, Wenkel E, et al. Investigation of aortocoronary artery bypass grafts by multislice spiral computed tomography with electrocardiographic-gated image reconstruction. Am J Cardiol 2001;88:792–5.

[18] Nieman K, Oudkerk M, Rensing BJ, et al. Coronary angiography with multi-slice computed tomography. Lancet 2001;357:599–603.

[19] Wackers FJ, Brown KA, Heller GV, et al. American Society of Nuclear Cardiology position statement on radionuclide imaging in patients with suspected acute ischemic syndromes in the emergency department or chest pain center. J Nucl Cardiol 2002;9:246–50.

[20] Klocke FJ, Baird MG, Lorell BH, et al. ACC/AHA/ASNC guidelines for the clinical use of cardiac radionuclide imaging—executive summary: a report of the American College of Cardiology/American Heart Association Task Force on Practice Guidelines. Circulation 2003;108:1404–18.

[21] Stowers SA, Eisenstein EL, Th Wackers FJ, et al. An economic analysis of an aggressive diagnostic strategy with single photon emission computed tomography myocardial perfusion imaging and early exercise stress testing in emergency department patients who present with chest pain but nondiagnostic electrocardiograms: results from a randomized trial. Ann Emerg Med 2000;35(1):17–25.

[22] Udelson JE, Beshansky JR, Ballin DS, et al. Myocardial perfusion imaging for evaluation and triage of patients with suspected acute cardiac ischemia: a randomized controlled trial. JAMA 2002;288:2693–700.

[23] Vilacosta I, San Roman JA. Acute aortic syndrome. Heart 2001;85:365–8.

[24] Macura KJ, Corl FM, Fishman EK, et al. Pathogenesis in acute aortic syndromes: aortic dissection, intramural hematoma, and penetrating atherosclerotic aortic ulcer. AJR Am J Roentgenol 2003;181:309–16.

[25] Pretre R, von Segesser LK. Aortic dissection. Lancet 1997;349:1461–4.

[26] Khan IA, Nair CK. Clinical, diagnostic, and management perspectives of aortic dissection. Chest 2002;122:311–28.

[27] Chirillo F, Marchiori MC, Andriolo L, et al. Outcome of 290 patients with aortic dissection. A 12-year multicentre experience. Eur Heart J 1990;11:311–9.

[28] Knaut AL, Cleveland Jr JC. Aortic emergencies. Emerg Med Clin North Am 2003;21:817–45.

[29] Hagan PG, Nienaber CA, Isselbacher EM, et al. The International Registry of Acute Aortic Dissection (IRAD): new insights into an old disease. JAMA 2000;283:897–903.

[30] Cigarroa JE, Isselbacher EM, DeSanctis RW, et al. Medical progress. diagnostic imaging in the evaluation of suspected aortic dissection: old standards and new directions. AJR 1993;161:485–93.

[31] Erbel R, Daniel W, Visser C, et al. Echocardiography in diagnosis of aortic dissection. The Lancet 1989;1:457–61.

[32] Nienaber CA, Kodolitsch YV, Nicolas V, et al. The diagnosis of thoracic aortic dissection by non-invasive imaging procedures. N Engl J Med 1993;328:1–9.

[33] Chung JW, Park JH, Im JG, et al. Spiral CT angiography of the thoracic aorta. Radiographics 1996;16:811–24.

[34] Sebastià C, Pallisa E, Quiroga S, et al. Aortic dissection: diagnosis and follow-up with helical CT. Radiographics 1999;19:45–60.

[35] Kapoor V, Ferris JV, Fuhrman CR. Intimomedial rupture: a new CT finding to distinguish true from false lumen in aortic dissection. AJR Am J Roentgenol 2004;183:109–12.

[36] Moore AG, Eagle KA, Bruckman D, et al. Choice of computed tomography, transesophageal echocardiography, magnetic resonance imaging, and aortography in acute aortic dissection: International Registry of Acute Aortic Dissection (IRAD). Am J Cardiol 2002;89:1235–8.

[37] Pruessmann KP, Weiger M, Scheidegger MB, et al. SENSE: sensitivity encoding for fast MRI. Magn Reson Med 1999;42:952–62.

[38] Vigen KK, Peters DC, Grist TM, et al. Undersampled projection-reconstruction imaging for time-resolved contrast-enhanced imaging. Magn Reson Med 2000;43:170–6.

[39] Mazaheri Y, Carroll TJ, Du J, et al. Combined time-resolved and high-spatial-resolution 3D MRA using an extended adaptive acquisition. J Magn Reson Imaging 2002;15:291–301.

[40] Yamada T, Tada S, Harada J. Aortic dissection without intimal rupture: diagnosis with MR imaging and CT. Radiology 1988;168:347–52.

[41] Choi SH, Choi SJ, Kim JH, et al. Useful CT findings for predicting the progression of aortic intramural hematoma to overt aortic dissection. J Comput Assist Tomogr 2001;25:295–9.

[42] Ledbetter S, Stuk JL, Kaufman JA. Helical (spiral) CT in the evaluation of emergent thoracic aortic syndromes: traumatic aortic rupture, aortic aneurysm, aortic dissection, intramural hematoma, and penetrating atherosclerotic ulcer. Radiol Clin North Am 1999;37:575–89.

[43] Murray JG, Manisali M, Flamm SD, et al. Intramural hematoma of the thoracic aorta: MR image findings and their prognostic implications. Radiology 1997;204:349–55.

[44] Kazerooni EA, Bree RL, Williams DM. Penetrating atherosclerotic ulcers of the descending thoracic aorta: evaluation with CT and distinction from aortic dissection. Radiology 1992;183:759–65.

[45] Kaji S, Nishigami K, Akasaka T, et al. Prediction of progression or regression of type A aortic intramural hematoma by computed tomography. Circulation 1999;100:281–6.

[46] Ide K, Uchida H, Otsuji H, et al. Acute aortic dissection with intramural hematoma: possibility of transition to typical dissection or aneurysm. J Thorac Imaging 1996;11:46–52.

[47] Beller CJ, Labrosse MR, Thubrikar MJ, et al. Role of aortic root motion in the pathogenesis of aortic dissection. Circulation 2004;109:763–9.

[48] Stanson AW, Kazmier FJ, Hollier LH, et al. Penetrating atherosclerotic ulcers of the thoracic aorta: natural history and clinicopathologic correlations. Ann Vasc Surg 1986;1:15–23.

[49] Hayashi H, Matsuoka Y, Sakamoto I, et al. Penetrating atherosclerotic ulcer of the aorta: imaging features and disease concept. Radiographics 2000;20:995–1005.

[50] Coady MA, Rizzo JA, Hammond GL, et al. Penetrating ulcer of the thoracic aorta: what is it? How do we recognize it? how do we manage it? J Vasc Surg 1998;27:1006–16.

[51] Ganaha F, Miller DC, Sugimoto K, et al. Prognosis of aortic intramural hematoma with and without penetrating atherosclerotic ulcer: a clinical and radiological analysis. Circulation 2002; 106:342–8.

[52] Sueyoshi E, Imada T, Sakamoto I, et al. Analysis of predictive factors for progression of type B aortic intramural hematoma with computed tomography. J Vasc Surg 2002;35:1179–83.

[53] Cho KR, Stanson AW, Potter DD, et al. Penetrating atherosclerotic ulcer of the descending thoracic aorta and arch. J Thorac Cardiovasc Surg 2004;127:1393–9.

[54] Fann JI. Descending thoracic and thoracoabdominal aortic aneurysms. Coron Artery Dis 2002;13: 93–102.

[55] Bickerstaff LK, Pairolero PC, Hollier LH, et al. Thoracic aortic aneurysms: a population based study. Surgery 1982;92:1103–8.

[56] Moon MR, Sundt TM. Aortic arch aneurysms. Coron Artery Dis 2002;13:85–92.

[57] Dalpont OE, Galla JD, Sadeghi AM, et al. The natural history of thoracic aortic aneurysms. J Thorac Cardiovasc Surg 1994;107:1323–33.

[58] Pressler V, McNamara JJ. Thoracic aortic aneurysm: natural history and treatment. J Thorac Cardiovasc Surg 1980;79:489–98.

[59] Long R, Guzman R, Greenberg H, et al. Tuberculous mycotic aneurysm of the aorta: review of published medical and surgical experience. Chest 1999;115:522–31.

[60] Muller BT, Wegener OR, Grabitz K, et al. Mycotic aneurysms of the thoracic and abdominal aorta and iliac arteries: experience with anatomic and extra-anatomic repair in 33 cases. J Vasc Surg 2001;33:106–13.

[61] Malouf JF, Chandrasekaran K, Orszulak TA. Mycotic aneurysms of the thoracic aorta: a diagnostic challenge. Am J Med 2003;115:489–96.

[62] Samore MH, Wessolossky MA, Lewis SM, et al. Frequency, risk factors, and outcome for bacteremia after percutaneous transluminal coronary angioplasty. Am J Cardiol 1997;79:873–7.

[63] Soravia-Dunand VA, Loo VG, Salit IE. Aortitis due to Salmonella: report of 10 cases and comprehensive review of the literature. Clin Infect Dis 1999;29:862–8.

[64] Macedo TA, Stanson AW, Oderich GS, et al. Infected aortic aneurysms: imaging findings. Radiology 2004;231:250–7.

[65] Castaner E, Andreu M, Gallardo X, et al. CT in nontraumatic acute thoracic aortic disease: typical and atypical features and complications. Radiographics 2003;S93–110.

[66] Goldhaber SZ, Visani L, De Rosa M. Acute pulmonary embolism: clinical outcomes in the International Cooperative Pulmonary Embolism Registry (ICOPER). Lancet 1999;353:1386–9.

[67] Laack TA, Goyal DG. Pulmonary embolism: an unsuspected killer. Emerg Med Clin North Am 2004;22:961–83.

[68] Lesur O, Delorme N, Fromaget JM, et al. Computed tomography in the etiologic assessment of idiopathic spontaneous pneumothorax. Chest 1990;98:341–7.

[69] Bense L, Eklung G, Wiman LG. Smoking and the increased risk of contracting spontaneous pneumothorax. Chest 1987;92:1009–12.

[70] Wright FW. Spontaneous pneumothorax and pulmonary malignant disease—a syndrome sometimes associated with cavitating tumours. Report of nine new cases, four with metastases and five with primary bronchial tumours. Clin Radiol 1976;27:211–22.

[71] Maeder M, Ullmer E. Pneumomediastinum and bilateral pneumothorax as a complication of cocaine smoking. Respiration 2003;70:407.

[72] Panacek EA, Singer AJ, Sherman BW, et al. Spontaneous pneumomediastinum: clinical and natural history. Ann Emerg Med 1992;21: 1222–7.

[73] Zylak CM, Standen JR, Barnes GR, et al. Pneumomediastinum revisited. Radiographics 2000;20: 1043–57.

[74] Janjua KJ. Boerhaave's syndrome. Postgrad Med J 1997;73:265–70.

[75] Fadoo F, Ruiz DE, Dawn SK, et al. Helical CT esophagography for the evaluation of suspected esophageal perforation or rupture. AJR Am J Roentgenol 2004;182:1177–9.

[76] White CS, Templeton PA, Attar S. Esophageal perforation: CT findings. AJR Am J Roentgenol 1993;160:767–70.

RADIOLOGIC
CLINICS
OF NORTH AMERICA

Radiol Clin N Am 44 (2006) 295–315

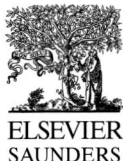

Acute Lung Infections in Normal and Immunocompromised Hosts

Stephen Waite, MD[1], Jean Jeudy, MD, Charles S. White, MD[*]

- Pneumonia
  - *Community acquired*
  - *Atypical pneumonia*
  - *Aspiration pneumonia*
  - *Viral pneumonia*
  - *Fungal pneumonia*
- Pneumonia in immunocompromised patients
  - *Imaging patterns of infection*
  - *AIDS*
  - *Pneumocystis jiroveci*
  - *Bacterial pneumonia in AIDS patients*
  - *Pyogenic airway disease in AIDS*
  - *Cryptococcus*
  - *Mycobacterial infections*
- Non-HIV immunocompromised patients
  - *Bone marrow transplant*
  - *Aspergillus pneumonia*
  - *Early-phase complications after bone marrow transplant*
  - *Late-phase complications after bone marrow transplant*
  - *Solid organ transplant infections*
  - *New/emerging infections*
  - *Anthrax*
  - *Severe acute respiratory syndrome*
- Summary
- References

Pulmonary infections are among the most common causes of morbidity and mortality worldwide and contribute substantially to annual medical expenditures in the United States. Despite the availability of antimicrobial agents, pneumonia constitutes the sixth most common cause of death and the number one cause of death from infection [1]. Pneumonia can be particularly life-threatening in the elderly, in individuals who have pre-existing heart and lung conditions, in patients who have suppressed or weakened immunity, and in pregnant women. Many of these patients present for emergency care, and radiologic imaging is critical in making the appropriate diagnosis, suggesting an etiologic microorganism, and monitoring response to therapy.

Microorganisms gain access to the respiratory system and cause infection in a variety of ways. The most common route of entry is inoculation of the tracheobronchial tree by the inhalation of aerosolized respiratory droplets. Other routes include aspiration of oropharyngeal secretions; hematogenous dissemination, such as in endocarditis; and contiguous extension of infection from adjacent areas, such as the abdomen [2].

Knowledge of the patient's underlying immune status is critical in arriving at an appropriate radiographic differential, and in some cases, suggesting a specific etiology. This article discusses some of the important causes of acute lung infections in normal and immunocompromised hosts.

Department of Diagnostic Radiology, University of Maryland School of Medicine, Baltimore, MD, USA
* Corresponding author. Department of Diagnostic Radiology, University of Maryland School of Medicine, 655 West Baltimore Street, Baltimore, MD 21201.
E-mail address: cwhite@umm.edu (C.S. White).
[1] *Present address:* Department of Radiology, State University of New York Downstate, Brooklyn, NY.

0033-8389/06/$ – see front matter © 2006 Elsevier Inc. All rights reserved.
radiologic.theclinics.com

doi:10.1016/j.rcl.2005.10.009

Pneumonia

Community acquired

Community-acquired pneumonia (CAP) is the most common cause of acute lung infection in immunocompromised and immunocompetent patients. Despite being common and potentially lethal, its importance is often underappreciated. Estimates of the incidence of CAP range from 4 to 5 million cases per year [3,4]. Eighty percent of patients are treated as outpatients, and their mortality is less than 1%. The remaining 20% of patients require inpatient management, and the overall mortality is approximately 12%. Risk factors for CAP include advanced age, chronic obstructive pulmonary disease, renal insufficiency, congestive heart failure, malignancy, diabetes, and alcoholism [5]. The etiologic organism in CAP is undetermined in 50% of cases [6]. Some of the more common organisms that cause CAP and the radiographic appearances are discussed below.

Streptococcus pneumoniae, a gram-positive coccus, is the most common bacterial cause of CAP. Classically, it causes a lobar pattern of consolidation that is characterized by the initial development of a peripheral opacity that rapidly becomes confluent. Air- bronchograms are common. Inflammation occurs predominantly at the level of the alveolar sac when the organism is inhaled. There is alveolar spread and the inflammatory response spreads throughout the lung through small channels—the canals of Lambert and the pores of Kohn. The spread of this process through collateral channels, rather than bronchioles, explains why this pattern of pneumonia often does not follow a segmental distribution. The infection easily crosses pulmonary segments and inflammation is limited by

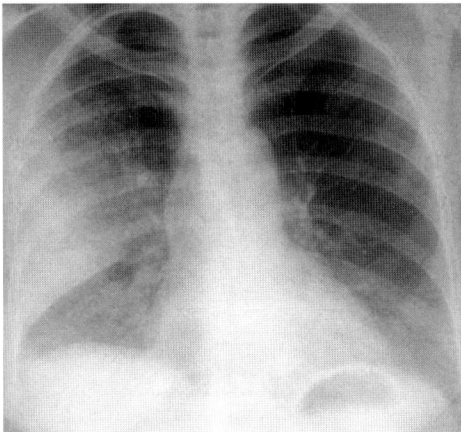

Fig. 2. Streptococcus pneumonia. CT scan of the chest in another patient demonstrates a classic appearance of lobar pneumonia with confluent homogenous opacification of the right middle lobe. Air-bronchograms are noted (*arrow*).

pleural boundaries. In addition to localized lobar consolidation, *Streptococcus pneumoniae*-associated pneumonia also has atypical appearances, such as bronchopneumonia or an interstitial pattern [2]. One study that investigated the radiographic appearances in 81 in-patients with culture-documented pneumococcal pneumonia demonstrated a lobar pattern of consolidation in 81% of the patients. Lobar consolidation was focal in 48% of patients and multifocal in 33%. A bronchopneumonia/lobular pattern of consolidation, often with peribronchial thickening, occurred in 19%. A bronchopneumonia pattern results when infections begin in bronchi and bronchioles and then extend into the contiguous airspace. It usually is patchy, multifocal, bilateral, heterogeneous, and nonconfluent. The radiographic pattern is not influenced by HIV status. Pleural effusions are uncommon, and in this study, were found in 11% of patients [Figs. 1 and 2] [7].

Staphylococcus aureus, another gram-positive coccus, is a less common cause of CAP and more often is acquired in the hospital. The frequency of *Staphylococcus aureus* infection ranges from 1% to more than 22% in severe CAP cases, and up to 5% of all CAP cases. Risk factors include intravenous drug abuse, diabetes, renal failure, and recent infection with viral influenza [5]. It usually causes a bronchopneumonia pattern that often predominates in the lower lobes. Volume loss is common. Pneumatoceles may occur and may contain air–fluid levels. Pleural effusions are found in more than 50% of cases, and can become superinfected [Figs. 3–5]. Abscesses are another common complication of bronchopneumonia [Fig. 6].

Haemophilus influenzae, a gram-negative coccobacillus, is another recognized cause of CAP. This organism frequently colonizes the upper respiratory tracts of individuals who have predisposing conditions, such as chronic obstructive pulmonary disease

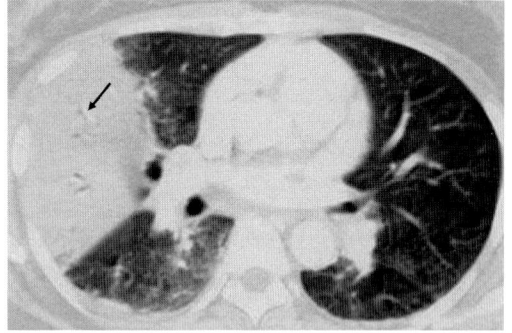

Fig. 1. Streptococcus pneumonia. Chest radiograph demonstrates classic lobar pneumonia in the right upper lobe. Air space disease is homogeneous and confluent and there is no evidence of volume loss.

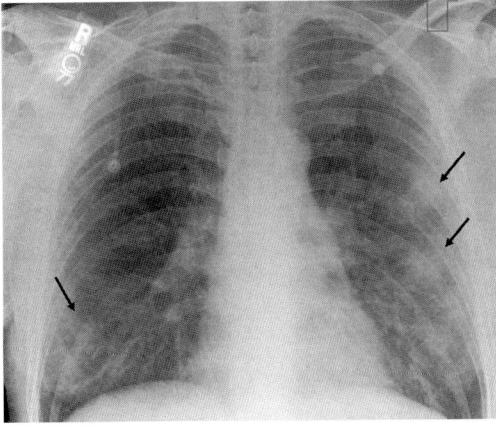

Fig. 3. *Staphylococcus aureus* pneumonia. Chest radiograph demonstrates multifocal opacities (*arrows*) predominantly in the left lung.

[5], and typically causes bronchitis. It usually produces a nonspecific bronchopneumonia pattern. Pleural and pericardial involvement is said to be common and affects up to 50% of patients [8].

Klebsiella pneumoniae, a gram-negative rod, is an important pathogen in nursing home–acquired pneumonia and in alcoholics. It is known for production of exudates that cause lobar consolidation and volume expansion that occasionally results in bowing of the fissures, although this appearance is seen less commonly with antibiotic use.

Atypical pneumonia

The term "atypical pneumonia" was coined in 1938 to describe cases of pneumonia without an obvious etiologic agent and with atypical signs and symptoms that failed to respond to standard treatments of that era [9]. *Mycoplasma pneumoniae* is the most common pathogen of this group. It also is one of the most commonly identified agents in CAP and

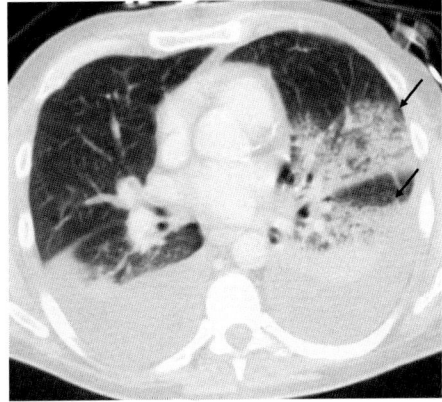

Fig. 5. Staphylococcus pneumonia. CT scan of the chest demonstrates multifocal inhomogeneous opacities consistent with bronchopneumonia (*arrows*) in addition to bilateral pleural effusions and secondary relaxation atelectasis.

causes 20% to 30% of infections [6]. *Mycoplasma* is the smallest free-living culturable organism and shares some similarities with bacteria; however, it lacks a cell wall. It causes infection by cytotoxicity and damage that is incurred from the host inflammatory response. Upper respiratory tract symptoms may precede overt *M pneumoniae* infection. Patients classically develop nonproductive cough, headache, malaise, fever, rhinorrhea, and chest pain.

Mycoplasma pneumonia has been known to produce segmental consolidation, sometimes with air trapping and mosaic perfusion. Pleural effusion and lymphadenopathy are uncommon. Using CT, Reittner and colleagues [10] demonstrated that 79% of patients who had mycoplasma pneumonia had consolidation and 86% had centrilobular nodules (as compared with 17% in bacterial pneu-

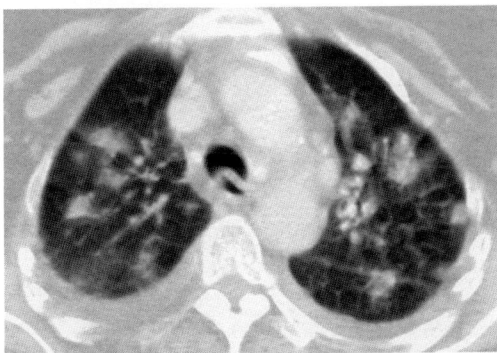

Fig. 4. *Staphylococcus aureus* bronchopneumonia. CT scan of the chest in another patient demonstrates bilateral multifocal opacities. Bronchopneumonia often is associated with pleural effusions as seen in this patient.

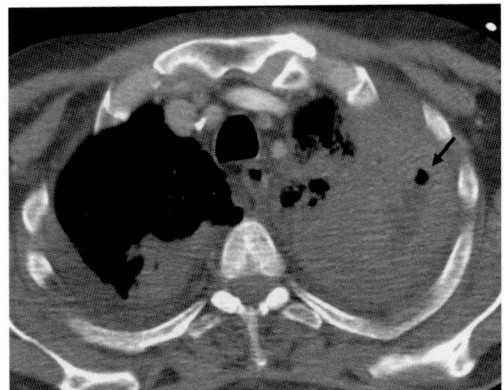

Fig. 6. Staphylococcus pneumonia. CT scan of the chest through the upper lobes of the same patient as in **Fig. 5** demonstrates dense consolidation in the left upper lobe containing a focal region of low attenuation and gas (*arrow*) that is consistent with necrosis and abscess formation.

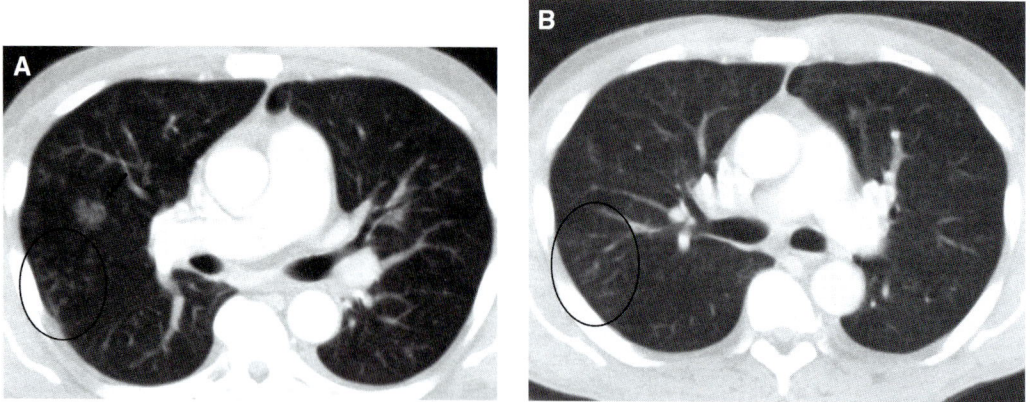

Fig. 7. *Mycoplasma pneumoniae*. CT scan of the chest demonstrates foci of ground glass attenuation (*arrow, A*). More inferiorly, CT scan of the chest demonstrates centrilobular nodules in a "tree-in-bud" pattern (*circles, A and B*).

monias). Focal areas of ground glass attenuation often were seen in association with these nodules [1,10]. Another retrospective study by Tomiyama and colleagues [11], using CT imaging, demonstrated centrilobular nodules in a patchy distribution in 96% of 13 patients who had mycoplasma infections versus 61% of patients who had bacterial pneumonia. Among patients in this study, 88% of patients had airspace consolidation, 100% had areas of ground glass attenuation, and 69% had centrilobular branching "tree-in-bud" structures compared with 34% in bacterial pneumonia. The "tree-in-bud" appearance represents dilated and fluid-filled (pus/mucus/inflammatory exudates) centrilobular bronchioles. It is characterized by a knobby bulbous appearance (the "bud") at the tip of branching impacted bronchioles (the "tree"). Overall, the combination of airspace consolidation, centrilobular nodules, and heterogeneous segmen-

tal distribution was found in 85% of patients who had mycoplasma pneumonia [Fig. 7] [11].

Chlamydia pneumoniae, another atypical pathogen, is an obligate intracellular parasite that is the etiologic agent in 2% to 16% of cases of CAP [6]. The illness usually is self-limited and rarely is fatal. It has the highest prevalence in the elderly, whereas *M pneumoniae* has the highest prevalence in the young [5]. The imaging appearance is nonspecific and includes a combination of consolidation and linear opacities. The radiographic appearance may progress to a multilobar distribution over time [2].

Legionella pneumophila resides in natural water sources and is indigenous to freshwater lakes and streams. Infection can occur when *Legionella* contaminates water systems such as air conditioners and condensers. Infections tend to be more severe than most infections with mycoplasma and *Chlamydia pneumoniae*, and it is estimated that

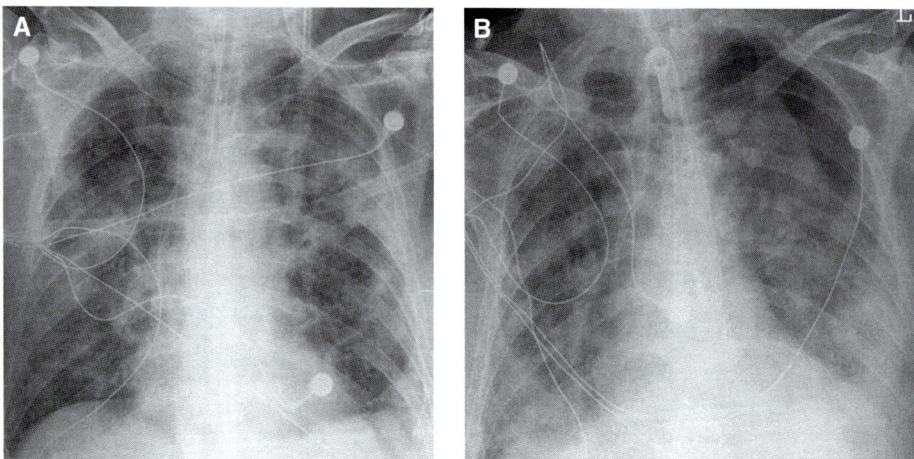

Fig. 8. Legionella pneumonia in a patient who presented with severe respiratory distress. (*A*) Chest radiograph demonstrates multifocal bilateral air space disease. (*B*) Within 2 weeks, the patient's respiratory status continued to decline and he developed a left-sided pneumothorax.

L pneumophila accounts for up to 6% of pneumonia that requires in-hospital management. The overall mortality in CAP that is attributed to *Legionella* is 14% [5]. *Legionella* often causes peripheral focal consolidation that rapidly progresses to involve an entire lobe or several lobes ipsilateral to the initial presenting site. Consolidation becomes bilateral in most patients, even with appropriate therapy. Pleural effusion occurs in 30% to 60% of patients and clears slowly compared with other bacterial pneumonias. Cavitation is common in immunocompromised patients [Fig. 8].

Aspiration pneumonia

Aspiration pneumonia is another important cause of consolidation in patients who present for emergency care. It characteristically occurs in dependent portions of the lung and is frequently bilateral. Material that is aspirated while the patient is upright tends to localize to the right lower lobe. In supine patients, aspirated material collects in the posterior segments of the upper lobes. Alcoholic patients and persons who have poor oral hygiene are at increased risk and these patients are particularly prone to develop infections after aspiration. Anaerobic organisms cause 90% of aspiration pneumonias. Radiologic findings vary depending on the material aspirated and the causative organism. Aspiration of infectious material often manifests as necrotizing consolidation and abscess formation [Fig. 9].

Viral pneumonia

Viral pneumonias are another important cause of lower respiratory tract infections in adults that may present acutely. Responsible viruses include influenza, adenovirus, measles, varicella zoster, and cytomegalovirus (CMV). Influenza viruses types A and B account for most viral pneumonias in immunocom-

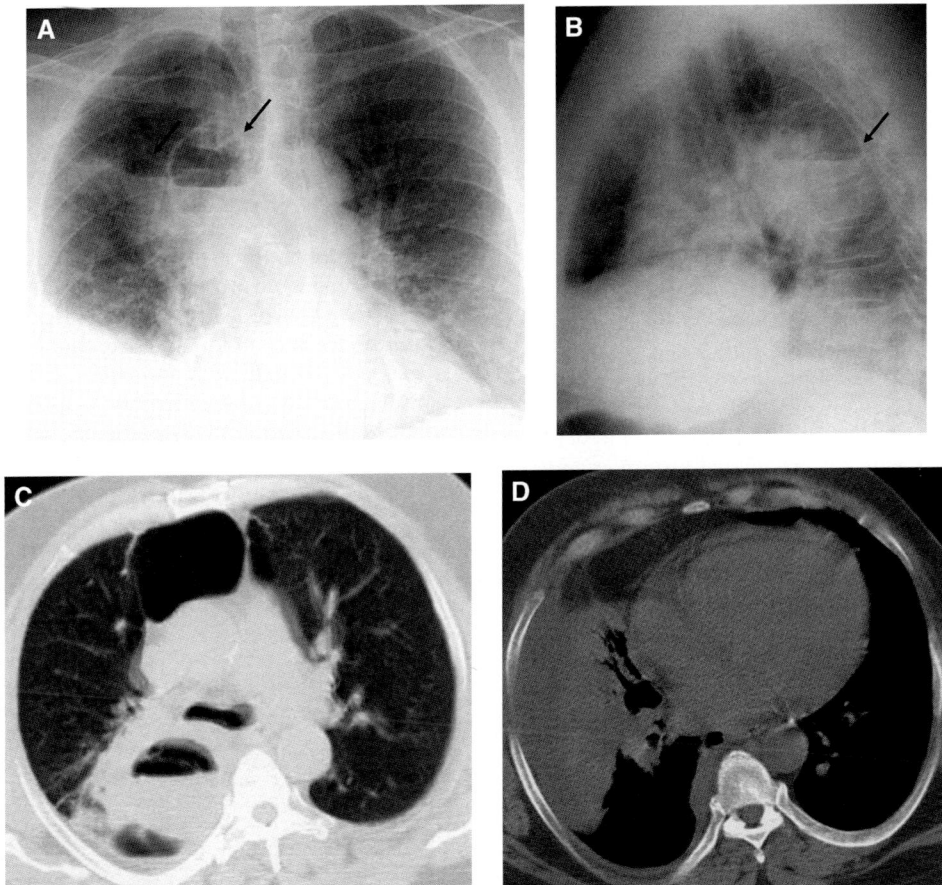

Fig. 9. Aspiration pneumonia in a 65-year-old alcoholic who had respiratory distress. (*A*) Admission chest radiograph demonstrates a right pleural effusion and multiple cavities containing air–fluid levels in the medial aspect of the right middle lung zone (*arrows*). (*B*) Lateral view localizes the cavities to the superior segment of the right lower lobe (*arrow*). (*C*) CT scan of the chest demonstrates multiple cavities in a dependent location in the medial aspect of the superior segment of the right upper lobe. (*D*) Images through the lung bases demonstrate right middle lobe consolidation and nondependent parapneumonic effusion.

petent adults. Immunocompromised patients are susceptible to CMV and other herpesvirus. Viruses can result in several forms of lower respiratory tract infections, including tracheobronchitis, bronchiolitis, and pneumonia.

Viral pneumonia is particularly severe in elderly and immunocompromised patients. Overall, patients who have viral pneumonia tend to have less severe illness than patients who have bacterial pneumonia, and they may complain of a dry hacking cough with minimal radiographic findings. Cultures often are necessary to make a definitive diagnosis.

The radiographic findings of viral pneumonia are nonspecific. Chest radiograph (CXR) can demonstrate reticular opacities that often are bilateral and diffuse in distribution. CT scan may show poorly defined air space nodules, patchy areas of peribronchial ground glass opacity, and consolidation. Hyperinflation commonly is present secondary to bronchiolitis. Uncommonly, viral pneumonias can be associated with thickened interlobular septa that results in Kerley B lines on CXR. Viral infections rarely are associated with complications or pleural effusion, but can lead to secondary bacterial pneumonia [Figs. 10–12] [12,13].

Fungal pneumonia

The endemic fungi, *Histoplasma capsulatum*, *Blastomyces dermatitidis*, and *Coccidioides immitis*, are regionally common causes of CAP in healthy individuals. These fungi reside in the soil where organic nitrogen allows optimum growth. Following inhalation of the infecting particles, a small area of pneumonitis develops. Only a minority of patients becomes symptomatic, and only a small fraction of symptomatic individuals visits a physician or requires treatment. The natural history of endemic

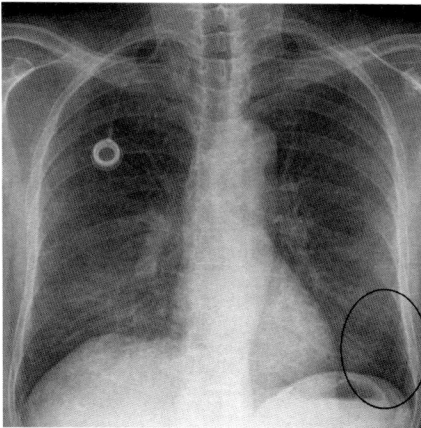

Fig. 11. Influenzae pneumonia. CT scan of the chest demonstrates patchy multifocal ground glass attenuation opacities (*arrows*).

fungal pneumonia is spontaneous resolution unless the inhaled infective dose is overwhelming or the patient is an abnormal host. Immunocompromised patients who present with the acute form of the disease require immediate treatment because of the high risk of progression that leads to ventilatory compromise and extrapulmonary dissemination.

Histoplasma capsulatum normally lives in soil that is contaminated with guano from bats or birds. Infection is endemic in the Ohio and Mississippi River valleys, and more than 70% of the population shows positive skin tests [2]. The initial polymorpholeukocytic response to the inhaled organism is ineffective in killing it, and lymphocytes and macrophages are recruited. Early in the disease, spread to lymph nodes is common and extrathoracic spread is frequent. Healing with formation of a fibrous capsule around the inflammatory focus frequently occurs with calcification. Symptomatic patients often present with respiratory problems, pulmonary opacities, hilar lymphadenopathy, and possibly,

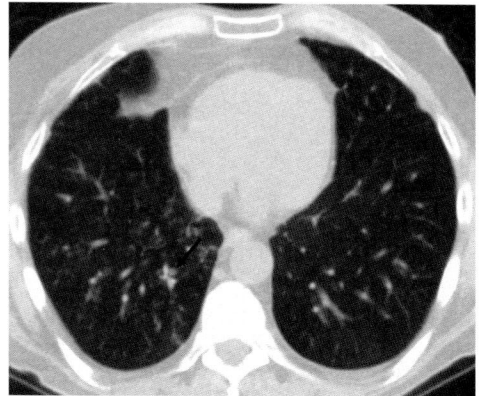

Fig. 10. Viral pneumonia. CXR demonstrates a diffuse bilateral reticular pattern consistent with viral infection. Note the presence of Kerley lines (*circle*), an uncommon feature in viral pneumonia.

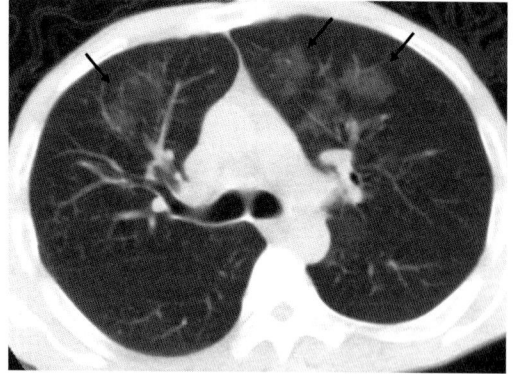

Fig. 12. Influenzae pneumonia. CT scan of another patient who has influenza pneumonia demonstrates areas of bronchial wall thickening (*arrow*) and airway disease.

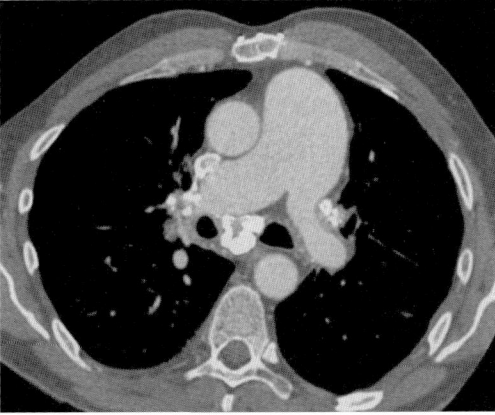

Fig. 13. Fibrosing mediastinitis in a 54-year-old man who had chronic histoplasmosis. CT scan of the chest demonstrates calcified mediastinal and hilar adenopathy. Note the narrowing of the left main pulmonary artery. The right main pulmonary artery is truncated and no right pulmonary veins are patent on imaging (incompletely seen).

organomegaly. In severe cases, the organism may cause overwhelming infection with hemoptysis, pericarditis, acute respiratory distress syndrome (ARDS), and death.

In most patients with histoplasma infection, the CXR is normal. It can manifest with a nonspecific pattern of multifocal air space consolidation or as multiple small nodules. Another pattern is that of a discrete pulmonary nodule, a histoplasmoma, which mimics carcinoma. These nodules can be large (≤3 cm). Adjacent "satellite" nodules are common, as is adenopathy that can be calcified. Occasionally, adenopathy may be the only finding which may cause atelectasis by compression of adjacent bronchi.

Chronic histoplasmosis can cause upper lobe linear opacities and fibrocavitary consolidation that resemble postprimary tuberculosis (TB). Infection of mediastinal lymph nodes can result in necrosis and fibrosis of the affected lymph nodes—"fibrosing mediastinitis"—with subsequent venous obstruction, bronchial stenosis, and narrowing of the pulmonary arteries. Fibrosing mediastinitis probably occurs most often in a genetically susceptible population [Fig. 13] [14]. The disseminated form of histoplasmosis usually occurs in very young children or in severely immunocompromised individuals, such as patients who have AIDS or transplant recipients. The radiographic appearance is a miliary pattern that can affect extrathoracic organs.

Coccidiomycosis immitis is a fungus that is endemic in the southwestern United States. Inhalation of the organism can produce varied appearances, including multifocal consolidation and multiple pulmonary nodules, sometimes with cavitation. Disseminated coccidiomycosis also can occur, which manifests in the chest as a miliary pattern that usually is associated with adenopathy [Fig. 14].

Blastomyces dermatitidis is an endemic fungus in the central and southeastern United States. As with the other endemic fungi, initial infection may be asymptomatic; symptomatic infection presents as a flu-like illness. Infection can be rapidly progressive with the development of multifocal bilateral air space opacities or even ARDS. Miliary disease also has been reported.

Pneumonia in immunocompromised patients

Immunocompromised patients frequently present to the emergency department with pneumonia. The etiologic agents that cause infections in immunocompromised hosts often are different from those that are found in immunocompetent individuals. Furthermore, the pattern of disease with the same organism often varies, depending on the immune

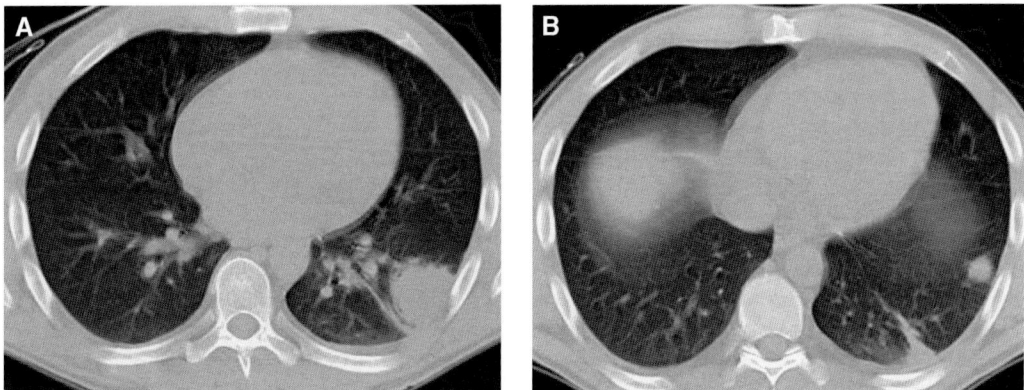

Fig. 14. *Coccidiodes immitis* was isolated at bronchoscopy in a 34-year-old Mexican patient who presented to the emergency department with mild respiratory symptoms. (*A* and *B*) CT scan at two levels through the bases demonstrates multiple nodular areas of consolidation in the left lower lobe.

status of the infected individual. An organized approach to the imaging evaluation of immuno-compromised patients is critical to ensure an accurate and timely diagnosis. In patients who have AIDS, the pattern and progression of abnormality should be correlated with the clinical scenario, including the CD4 count; in patients who have undergone transplants, the amount of time that has elapsed since institution of chemotherapy or transplant is important.

Imaging of immunosuppressed patients usually starts with chest radiography. Although radiographic findings often are nonspecific, they play an important role in triage. Follow-up radiography can help to monitor response to treatment. Recognizing basic patterns may help to establish the differential diagnosis.

Imaging patterns of infection

Infected immunosuppressed patients with focal air space opacities are most likely to have a bacterial infection. TB also should be a consideration in patients who have low CD4 levels. Multifocal air space opacities have a broader differential diagnosis and include bacterial infections, *Pneumocystis jiroveci* (PCP), and fungi (eg, *Cryptococcus* and *Aspergillus*). Mycobacterial infection is less likely. A pattern of nodular densities suggests fungal or mycobacterial infections. Cavitation usually is not found in viral infections. Franquet and colleagues [15] analyzed high-resolution CT (HRCT) scans in 78 immuno-compromised patients with nodules and found that only 15% of the patients with nodules had a viral infection. Nodules were always multiple, 83% were less than 1 cm, and none was cavitary [15]. A diffuse or interstitial pattern is particularly concerning for viral infections and PCP. Less frequently can appear in this fashion bacterial infections, mycobacterium, or fungi [16].

AIDS

Respiratory disease is an important cause of morbidity and mortality in HIV-infected individuals; most patients encounter a pulmonary complication during the course of their illness. A variety of these infections has been classified as AIDS-defining illnesses, including cryptococcus, CMV, PCP, non-TB mycobacterium, mycobacterium TB, recurrent pneumonia, and disseminated histoplasmosis [17]. The epidemiology of thoracic manifestations of AIDS has changed because of antibiotics, with a reduction in the number of cases of PCP and an increase in the number of cases of *Mycobacterium avium* complex (MAC) and CMV. Because there is considerable overlap between the radiologic findings of numerous infections and neoplastic entities that are known to occur with increased frequency in patients who have AIDS; clinical information, including the acuity of the illness, CD4 count, and current drug therapy, is valuable in limiting the differential diagnosis.

Regardless of the radiologic appearance, opportunistic infections generally do not occur before a decrease in the $CD4^+$ count to less than 200×10^6 cells/L. Several other disease processes tend to be encountered only when the $CD4^+$ count decreases to less than certain threshold levels as listed below [17]:

$CD4^+$ *greater than* 200×10^6 *cells/L:* bacterial pneumonia, TB (reinfection)
$CD4^+$ *50 to* 200×10^6 *cells/L:* bacterial pneumonia, primary TB, PCP, fungal infections
$CD4^+$ *less than* 50×10^6 *cells/L:* bacterial pneumonia, atypical appearances of TB, PCP, fungal infections, MAC, CMV

Pneumocystis jiroveci

Pneumocystis jiroveci, previously known as *P carinii*, was initially classified as a protozoan but is now believed to be a fungus. The prevalence of PCP has been decreasing with antibiotic prophylaxis. The diagnosis is suggested strongly by typical history, low CD4 count, and hypoxia. Induced sputum can establish the diagnosis, or alternatively, bronchoscopy with bronchoalveolar lavage can be used in patients who are at risk but who have a negative sputum induction result.

The radiographic appearance of PCP demonstrates considerable variation. The CXR can be normal; typical radiographic findings include bilateral perihilar air space disease or reticular markings [Fig. 15]. On CT, acute infection classically results in perihilar ground glass opacification, often in a geographic distribution with areas of affected lung interspersed by normal lung parenchyma. A linear or reticular pattern is demonstrated frequently with thickening of the interlobular septa causing a "crazy paving" pattern [Fig. 16] [18–20]. Some patients develop thin-walled cystic areas (pneumatoceles) that have an upper lobe distribution. Typically, these cysts do not contain fluid or other material. The exact etiology of pneumatoceles is unclear although a variety of mechanisms has been suggested, including check valve obstruction of small airways, pulmonary infarction, and production of proteases or elastases with lung digestion. Pneumatoceles may predispose to pneumothorax or pneumomediastinum [Fig. 17]. Atypical manifestations of PCP include focal consolidation, mass lesions, cavitation, and adenopathy [Fig. 18]. Multifocal air space consolidation can be seen if the patient has been ill for some time. Characteristically, pleural effusions are absent [2]. HRCT is highly sen-

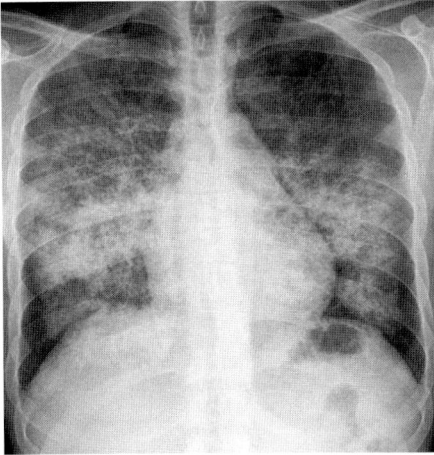

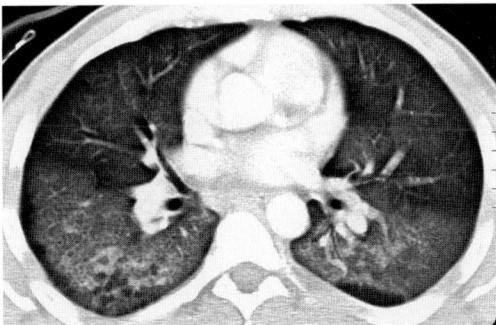

Fig. 17. PCP pneumonia. CT scan of the chest demonstrates cystic air spaces of varying sizes that are consistent with pneumatoceles.

Fig. 15. PCP pneumonia in a young HIV-positive patient. CXR demonstrates predominantly central airspace disease with peripheral sparing.

sitive and in a study by Hidalgo and colleagues [21], 10% of HIV-positive patients who had PCP and a normal CXR had an abnormal HRCT. Ground glass areas were found in all of the patients. A normal HRCT is said to rule out PCP pneumonia [22].

Bacterial pneumonia in AIDS patients

Although the major immune deficiency in AIDS patients impacts T-cell function, B-cell and antibody production are also affected and increase the susceptibility to pyogenic organisms. Bacterial pneumonia tends to occur throughout the course of HIV illness and becomes increasingly common with a decreasing CD4$^+$ count. Two or more episodes of bacterial pneumonia within a 1-year period constitute an AIDS-defining illness. The prevalence of bacterial pneumonia is six times greater than in the general population, and the development of pneumococcal septicemia is 100-fold greater [23]. Similar to that in the general population, bacterial pneumonia in HIV-infected individuals is usu-

ally community acquired. *Streptococcus pneumoniae* is the most common infecting organism; *Haemophilus influenzae, Staphylococcus aureus, Escherichia coli,* and *Pseudomonas* account for the majority of remaining cases. The clinical presentation of pneumonia is generally the same as in the HIV-negative population; however, there is an increased tendency for rapid progression, cavitation, parapneumonic effusion, and empyema formation.

The most common radiographic finding in bacterial pneumonia in AIDS patients is focal consolidation, and the combination of focal consolidation and clinical symptoms of fewer than 7 days' duration is highly specific for the diagnosis of bacterial pneumonia. Almost one half of cases demonstrate a radiographic pattern other than focal consolidation that can mimic infections by nonbacterial pathogens such as PCP [23]. Bacterial infections also can present as nodules that can cavitate. A study of cavitary nodules in HIV patients by Aviram and colleagues [24], found a bacterial cause in 85% of the cases; more than one pathogen was

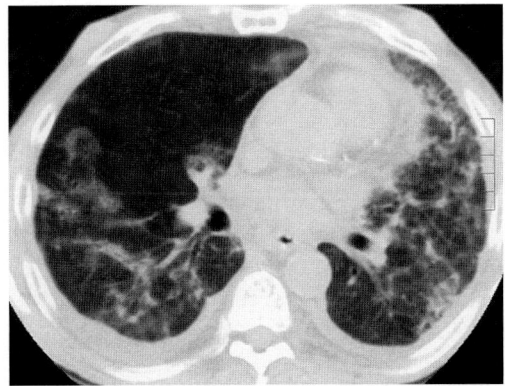

Fig. 16. PCP pneumonia in another young HIV-positive patient. CT scan demonstrates a mixed pattern of ground glass attenuation and superimposed prominent septal lines in a "crazy-paving" pattern.

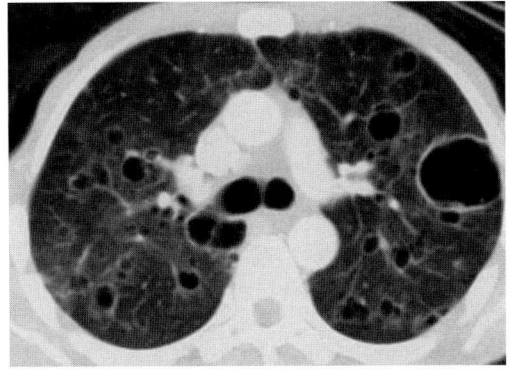

Fig. 18. PCP pneumonia in an HIV-positive patient who had hypoxia. CT scan of the chest demonstrates an atypical pattern with scattered irregular heterogeneous densities and areas of bronchial wall thickening.

identified in most patients. The most frequently identified organisms were *Pseudomonas aeruginosa* and *Staphylococcus aureus*. In most bacterial infections, mildly enlarged lymph nodes are seen frequently on CT imaging but usually not on CXR. Visibly enlarged nodes on CXR in HIV-positive patients with CD4 counts of less than 200 × 10^6 cells/L suggests TB. Pleural effusions are uncommon in patients who have PCP, but are seen more typically in patients who have pyogenic bacterial infections.

Pyogenic airway disease in AIDS

HIV-infected patients are at an increased risk for developing airway disease such as bacterial tracheobronchitis, in addition to pneumonia. The most common infectious organisms include *Haemophilus influenzae, Pseudomonas aeruginosa*, and *Streptococcus pneumoniae*. Airway infection leads to inflammation with subsequent bronchial wall thickening and dilatation. These changes can be irreversible if they are not treated early with antimicrobial agents. Bronchiolitis may create an interstitial pattern of reticulonodular opacities that represent impacted bronchioles; however, the CXR can be normal. The characteristic findings of infectious bronchiolitis are centrilobular nodules and "tree-in-bud" structures. Focal regions of air trapping may be evident on expiratory CT scans [17,23].

Cryptococcus

Cryptococcus is the most common fungal pulmonary infection in patients who have AIDS, and it usually coexists with cryptococcal meningitis. Infection may be asymptomatic, but clinically apparent pneumonia occurs in approximately 30% of patients. It tends to affect patients who have CD4 counts that are less than 100 × 10^6 cells/L [17]. In healthy patients, cryptococcal infection usually manifests as one or more peripheral circumscribed nodules, usually without cavitation [25]. In patients who have AIDS, cryptococcal pneumonia may have a variety of appearances. It has been known to demonstrate a diffuse reticular or reticulonodular pattern that resembles PCP, lobar or segmental consolidation, or multiple nodules that have a propensity to cavitate [26]. Disseminated disease can occur and manifests as a miliary pattern that may be associated with lymphadenopathy or pleural effusion [Fig. 19] [2].

Mycobacterial infections

Mycobacteria are aerobic, nonspore-forming rods with unusually long doubling times. Two broad groups cause human disease: TB complex and the non-TB/atypical mycobacteria complex (NTMB).

Tuberculosis

TB has been an infection of importance throughout human history and can be a serious diagnostic dilemma in the emergency department setting. It has become increasingly important with the emergence of HIV and is one of the leading causes of death among HIV-infected individuals. Numerous factors influence the likelihood of contracting TB. Homeless individuals, intravenous drug users, and immunocompromised patients are at an increased risk compared with the rest of the population. TB becomes increasingly common in patients toward the later stages of immunosuppression, but as with

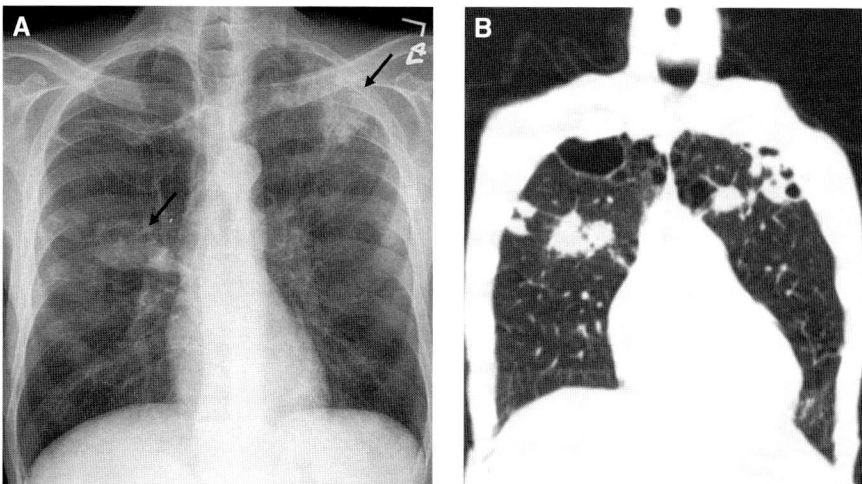

Fig. 19. (*A*) Cryptococcus infection in an HIV-positive patient who had respiratory distress. CXR demonstrates multiple bilateral foci of consolidation (*arrows*), some of which appear nodular and cavitary. Emphysematous changes are identified at the apices, especially on the right. (*B*) Accompanying CT coronal image demonstrates upper lobe cystic air space disease. Bilateral upper lobe nodules, cavitary in the left upper lobe, are demonstrated.

bacterial pneumonia, infection may occur at relatively high CD4 counts. Very young and elderly patients also are at higher risk of infection. Infection begins with the inhalation of airborne respiratory droplets that contain the organisms. Person-to-person contact is more likely if exposure occurs in a poorly ventilated area, or if contact with the infected person is prolonged.

Primary tuberculosis Primary TB is said to occur when clinical infection occurs after the first exposure to the organism. TB is able to survive dormant within host macrophages for long periods of time and incite a delayed hypersensitivity response by the infected host. Under normal circumstances, the host sequesters the organism by forming caseating granulomas. This initial infection has been termed the "Ghon focus" and usually heals by developing a fibrous capsule around the focus of infection which often calcifies. Organisms may spread through the lymphatics to hilar and mediastinal lymph nodes where a similar reaction occurs; the combination of lung and hilar infection is called the "Ranke complex." Usually, host defenses are sufficient to prevent overt infection. Organisms remain viable and may serve as the nidus for reactivation when conditions become more favorable [2].

Most often, patients who have primary TB show no radiologic abnormalities. If there is overt infection, the pattern is one of air space consolidation with no zonal predominance. Cavitation is uncommon. Adenopathy is common in children and can be striking; occasionally, it causes atelectasis by airway compression. Usually, hilar lymph nodes are involved, and mediastinal lymph nodes, particularly in the right paratracheal region, may be enlarged as well. Unilateral adenopathy is more common than bilateral disease. After administration of intravenous contrast, enlarged lymph nodes may have central areas of low attenuation with peripheral enhancement, which reflect the presence of necrosis [Fig. 20]. Unilateral pleural effusion is another less common presentation and these effusions can be large [27].

Progressive and postprimary tuberculosis Primary TB infection can progress rapidly and cause extensive consolidation and cavitation at the site of the initial pulmonary parenchymal focus of infection or in the apical and posterior segments of the upper lobes. This pattern of progression of primary TB is called *progressive TB* and radiographically resembles postprimary TB infection.

Postprimary (reactivation) TB occurs as a result of previously latent infection. During the initial infection, organisms may be transported by the bloodstream to the apical and posterior segments of the upper lobes and to the superior segments of the lower lobes. Reactivation in these regions may be favored by high oxygen tension and tends to occur when host defenses become impaired. Latent organisms become active and overt infection develops. Unlike the healing that commonly occurs with primary *Mycobacterium tuberculosis* (MTB) infection, postprimary TB infection is often associated with progressive disease. As inflammation mounts, tissue destruction occurs, caseous material liquefies, and communication with the tracheobronchial tissue can ensue. This produces cavitation, the characteristic pathologic and radiologic finding of postprimary MTB. Cavitation creates the opportunity for endobronchial spread of infection and communication to other individuals. If host defenses triumph, these cavities usually heal by scar formation with bronchiectasis, volume loss, and areas of emphysema. Chronic thin-walled cavities may persist. Typical clini-

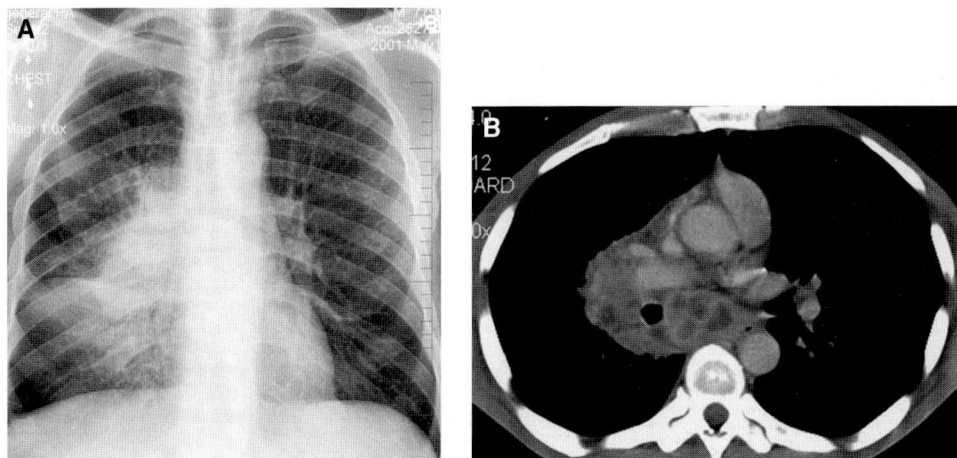

Fig. 20. Primary TB. (*A*) CXR demonstrates prominent unilateral right hilar adenopathy. (*B*) CT scan demonstrates necrotic subcarinal and right hilar adenopathy.

cal manifestations of postprimary TB include failure to thrive, fatigue, night sweats, weight loss, and low-grade fever. Bronchiectasis may result in hemoptysis [2].

Radiographic findings of postprimary TB include consolidation in apical and posterior segments of the upper lobes, and, to a lesser extent, the superior segments of the lower lobes. Areas of cavitation develop in 20% to 45% of patients. Often small, poorly defined "satellite" nodules are seen at the periphery of the dominant foci of consolidation. Commonly there are poorly defined nodules in a centrilobular location and branching structures in a "tree-in-bud" pattern. Lymphadenopathy and effusions are uncommon [Fig. 21].

Miliary tuberculosis   In fewer than 5% of patients who have TB, the mycobacterial infection spreads hematogenously and causes a "miliary" pattern of nodularity on CXR. It can occur with primary or postprimary TB infection. HIV-positive individuals have a higher frequency of miliary and extrapulmonary disease [28]. The characteristic radiographic findings of miliary TB consist of innumerable 1- to 3-mm noncalcified nodules that are scattered throughout both lungs. Associated radiographic findings, which may suggest the diagnosis of TB and are present in up to 30% of affected persons, include consolidation, cavitation, calcified lymph nodes, and lymphadenopathy. On thin-section CT nodules are found in a diffuse, random fashion. After acute infection, the radiograph may return to normal rapidly or scattered residua of the nodules may persist [Fig. 22].

In general, previous radiographs are needed for comparison to determine disease activity. Stability for longer than 6 months suggests inactivity. Other findings that are associated with inactive disease include bronchiectasis, linear opacities, and calcified nodules [28]. Consolidation, endobronchial spread, a miliary pattern, and cavities suggest active disease. The "tree-in-bud" pattern is the most characteristic CT feature of active endobronchial spread and can be found in 72% of patients who have active disease. In a study of patients who had active TB (based on acid-fast bacilli in sputum), Im and colleagues [29] found centrilobular lesions (nodules or a "tree-in-bud" pattern) in 95% of patients. Most of these nodules disappeared with treatment.

Tuberculosis in AIDS patients   The radiographic manifestation of TB in AIDS patients depends on the patient's CD4 count. Patients who have preserved immunity and CD4 counts greater than 200×10^6 cells/L usually present with a pattern of disease that resembles postprimary MTB infection. Patients with CD4 counts that are less than 200×10^6 cells/L present with a pattern of disease that resembles primary MTB infection with lymphadenopathy, pleural disease, and a tendency for dissemination [17]. Culture-positive pulmonary TB with a normal CXR is not uncommon and in a study by Greenberg and colleagues [30], 21% of 48 patients with active TB and CD4 counts less than 200×10^6 cells/L had a normal CXR. Extrapulmonary dissemination is more frequent in immunocompromised patients than in immunocompetent patients.

Nontuberculosis mycobacterial pneumonia
NTMB includes at least 20 organisms, of which only a fraction is important in causing lung infection. They are classified by pigment production and growth rate. NTMB pulmonary infections in immu-

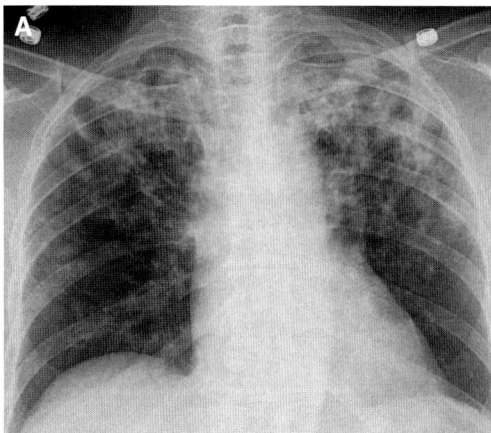

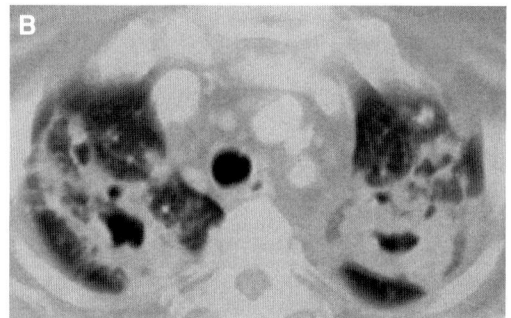

Fig. 21. Postprimary TB in an immunocompromised patient who had weight loss and night sweats. (*A*) CXR demonstrates biapical cavitary consolidation. (*B*) CT scan confirms the cavitary nature of upper lobe opacities.

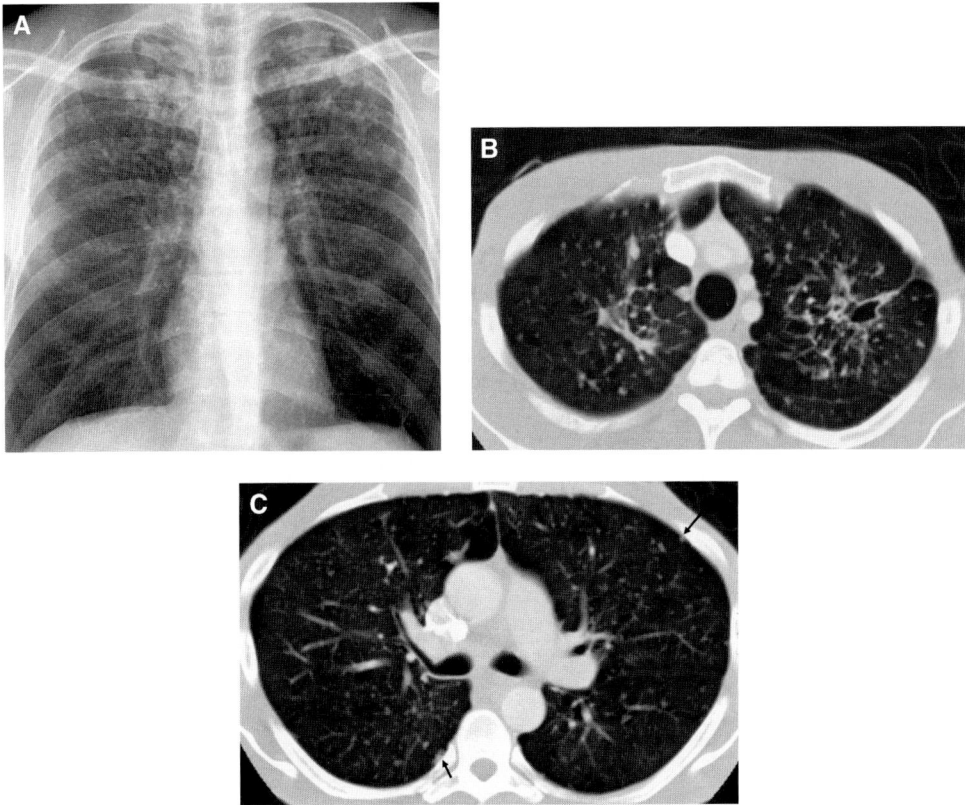

Fig. 22. Miliary TB. Culture proven miliary TB in an HIV-positive patient with several weeks' duration of constitutional symptoms, fever, and weight loss. (*A*) CXR demonstrates biapical cavitary lesions and superimposed innumerable diffuse well-defined subcentimeter nodules. (*B* and *C*) CT scan confirms presence of upper lobe consolidation and innumerable randomly distributed subcentimeter nodules consistent with a miliary distribution. Some nodules (*arrows*, *C*) are on pleural surfaces, an important differentiation from airway nodules which are separate from the pleura.

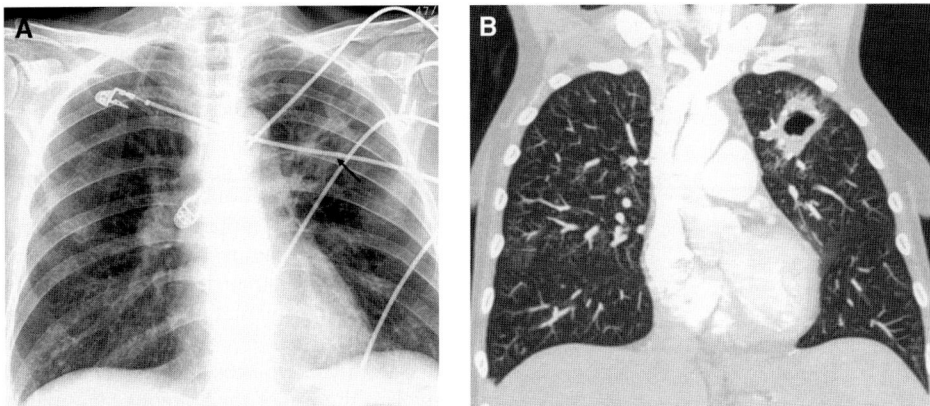

Fig. 23. Mycobacterium avium–intracellularae pneumonia in a middle-aged man who had fever. (*A*) CXR demonstrates cavitary consolidation in the left upper lung zone (*arrow*). (*B*) Coronal CT confirms the presence of a thick-walled cavitary lesion in the left upper lobe. Imaging is indistinguishable from postprimary TB.

nocompetent hosts have two distinct radiologic manifestations: an upper lobe cavitary form and a nodular bronchiectatic form.

The characteristic findings of the upper lobe cavitary form are heterogeneous nodular and cavitary opacities. Often there is a combination of consolidation, cavities, and scar formation that is indistinguishable from postprimary TB. This form is encountered most often in older men who have mild immunocompromised states, such as chronic obstructive pulmonary disease, and is seen most often in infection by *M avium–intracellulare* complex [Fig. 23].

The second pattern is a nodular bronchiectatic form which often occurs in middle-aged women who do not have underlying lung disease called "Lady Windemere syndrome." This pattern consists of bronchiectasis and centrilobular nodules that predominate in the right middle lobe and lingula. A study by Jeong and colleagues [31], of 22 patients who had NTMB pulmonary infection, found that 87% had nodules that were smaller than 10 mm, 58% had a branching centrilobular "tree-in-bud" pattern, and 81% had cylindrical bronchiectasis. Large nodules (>1 cm) were seen in some patients. Findings often can be extensive and a study by Koh and colleagues [32] demonstrated that 34% of 105 HIV-negative patients who had a combination of bilateral multifocal bronchitis (centrilobular nodules and "tree-in-bud" structures) and bronchiectasis had a subsequent positive diagnostic work-up for NTMB [Figs. 24 and 25].

The prevalence of NTMB infection increases as the CD4 count decreases and most patients who have clinically overt infection have CD4 cell counts that are less than 50 cells/μL. The immunocompromised patient who has NTMB presents in a

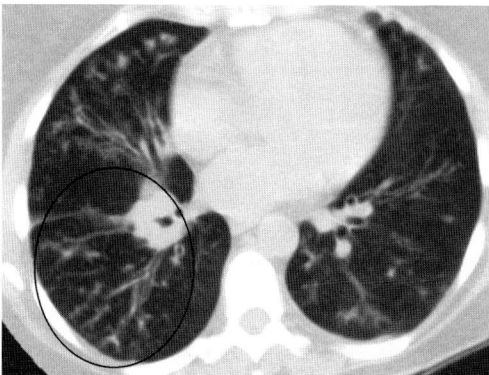

Fig. 25. *Mycobacterium avium–intracellularae* pneumonia in another patient. CT scan of the chest demonstrates bronchiectasis and bronchial wall thickening in the right middle lobe (*arrow*) and "tree-in-bud" structures in the lower lobes.

manner that is entirely different from the patterns described above. They may have no radiographic abnormalities, presumably because of inadequate inflammatory response. When present, radiographic findings include small, usually centrilobular, nodules combined with air space consolidation. Lymphadenopathy and pleural effusions may be the only abnormalities with no evidence of parenchymal disease. Mediastinal lymph node enlargement may show central areas of low attenuation, although this finding is seen more commonly in patients who have TB [33].

Atypical organisms, such as *Nocardia*, always should be considered in HIV-infected individuals who have advanced immune suppression. Cavitating masses, consolidation, and pleural effusions are common features [17].

Non-HIV immunocompromised patients

Bone marrow transplant

Patients who are immunocompromised secondary to chemotherapy and bone marrow transplant recipients are susceptible to different organisms than are HIV-infected patients. Bone marrow transplant (BMT) or hematopoietic stem cell transplantation involves the intravenous infusion of hematopoietic progenitor cells to replace the malignant or ablated bone marrow cells. It is used in the treatment of hematologic malignancies and certain solid tumors. Allogeneic transplantation refers to the transfer of marrow from a donor to a recipient who is not an identical twin, whereas autologous transplantation involves the use of the patient's own marrow. Pulmonary complications occur in 40% to 60% of patients who undergo BMT and are a common cause of morbidity and mortality [34].

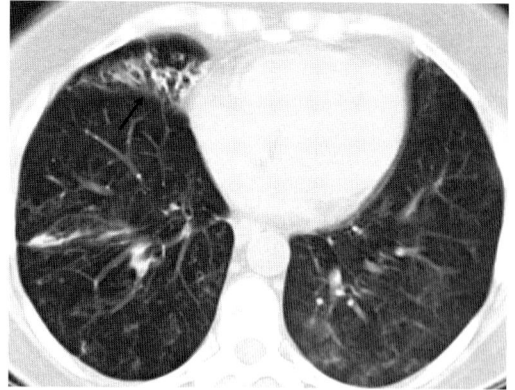

Fig. 24. *Mycobacterium avium–intracellularae* pneumonia in a middle-aged woman. CT scan demonstrates evidence of small airway disease with scattered bilateral centrilobular "tree-in-bud" structures (*circle*). Bronchial wall thickening is seen in the right middle lobe.

There is a predictable time course of neutropenia, immunosuppression, and recovery that allows for the development of a post-BMT timeline in patients who receive allogeneic transplants. Knowledge of this timeline is of critical importance when confronted with an abnormal CXR in a patient who has undergone BMT. This issue is especially important as the prognosis is grim for immunosuppressed patients who have pulmonary complications. The mortality in immunosuppressed patients who require mechanical ventilation exceeded 80% [35]. A study of 200 non-HIV immunocompromised patients demonstrated that a delay of greater than 5 days in identifying the etiology of infectious "infiltrates" was associated with a more than threefold risk of death [36]. The radiologist's role in helping to narrow the differential diagnosis in these patients is critical. Pulmonary complications can be classified chronologically as occurring in the neutropenic or pre-engraftment period (0–30 days after BMT), in the early post-engraftment period (31–100 days after BMT), or in the late post-engraftment period (>100 days after BMT). CMV and *Aspergillus* were the most common pathogens overall in one study [37].

Neutropenic phase complications after bone marrow transplant

During the neutropenic phase, patients are particularly susceptible to bacterial and candidal infections and invasive aspergillosis [37]. Bacterial infections during this time period are related to severe granulopenia and often are caused by gram-negative bacteria. Usually the appearance is similar to that in an immunocompetent patient, with focal or multifocal consolidation. Candida pneumonia manifests as a focal or multilobar consolidation occasionally with a linear interstitial component. Cavitation and adenopathy are not features. Patients also may have multiple nodules with areas of ground glass opacity [2].

Aspergillus pneumonia

Aspergillus is a ubiquitous fungus, found throughout nature which may cause disease in susceptible hosts when inhaled. The risk groups for invasive aspergillosis are patients who have severe, prolonged granulocytopenia secondary to hematologic malignancy; hematopoietic stem cell/solid organ transplant recipients; and patients who are taking high-dose corticosteroids. Rarely, persons who have HIV infection develop aspergillosis. *Aspergillus fumigatus* is the most important species that causes infection in humans.

Angioinvasive aspergillosis results when *Aspergillus* invades the pulmonary vasculature and causes thrombosis, pulmonary hemorrhage, and infarction. It is characterized at histologic analysis by the invasion and occlusion of small- to medium-sized pulmonary arteries by fungal hyphae that lead to the formation of necrotic hemorrhagic nodules or pleural-based, wedge-shaped, hemorrhagic infarcts [38]. CXRs often are abnormal, but nonspecific, and reveal patchy segmental or lobar consolidation or multiple, ill-defined nodular opacities. Characteristic CT findings consist of nodules that are surrounded by a halo of ground glass attenuation ("halo sign") or pleural-based, wedge-shaped areas of consolidation. These findings correspond to hemorrhagic infarcts. In severely neutropenic patients, the halo sign is highly suggestive of angioinvasive aspergillosis; however, a similar appearance has been described in several other conditions, such as candida, mucor, herpes simplex, CMV, and Kaposi's sarcoma [Fig. 26] [39].

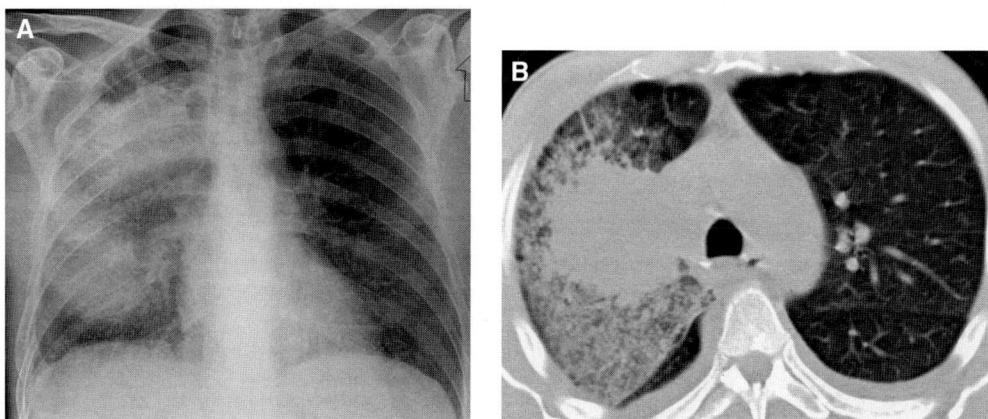

Fig. 26. Acute aspergillus infection in a neutropenic patient. (*A*) CXR demonstrates large foci of nodular consolidation with "shaggy" borders in the right lung. (*B*) Corresponding CT scan confirms large nodular consolidation in the right upper lobe with surrounding heterogeneous ground glass attenuation. Findings are consistent with a "halo" sign.

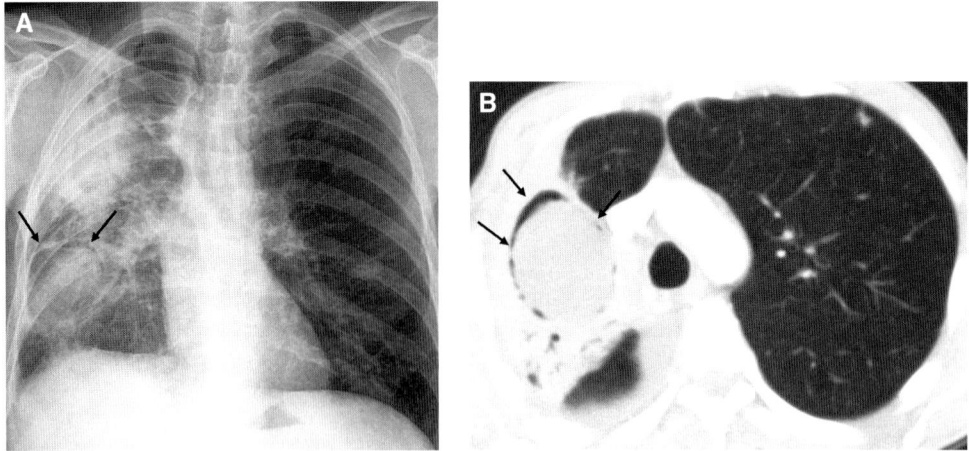

Fig. 27. (*A*) CXR of the patient in Fig. 26 a couple of weeks later demonstrates that the previously identified nodules are better defined and have developed a peripheral crescent of air (*arrows*). (*B*) Corresponding CT scan demonstrates cavitary consolidation containing air-bronchograms and an "air crescent" sign (*arrow*). The "air crescent sign" results when air fills the space between devitalized tissue and surrounding parenchyma. In the appropriate clinical setting, this finding is specific for aspergillus infection.

As the patient's immune system recovers, about 2 weeks after the onset of infection, CXR or CT may demonstrate an "air crescent sign," corresponding to necrotic lung around retracted infarcted lung. Although this finding is not specific for angioinvasive aspergillosis, it is highly characteristic in the proper clinical setting, especially when the initial lesion is consolidation or a mass [38]. Air crescent formation was shown to be associated with improved survival [Fig. 27] [40].

Predominant airway involvement by *Aspergillus* organisms, termed "airway-invasive aspergillosis," occurs most commonly in immunocompromised neutropenic patients and in patients who have AIDS [38,41]. Radiologic findings include patchy centrilobular nodules, "tree-in-bud" centrilobular structures, and a bronchopneumonia pattern. Bronchial wall thickening also may occur [38].

Early-phase complications after bone marrow transplant

Later, in the postengraftment or early phase, the predominant infectious risk is viral, most commonly from CMV. Respiratory syncytial virus and parainfluenza commonly cause upper respiratory symptoms during this time as well and progress to clinically significant pneumonia in 30% to 40% of cases [34,42]. CMV pneumonia occurs in approximately 15%–30% of patients who receive allogeneic BMT, usually between 6 and 12 weeks after transplantation [34]. Infection most commonly occurs from reactivation of latent endogenous virus [34,43]. It is uniformly fatal if not treated [43].

The radiographic manifestations of CMV are nonspecific and can be normal. CT may reveal multifocal, bilateral ground glass opacities and foci of air space consolidation accompanied occasionally by small centrilobular nodules. Franquet and colleagues [44] demonstrated areas of ground glass opacities on CT in 66% of 32 HIV-negative immunocompromised patients who had CMV pneumonia. Multiple, subcentimeter nodules were identified in 59% of the cases, and a halo of ground glass attenuation was seen in 37% of the cases. Fifty-nine percent of the patients also had areas of air space consolidation. A study by Gasparetto and colleagues [45], of 13 patients who had undergone BMT and who had CMV pneumonia, similarly demonstrated ground glass opacities as the predominant abnormality in 69% of patients. Small centrilobular nodules were found in 69% of patients and air space opacities were found in 54% of patients. In both studies, findings were almost always bilateral [Fig. 28].

Late-phase complications after bone marrow transplant

Late-phase complications occur 100 days or more after BMT, and the patient's immune system is near normal by 1 year. The most common infections in this phase are bacterial, although mycobacterial infections also should be considered.

Solid organ transplant infections

Solid organ transplant recipients are susceptible to infections similar to those following BMT. In organ transplant patients there are three important periods. In the first month, infections are second-

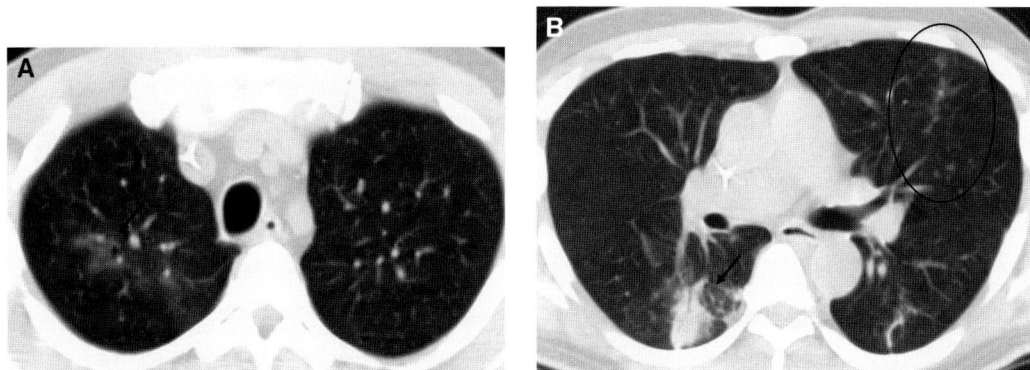

Fig. 28. CMV pneumonia in a bone marrow transplant recipient. CT scan of the chest demonstrates ground glass attenuation and consolidation (*arrow, A* and *B*). Centrilobular air space nodule consistent with an airway distribution is identified in the lingula (*circle, B*). CMV was isolated at bronchoscopy.

ary to nosocomial bacteria. At 1 to 6 months after transplantation, viruses, such as CMV, Epstein-Barr virus, and herpes simplex, become more important potential causes of lung infection. In addition, because these viruses can impair immunity, they can predispose the host to opportunistic pneumonia by PCP or *Aspergillus fumigatus*. Beyond 6 months after transplantation, patients with adequate graft function develop infection only occasionally, and the infecting organisms tend to be those of the non-transplant population [16].

New/emerging infections

Anthrax and severe respiratory syndrome (SARS) cause acute respiratory distress and are emerging conditions the emergency radiologist needs to recognize in order to assist referring clinicians in making an appropriate diagnosis.

Anthrax

Anthrax is caused by the bacterium *Bacillus anthracis*. It is a gram-positive aerobic spore-forming micro-organism. Infection occurs by three different portals of entry: the skin, the gastrointestinal tract, and the lungs. The inhalational form has the highest mortality. When dispersed in the air and inhaled, anthrax spores are deposited into the alveolar ducts or alveoli where they are engulfed by macrophages that carry them to peribronchial and mediastinal lymph nodes. They germinate in the lymph nodes and cause a large amount of toxin production and secondary edema, necrotizing lymphadenitis, hemorrhagic mediastinitis, mediastinal enlargement, and bacteremia [46,47]. The bacillus does not cause a true pneumonia in most cases; however, retrograde migration through lymphatics can occur resulting in an interstitial perihilar pneumonia [47].

Anthrax was largely unknown in the United States until shortly after the terrorist attacks on the World Trade Center and Pentagon on September 11, 2001. In late 2001, 23 cases of anthrax were reported, 11 of which were inhalational. Five of the patients who had the inhalational form died [46]. The possibility of terrorism still exists and, it is important for health care providers to consider anthrax in the appropriate differential diagnosis because the clinical manifestations of early disease are nonspecific and the predicted case fatality of inhalational anthrax, based on historical data, is approximately 90% [48]. Timely diagnosis can reduce mortality substantially and initiate public health and law enforcement measures.

All recent patients who had inhalational anthrax had abnormal findings on CXR. Manifestations include mediastinal widening due to bulky lymphadenopathy and pleural effusions. Hilar adenopathy also may be present. Consolidation can be present often secondary to pulmonary hemorrhage [49]. CT findings include high attenuation mediastinal and hilar adenopathy, pleural effusions that can be hemorrhagic, and mediastinal widening. Ring-like nodal enhancement also is described [Fig. 29] [47,49].

Anthrax should be considered in the differential diagnosis of a patient with possible exposure and the above radiographic findings in the absence of trauma, dissection, or bleeding diathesis.

Severe acute respiratory syndrome

SARS is an infectious pulmonary disease that seems to have originated in southern China in the fall of 2002. Sophisticated isolation methods demonstrated that the causative agent is a coronavirus that is spread by respiratory droplets. It spread to other parts of Asia, Europe, and North America; more than 8422 cases were reported from November

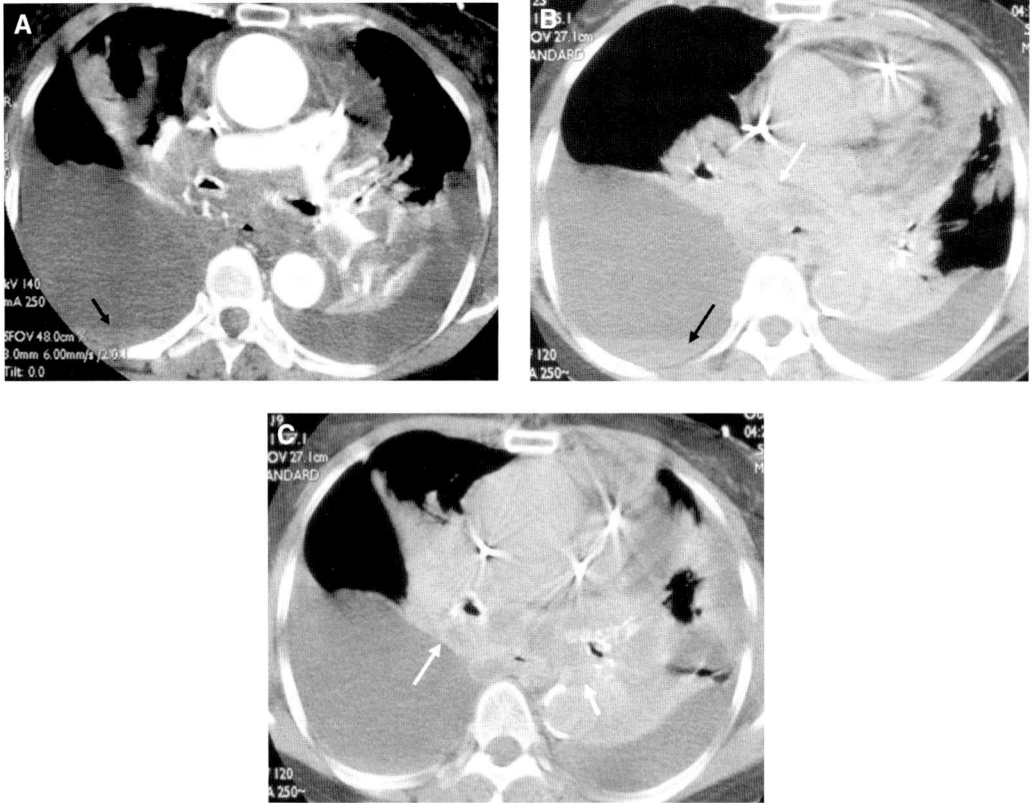

Fig. 29. Anthrax. Blood culture confirmed case of inhalational anthrax in a 61-year-old postal worker who presented to the emergency room after 3 days of experiencing general malaise and chills. (*A*) Contrast-enhanced CT scan demonstrated diffuse mediastinal infiltration and large bilateral pleural effusions. Right pleural effusion has a fluid-fluid level with layering high attenuation fluid; consistent with hemorrhage (*black arrows, A* and *B*). (*B* and *C*) Delayed CT scan of the chest demonstrates high attenuation mediastinal and hilar adenopathy; consistent with hemorrhage (*white arrow, C*). Anthrax infection should be considered in cases with high-attenuation adenopathy without intravenous contrast administration. (Courtesy of Jeffrey Galvin, MD, Baltimore, MD and the Armed Forces Institute of Pathology).

2002 to August 2003 and the death toll reached 916 (11%) individuals [50]. As of this writing, the world is in an interepidemic period and the last human chain of transmission has been broken [51].

The clinical presentation of SARS includes fever, dyspnea, nonproductive cough, chills or rigors, malaise, and myalgias. The natural clinical history ranges from febrile respiratory symptoms without hypoxemia to fatal respiratory distress. The World Health Organization defines SARS as "suspect" or "probable." Clinical presentation and the patient's level of contact with a SARS person who has SARS define a "suspect" case [52]. A "probable" case involves a "suspect" case with the additional finding of "infiltrates" on radiography.

Radiographically, abnormalities appear approximately 12 days after viral exposure or 5 days after the onset of fever. In a study of 40 patients in Canada, Grinblat and colleagues [52] found that 40% of patients initially had a normal CXR. In a report by Hui and colleagues [50], 78.3% of

138 patients presented with consolidation. In both series, all patients ultimately developed consolidation. Usually consolidation is peripheral and distributed in the lower lung zones. Hui and colleagues [50] found that patients who had more extensive consolidation, including bilateral distribution at presentation, were more likely to have an adverse outcome, including death and ICU admission, than were those who had unilateral pneumonia. The disease can progress rapidly. SARS is not associated with adenopathy or pleural effusion.

In one CT study of patients who had SARS, an area of ground glass opacification with or without consolidation was seen in 83.2% of patients. Consolidation without ground glass opacity was uncommon (16.8%). Affected segments were predominantly in the lower lobes (61.1%). Consolidation tended to be peripheral (71.8%) or central and peripheral (19.5%). Other findings included thickening of interlobular septa, which occurred only when superimposed on ground glass opacification

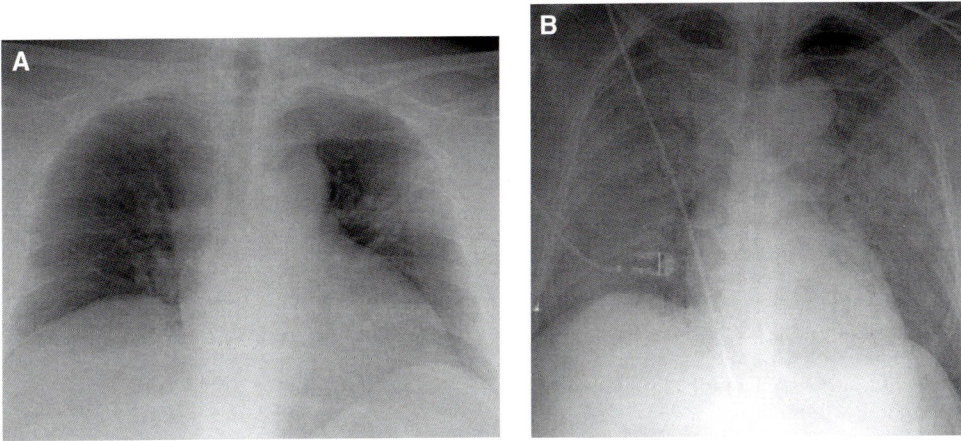

Fig. 30. SARS in a 54-year-old Asian physician who was living in Toronto, Canada. (*A*) Initial radiograph demonstrates foci of consolidation in the left upper lobe. (*B*) Within 3 days there was marked progression with diffuse bilateral air space disease, and the patient required mechanical ventilation. A rapid progression is typical of SARS pneumonia. (Courtesy of Jeffrey Galvin, MD, Baltimore, MD and the Armed Forces Institute of Pathology).

to produce a "crazy-paving pattern." None of the CT features of SARS is diagnostic [Fig. 30] [53].

Summary

Although imaging in patients who have acute lung infections rarely is specific, the combination of clinical information and input regarding the radiographic appearance can help the emergency room physician to refine the differential diagnosis, and in some cases, suggest a specific etiology.

References

[1] Reittner P, Ward S, Heyneman L, et al. Pneumonia: high-resolution CT findings in 114 patients. Eur Radiol 2003;13(3):515–21.

[2] Webb WR, Higgins CB. Thoracic imaging-pulmonary and cardiovascular radiology. Philadelphia: Lippincott Williams and Wilkens; 2005.

[3] American Thoracic Society. Guidelines for the initial management of adults with community acquired pneumonia: diagnosis, assessment of severity, and initial antimicrobial therapy. Am J Respir Crit Care Med 2001;163:1730–54.

[4] National Center for Health Statistics. National hospital discharge survey: annual summary 1990. Vital Health Stat 1998;13:1–225.

[5] Mandell LA. Epidemiology and etiology of community acquired pneumonia. Infect Dis Clin North Am 2004;18:761–76.

[6] Marrie TJ. Empiric treatment of ambulatory community acquired pneumonia: always include treatment for atypical agents. Infect Dis Clin North Am 2004;18:829–41.

[7] Shah RM, Gupta S, Angeid-Backman E, et al. Pneumococcal pneumonia in patients requiring hospitalization: effects of bacteremia and HIV

seropositivity on radiographic appearance. AJR Am J Roentgenol 2000;175(6):1533–6.

[8] Schleiss MR. *Haemophilus influenzae* infections. eMedicine. 2/18/2005. Available at: http://www.emedicine.com. Accessed June 1, 2005.

[9] Reiman H. An acute infection of the respiratory tract with atypical pneumonia. JAMA 1938;26:2377–84.

[10] Reittner P, Muller NL, Heyneman L, et al. Mycoplasma pneumoniae pneumonia: radiographic and high resolution CT features in 28 patients. AJR Am J Roentgenol 2000;174:37–41.

[11] Tomiyama N, Müller N, Johkoh T, et al. Acute parenchymal lung disease in immunocompetent patients: diagnostic accuracy of high-resolution CT. AJR Am J Roentgenol 2000;174:1745–50.

[12] Kim EA, Lee KS, Primack SL, et al. Viral pneumonias in adults: radiologic and pathologic findings. Radiographics 2002;22:S137–49.

[13] Oikonomou A, Muller NL, Nantel S. Radiographic and high-resolution CT findings of influenza virus pneumonia in patients with hematologic malignancies. AJR Am J Roentgenol 2003;181(2):507–11.

[14] Rossi S, Page McAdams H, Rosado-de-Christenson ML, et al. Fibrosing mediastinitis. Radiographics 2001;21:737–57.

[15] Franquet T, Muller NL, Gimenez A, et al. Infectious pulmonary nodules in immunocompromised patients: usefulness of computed tomography in predicting their etiology. J Comput Assist Tomogr 2003;27(4):461–8.

[16] Oh YW, Effmann EL, Godwin JD. Pulmonary infections in immunocompromised hosts: the importance of correlating the conventional radiologic appearance with the clinical setting. Radiology 2000;217(3):647–56.

[17] King LJ, Padley SPG. Imaging of the thorax in AIDS. Imaging 2002;14:60–76.

[18] Kuhlman JE, Kavuru M, Fishman EK, et al.

Pneumocystis carinii pneumonia: spectrum of parenchymal CT findings. Radiology 1990;175: 711–4.

[19] Bergin CJ, Wirth RL, Berry GJ, et al. *Pneumocystis carinii* pneumonia: CT and HRCT observations. J Comput Assist Tomogr 1990;14(5):756–9.

[20] Richards PJ, Riddell L, Reznek RH, et al. High resolution computed tomography in HIV patients with suspected *Pneumocystis carinii* pneumonia and a normal chest radiograph. Clin Radiol 1996;51(10):689–93.

[21] Hidalgo A, Falco V, Mauleon S, et al. Accuracy of high-resolution CT in distinguishing between *Pneumocystis carinii* pneumonia and non-*Pneumocystis carinii* pneumonia in AIDS patients. Eur Radiol 2003;13(5):1179–84.

[22] Raoof S, Raoof S, Naidich DP. Imaging of unusual diffuse lung diseases. Curr Opin Pulm Med 2004;10(5):383–9.

[23] Brecher CW, Aviram G, Boiselle PM. CT and radiography of bacterial respiratory infections in AIDS patients. AJR Am J Roentgenol 2003; 180(5):1203–9.

[24] Aviram G, Fishman JE, Sagar M. Cavitary lung disease in AIDS: etiologies and correlation with immune status. AIDS Patient Care STDS 2001; 15(7):353–61.

[25] Murayama S, Sakai S, Soeda H, et al. Pulmonary cryptococcosis in immunocompetent patients: HRCT characteristics. Clin Imaging 2004;28(3): 191–5.

[26] McGuinness G. Changing trends in the pulmonary manifestations of AIDS. Radiol Clin North Am 1997;35(5):1029–82.

[27] Stern EJ, White CS. Chest radiology companion. Philadelphia: Lippincott Williams & Wilkins; 1999.

[28] Leung AN, Brauner MW, Gamsu G, et al. Pulmonary tuberculosis: comparison of CT findings in HIV-seropositive and HIV-seronegative patients. Radiology 1996;198(3):687–91.

[29] Im JG, Itoh H, Shim YS, et al. Pulmonary tuberculosis: CT findings–early active disease and sequential change with antituberculous therapy. Radiology 1993;186(3):653–60.

[30] Greenberg SD, Frager D, Suster B, et al. Active pulmonary tuberculosis in patients with AIDS: spectrum of radiographic findings (including a normal appearance). Radiology 1994;193(1): 115–9.

[31] Jeong YJ, Lee KS, Koh WJ, et al. Nontuberculous mycobacterial pulmonary infection in immunocompetent patients: comparison of thin-section CT and histopathologic findings. Radiology 2004;231(3):880–6.

[32] Koh WJ, Lee KS, Kwon OJ, et al. Bilateral bronchiectasis and bronchiolitis at thin-section CT: diagnostic implications in nontuberculous mycobacterial pulmonary infection. Radiology 2005;235:282–8.

[33] Agrawal A. Lung, nontuberculous mycobacterial infections. Available at: http://www.emedicine.com/radio/topic413.htm.

[34] Gosselin MV, Adams RH. Pulmonary complications in bone marrow transplantation. J Thorac Imaging 2002;17(2):132–44.

[35] Shorr AF, Kollef MH. The quick and the dead: the importance of rapid evaluation of infiltrates in the immunocompromised patient. Chest 2002; 122(1):9–12.

[36] Rano A, Agusti C, Benito N, et al. Prognostic factors of non-HIV immunocompromised patients with pulmonary infiltrates. Chest 2002; 122(1):253–61.

[37] Leung AN, Gosselin MV, Napper CH, et al. Pulmonary infections after bone marrow transplantation: clinical and radiographic findings. Radiology 1999;210(3):699–710.

[38] Franquet T, Muller NL, Gimenez A, et al. Spectrum of pulmonary aspergillosis: histologic, clinical, and radiologic findings. Radiographics 2001;21(4):825–37.

[39] Primack SL, Hartman TE, Lee KS, et al. Pulmonary nodules and the CT halo sign. Radiology 1994;190(2):513–5.

[40] Gefter WB, Albelda SM, Talbot GH, et al. Invasive pulmonary aspergillosis and acute leukemia. Limitations in the diagnostic utility of the air crescent sign. Radiology 1985;157(3):605–10.

[41] Collins J, Blankenbaker D, Stern EJ. CT patterns of bronchiolar disease: what is "tree-in-bud"? AJR Am J Roentgenol 1998;171(2):365–70.

[42] Ghosh S, Champlin RE, Englund J, et al. Respiratory syncytial virus upper respiratory tract illnesses in adult blood and marrow transplant recipients: combination therapy with aerosolized ribavirin and intravenous immunoglobulin. Bone Marrow Transplant 2000;25(7):751–5.

[43] McGuinness G, Gruden JF. Viral and *Pneumocystis carinii* infections of the lung in the immunocompromised host. J Thorac Imaging 1999; 14(1):25–36.

[44] Franquet T, Lee KS, Muller NL. Thin-section CT findings in 32 immunocompromised patients with cytomegalovirus pneumonia who do not have AIDS. AJR Am J Roentgenol 2003;181(4): 1059–63.

[45] Gasparetto EL, Ono SE, Escuissato D, et al. Cytomegalovirus pneumonia after bone marrow transplantation: high resolution CT findings. Br J Radiol 2004;77(921):724–7.

[46] Mina B, Dym JP, Kuepper F, et al. Fatal inhalational anthrax with unknown source of exposure in a 61-year-old woman in New York City. JAMA 2002;287(7):858–62.

[47] Krol CM, Uszynski M, Dillon EH, et al. Dynamic CT features of inhalational anthrax infection. AJR Am J Roentgenol 2002;178(5): 1063–6.

[48] Inglesby TV, O'Toole T, Henderson DA, et al. Working Group on Civilian Biodefense. Anthrax as a biological weapon, 2002: updated recommendations for management. JAMA 2002; 287(17):2236–52.

[49] Wood BJ, DeFranco B, Ripple M, et al. Inhala-

tional anthrax: radiologic and pathologic findings in two cases. AJR Am J Roentgenol 2003; 181(4):1071–8.

[50] Hui DS, Wong KT, Antonio GE, et al. Severe acute respiratory syndrome: correlation between clinical outcome and radiologic features. Radiology 2004;233(2):579–85.

[51] WHO guidelines for the global surveillance of severe acute respiratory syndrome (SARS). Updated recommendations, October 2004. Available at: http://www.who.int/csr/resources/publications/en/WHO_CDS_CSR_ARO_2004_1.pdf.

[52] Grinblat L, Shulman H, Glickman A, et al. Severe acute respiratory syndrome: radiographic review of 40 probable cases in Toronto, Canada. Radiology 2003;228(3):802–9.

[53] Wong KT, Antonio GE, Hui DS, et al. Thin-section CT of severe acute respiratory syndrome: evaluation of 73 patients exposed to or with the disease. Radiology 2003;228(2):395–400.

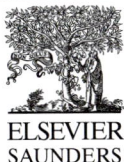

RADIOLOGIC
CLINICS
OF NORTH AMERICA

Radiol Clin N Am 44 (2006) 317–322

Index

Note: Page numbers of article titles are in **boldface** type.

0033-8389/06/$ – see front matter © 2006 Elsevier Inc. All rights reserved.
radiologic.theclinics.com

doi:10.1016/S0033-8389(06)00019-4

Changing Your Address?

Make sure your subscription changes too! When you notify us of your new address, you can help make our job easier by including an exact copy of your Clinics label number with your old address (see illustration below.) This number identifies you to our computer system and will speed the processing of your address change. Please be sure this label number accompanies your old address and your corrected address—you can send an old Clinics label with your number on it or just copy it exactly and send it to the address listed below.

We appreciate your help in our attempt to give you continuous coverage. Thank you.

W. B. Saunders Company

SHIPPING AND RECEIVING DEPTS.
151 BENIGNO BLVD.
BELLMAWR, N.J. 08031

SECOND CLASS POSTAGE
PAID AT BELLMAWR, N.J.

This is your copy of the
CLINICS OF NORTH AMERICA

00503570 DOE—J32400   101   NH   8102

JOHN C DOE MD
324 SAMSON ST
BERLIN   NH   03570

XP-D11494

JAN ISSUE

Your Clinics Label Number

Copy it exactly or send your label
along with your address to:
W.B. Saunders Company, Customer Service
Orlando, FL 32887-4800
Call Toll Free 1-800-654-2452

Please allow four to six weeks for delivery of new subscriptions and for processing address changes.